THE NEW
1996
BOOK
OF
HEALTH.©

IMPORTANT NOTICE

This manual is intended as a reference volume only, not as a medical guide or a reference for self treatment. You should always seek competent medical advice from a doctor if you suspect a problem.

This book is intended as educational device to keep you informed of the latest medical knowledge. It is not intended to serve as a substitute for changing the treatment advice of your doctor. You should never make medical changes without first consulting your doctor.

Printed in the United States of America 0 9 8 7 6 5 4 3 2 1

THE NEW 1996
BOOK OF HEALTH

TABLE OF CONTENTS

Allergy Relief Tips

Allergy sufferers are especially vulnerable during "ragweed" season as the watery-eyed and congested will attest. A string of warm, sunny days brings up the ragweed pollen, followed by allergic reactions. While there doesn't seem to be any miracle cure for this type of allergy, there are ways to avoid the conditions that trigger allergic reactions. Here are some tips to help allergy sufferers:

1) Keep your windows closed in both your home and your car.

2) Avoid exercising during the peak pollen hours (5-10 a.m.)

3) Use your air conditioner or furnace fans to trap pollen in filters.

4) Be sure to shower and wash hair nightly to remove pollen.

5) Don't dry your clothes outdoors.

6) Keep your lawn cut low, and wear a mask when cutting

7) Always wash your hands after being outside.

4 Little Known Foods That Can Cause Allergies

Certain foods and some food additives are known agents of allergic reactions. Even such "innocent" items as chewing gum, cake mixes, salted peanuts, and potato chips can trigger allergies because of the additive BHT (butylated hydroxytoluene). BHT can cause a sudden inflammation of the blood vessels, triggering allergic reactions in some people. If you develop a sudden skin rash or other allergic reactions, the culprit may be in some product you've been using or food you've been eating. Skip each food you suspect for a week to see if it helps.

New Anti-Gas Tablet Works Better And Safer Than Medicines

People who have a problem with intestinal gas may find relief in the new CHARCOAL PLUS. The new product is an anti-gas tablet that has two active ingredients which combat the pain and bloating caused by stomach or intestinal gas.

CHARCOAL PLUS fights gas in both the stomach and intestines with two potent anti-gas agents— Simethocone for stomach gas, and Activated Charcoal for intestinal gas. You can get CHARCOAL PLUS without a prescription at your pharmacy, or you can have your pharmacy contact Kramer Laboratories, 8778 S.W. 8 St., Miami, FL 33174.

The Delicious Candy That Is Good For You

According to some recent studies, peppermint may help relieve stomach gas and indigestion. Researchers say that the intake of peppermint can help the sphincter muscle to relax which can in turn help relieve the discomfort of indigestion. Some specialists recommend using spirit of peppermint drops, which are available from your pharmacist, drinking peppermint tea, or eating peppermint candy made with real oil of peppermint.

Another candy, licorice, may, according to some studies, have therapeutic potential for treating some viral infections, such as chronic viral hepatitis, and for treating some ulcers. Real licorice has been used in China for thousands of years as a treatment for various ulcers, sore throats, coughs, and other health problems.

A Sore Throat And Cold Relief Secrets

Evidence—which is yet to be defined as conclusive— suggests that honey helps to alleviate both sore throats and symptoms of the common cold. While experts generally agree that honey seems to be effective in relieving a sore throat, they are currently at a loss as to exactly why.

New Study Reveals
The Most Dangerous Time Of Day

Getting out of bed after a good night's sleep may be one of the most dangerous things you do all day. That's because the first two hours or so after waking you are up to three times more likely to suffer a heart attack or a stroke. On the other hand, late evening is the safest cardio-vascular time of the day, according to researchers at the Scripps Clinic and Research Foundation in La Jolla, California. The researchers say their study also shows that 6 a.m. to 10 a.m. is, on average, the time of day people are most vulnerable to many other leading causes of death including cancer, emphysema, asthma, bronchitis, and ischemic heart disease.

Recent research reveals that while you sleep many changes are taking place inside your body— your blood pressure falls, your tempera-ture drops more than one degree from its normal afternoon high and some blood collects in your body's extremities. When you wake, your body makes the transition by producing a surge of "stimulation" chemicals called catecholamines. This causes the heart rate to increase and blood vessels to constrict, resulting in higher blood pressure and reduced blood flow to heart muscle. Such a "condition" could lead to angina, or ischemia, as well as myocardial infarction.

While this less-than-cheerful bit of news may make you want to stay in bed and avoid the potential danger as long as you can, you do have other more realistic options. For example, you can set your alarm clock 10 to 15 minutes earlier in order to give yourself time to stretch your arms and legs slowly while you are still in bed. This helps get the pooled blood in your extremities circulating. You should also avoid taking a very hot or a very cold shower. Either extreme is likely to result in a thermal shock which could cause your blood pressure to rise. It is also important that you eat a good breakfast. According to medical experts, skipping breakfast may lead to an increase in platelet activity and possibly contribute to heart attacks and stroke during the first few hours of the morning.

In some cases, aspirin and some prescription drugs can help reduce the risk of morning heart attacks. Results from one major study revealed that men who took an aspirin every other day reduced their overall occurrence of heart attack by almost 45 percent and morning risk by almost 60 percent. However, you should not begin taking aspirin to "protect" yourself from heart attacks without first consulting your doctor.

Doctors say that by understanding how our bodies work, even when we are asleep we can be better prepared to take the necessary steps to reduce many health risks and promote our survival.

Be Careful On Monday - "The Heart Attack Day"

Having to return to work after two days of "rest and relaxation" is not the only reason to dislike Mondays. Researchers in Germany say that the risk of suffering a heart attack, among people who work, may be as much as 50 percent greater on Monday than on any other day of the week.

The researchers studied almost 6,000 people who had suffered heart attacks and found that among working people Mondays were especially dangerous, accounting for about 18 percent of all heart attacks.

Compared with the rest of the week, Mondays had a 40 percent higher risk of heart attacks. Thursday was the second riskiest day, followed by Saturday, Tuesday, Wednesday, and Friday. Sunday was the safest day, accounting for 12 percent of all heart attacks.

The researchers also noted in their report, which was presented at the annual scientific meeting of the American Heart Association, that for retirees and others who were not employed, there seemed to be no significant difference when heart attacks happened.

New Pill Could End Insomnia And Jet Lag

A low-dosage hormone pill, known as melatonin, may reset the body's internal time clock and help cure "night owl" insomnia. The pill may also serve as a prevention for jet lag.

According to researchers, the hormone melatonin brings on drowsiness and is secreted by the brain naturally overnight. However a pill with 0.5 milligram of melatonin, taken during the day, may "trick" the body clock into thinking that it is nighttime.

When the pill is taken in the late afternoon, the body tends to think that night time has come on, and begins to get sleepy.

In order to prevent jet lag, the hormone pill would most likely be taken for a few days beginning the day before departure. Its use would be combined with exposure to outdoor light at the travelers destination.

Still in the experimental stages, the hormone pill is not yet available. However, researchers say that if their findings continue to be positive, it could be available on the market in a few years.

The study, reported in Archives of Ophthalmology, while not conclusive, does lend more support to the importance of proper lens care.

Water Coolers May Make You Sick

Drinking water from a frequently used water cooler may not be especially good for you. In fact, there is a chance you'll come into contact with enough nasty bacteria to cause nausea and diarrhea.

That pleasant bit of news comes from scientists who checked out the contents of ten water coolers at Northeastern University in Boston and discovered four times the federal government's recommended bacterial content limit. The organism count in frequently used water coolers was as much as 2,000 times the limit. Researchers say bacterial levels that high could pose a problem for infants, the elderly and those people with especially vulnerable immune systems.

The problem appears to stem from the cooler itself. Apparently, the small amount of bacteria in each bottle of water—well below federal limits— adheres to the cooler's reservoir and spigots. As more and more water bottles are used, the bacteria accumulates.

The researchers advise cleaning water coolers once a month by running at least a half gallon of household bleach through the reservoir and spigots. You can remove any bleach residue by using at least 4 gallons of tap water to rinse out the cooler.

How The Weather Affects Your Health

Medical experts say that climate has a definite impact on a person's physical well-being. For example, many people often feel lethargic during the hottest days of summer because of changes in the body's circulation. In order to keep the body cool, the heart has to send more blood to the skin where its heat can evaporate more easily. The result is that less blood is available to fuel the muscles and other organs, leading to weakness, fatigue and lethargy.

Many people get sick whenever the weather changes. Scientists now think that's because of a fluctuating balance of positive and negative ions in the air. The scientists speculate that the electrically charged particles affect brain chemistry by altering the secretion of cortisol, which is the body's natural steroid that prevents inflammation. That may explain why people with painful joints are especially sensitive to changes in the weather. Scientists also say that the ions can cause migraine headaches in some people.

8 Things You Can Do For Your Dog Or Cat So They Will Enjoy Good Health And Live Longer

Anyone who has ever had a dog or a cat knows such pets need adequate "health care" if they are to stay healthy. There are several things you can do to help your pet remain in good health and live a longer life.

1) Have your dog or cat tested by a competent D.V.M. for worms, including hookworm and tapeworm.

2) Make sure your dog or cat gets all the required vaccinations. These include shots for rabies and distemper. Consult your vet about what vaccinations your dog and/or cat should have, and how often.

3) Proper diet is an important part of a dog or cat's health maintenance. Your vet can recommend what sort of diet is best for your pet.

4) There are several ways to relieve your pet's misery from an infestation of fleas. Many veterinarians recommend "traditional" insecticide dips as the most effective way to rid your dog or cat of fleas. Ask your

vet for advice about the appropriate dip for your pet.

Some sprays and powders can also be helpful if the flea infestation isn't too heavy. It is also important that you treat the animal's bedding with an appropriate dip, spray or powder.

5) Ticks, while extremely nasty, are easier to control than an infestation of fleas. If your pet spends a great deal of time outdoors, especially in fields or wooded areas, you should give it frequent "tick inspections". One good way to do this, and to remove any ticks that haven't attached themselves yet, is to brush your pet with a fine-toothed flea comb. You should pay particular attention to the animal's neck and under its ears.

Many flea dips will also kill ticks, so you may be able to rid your dog or cat of ticks and fleas at the same time.

6) Ridding your dog or cat of pesky ear mites usually requires prescription medication that is placed into the animal's ears. While your pet may not enjoy the treatment, it will certainly be better off without the parasitic mites.

7) Bothersome skin conditions, such as "hot spots" on dogs, are usually caused by a "flea allergy". The reaction results from the flea's saliva and causes your dog to irritate its skin trying to relieve excessive itching. The best way to eliminate skin conditions resulting from flea allergy is to eliminate the fleas. This can be done in several ways, as noted earlier. You can also help to ease the animal's discomfort by treating the affected area. Trim the hair away from the "hot spot", then clean the area with warm water and apply a powder to dry it out. Many vets recommend Domeboro which is available over- the-counter.

8) Keep your pets well-groomed. A well-groomed dog or cat is less likely to have health menacing parasites such as fleas, ticks and mites.

Little-Known Ways To get Rid Of Dry, Scratchy Eyes

Experts agree that there are several things you can do to alleviate the discomfort of dry, scratchy eyes and to prevent serious eye and vision problems. Here are some common-sense suggestions and advice everyone should heed and follow:

1) If your eyes are frequently focused on close work—reading, doing paperwork, sewing, etc.—take a five minute break every hour and re-focus on distant objects. The advice is just the opposite when you've been focusing on distant objects. Give your eyes a five minute break on a regular basis and re-focus on close objects.

2) Computer users are subject to the discomfort of dry, scratchy eyes more than non-users. Experts say that's because staring at the screen of a computer monitor for long periods of time causes your eyes to blink less than is normal. Since blinking allows the tear glands to moisten the eyes, the absence of blinking results in a lack of lubrication which can cause dry, scratchy eyes. One way to prevent the condition is to take a break and blink rapidly to activate the tear glands. You can also get tear substitutes from most eye doctors. If nothing else, you can try bathing your eyes, gently, in clear cold water.

3) Use only one type of eye medication at a time. Mixing eye medicines may cause them to be less effective and result in increased irritation.

4) Astringent drops are effective, but not if they are overused. Don't use astringent drops every day or your eyes may become red and dry. If used properly, a preparation containing tetrahydrozoline will help reduce any swelling and redness and ease eye discomfort. You can buy astringent drops at most drugstores for about $3.

5) Dry eyes can be treated quite effectively with drops containing methylcellulose or polyvinyl alcohol. Such drops, commonly known as "artificial tears" help lubricate dry eyes. If your eyes are supersensitive, or if you use artificial tears more than four times a day, you should get a product labeled "preservative free". The preservatives in your regular artificial tears may be irritating your eyes. Artificial tears are available for about $8 at most drugstores.

6) If your eyes are infected or irritated, you shouldn't use eye makeup. Eye pencils or brushes can transfer an infection and make the condition worse. To be safe, and possibly prevent eye infections, it's a good idea to replace your supply of eye makeup at least twice a year.

7) If you develop a sty, applying hot compresses 3 or 4 times for ten to fifteen minutes each time can help alleviate the problem. Also, if a sty develops, you should stop using your present eye makeup.

8) A cool compress can clear up red eyes. Placing a compress over closed eyes constricts small blood vessels in the membrane that covers the eye. The result is that reddened eyes look temporarily whiter.

How To Save Over Seventy Percent On Your Contact Lenses

It isn't always necessary to consult an eye doctor if you want to replace your contact lenses with the same brand, type and prescription. Several mail-order firms offer over 70% off most brands and types of contact lenses. However, many experts are opposed to this type of lens buying because they feel that mail-order customers will stop seeing their doctor for regular vision checkups.

You can find about mail-order discounts for contact lenses by calling LenSmart (800- 231-LENS), The Ultimate Contact (800-432-LENS), Lens Express (800-666-LENS), and General Lens Corporation (800-333-LENS).

Disposable Contacts May Increase Risk Of Eye Ulcers

Findings from a new study suggest that people who wear disposable contact lenses may be up to 14 times more likely to get sight-threatening eye ulcers than those people who wear non-disposable soft lenses.

Researchers say, however, that the condition may not be due to the lenses, but rather to improper care by wearers. Apparently, many people fail to heed the limits stated on the recommended wearing times for the lenses.

The study was focused on 42 cases of eye ulcers associated with contact lens wear. The results showed that compared with people who use d daily-wear soft lenses, disposable soft lens users had a 14-times greater risk of developing a potentially dangerous eye ulcer called ulcerative keratitis. The ulcers can be treated effectively by antibiotics , but if left untreated, can cause scars and blindness. Key: Don't wear your contact lenses longer than you are supposed to.

Vitamin A and Hearing Loss

According to recent research, some istances of hearing loss may be associated with a vitamin a deficiency in vitamin A apperars to make the ear more senstitber to sound, which can increase the chances of hearing loss due to frequent and sustained exposure to loud noises. If you are experiencing any problems with your hearing, try increasing your vitamin a foods or take supplements to see if it helps.

How To Have A Whiter, Brighter Smile Without A Dentist Or Dangerous Products

The way to have cleaner and whiter teeth, is by brushing them in the morning and evening (after each meal, if possible) with fluoride toothpaste and by flossing every day. These steps remove unsightly plaque, which can lead to cavities and gum disease. There are many effective fluoride toothpastes on the market. Quitting smoking will also make your teeth whiter and brighter.

5 Insiders Secrets For Beautiful, Natural Nails

1) You can make your nails temporarily softer and more pliant by soaking them in water and then coating them with olive oil. This "treatment" should also keep your nails from splitting. Plain petroleum jelly is also effective as a protective coating.

2) Avoid having brittle nails that frequently break by wearing rubber gloves when doing work that requires getting your hands wet. You can also rub your nails with a rich moisturizer.

3) Strengthen your nails by filing them with with a fine-grain

emery board instead of a metal one. You should also file in one direction to prevent tiny, invisible tears.

4) Have a weekly manicure, supplemented by a nourishing cream rich in vitamin E and collagen. This will help to protect against splitting and to maintain toughness. Massage the cream into your cuticles and nails.

5) To keep your nail tips beautiful and chip-free, apply a moisturizing base coat which will help nail color last longer. Always apply a topcoat over polish in order to minimize chips.

New Shoes Help Aching Feet

A new, space-age designed innersole by Air Pro-Tec seems to stop foot pain in its tracks! The innersoles cushion and massage your feet as you walk, resulting in less pain and much more comfort. Medical Specialists created Air Pro-Tec innersoles, which have a high-tech value system that lets you adjust instantly to the proper amount of cushion and comfort. These innersoles are also much less expensive than the current "air-pump" shoes.

The Air Pro-Tec Innersoles are reportedly effective in reducing pain caused by shin splints. They also provide relief from arthritis in feet, legs and back. The innersoles are priced at about $20.00 and are available from Air Pro-Tec, P.O. Box 1809, Vista, CA 92085.

Inexpensive Home Treatments And Cures For Blisters, Bunions And Corns

Here are several expert tips for relieving pain and avoiding complications from blisters, bunions and corns:

1) To cushion a blister that has developed between your toes, use a tuft of genuine lamb's wool. You can get lamb's wool at any drugstore for under $3.

2) To reduce the inflammation and pain of bunions, soak the area

in a kosher salt solution. A soaking in kosher salt works even better than epsom salt in easing the discomfort from bunions. Use two cups of coarse kosher salt for every gallon of lukewarm water. You can get kosher salt for about $1.25 at your local grocery store.

3) Unless your blister is in a painful or weight-bearing area—like the bottom of your foot—don't break it open. Popping a blister creates an open wound which is susceptible to infection.

4) If you do break open a blister, make sure you use a sterile sewing needle. Hold the needle over a burning match until the tip glows, then let it cool. It is also a good idea to leave the drained flap of skin as is instead of removing it.

5) Clean the area with alcohol, apply an antibiotic cream and then use some type of sterile dressing to cover and protect the area.

6) Use a pumice stone—an abrasive stone that fits comfortably in the palm of your hand—to remove the buildup of dead skin that makes up a corn. Such stones are available at most drug stores for about $4.

7) To soften hard corns and calluses, use lanolin, glycerin or urea-containing lotions or bath oils. These items are priced from about $2 and up at most drug stores.

8) In the evening, a 20 minute application of ice—wrapped in cloth—directly on a bunion, may help numb the nerves that make you feel pain.

9) Shoes with rounded toes are usually roomier than pointed styles, and are much better for people who have bunions. Even though bunions may be hereditary, tight-fitting shoes make make them worse.

Sleep One Hour Less Every Night And Still Wake Up Fully Rested

While it may be impossible for you to get eight hours of sleep every night, there are ways to provide yourself with extra energy in the mornings. Here are six ways experts say you can wake up refreshed in the morning, even if you sleep one hour less than usual:

1) Don't eat or snack right before you go to bed. That turns on the digestive system and could keep you awake.

2) Make an effort to get no less than six hours of sleep and no more than eight hours every night. Either too little or too much sleep can make you feel tired in the morning.

3) Don't go to bed until you are exhausted. That will ensure that you get a deep, restful sleep. And as soon as you are wide awake in the morning, get out of bed.

4) After you get up, exercise for a few minutes to stimulate your body. A ten minute shower should then get rid of whatever weariness remains.

5) Eat a good breakfast, including a high-fiber cereal and fruit. A glass of fruit juice is also a good body energizer.

6) Take five-minute breaks while you're at work. Divert your attention during these breaks and think of restful things that have nothing to do with work.

New Sleep Video Helps You Sleep Better Without Dangerous Drugs

A new video program called "The Sleep Tape" has been billed as "an effective treatment for insomnia". That's good news for the almost 80 million Americans who suffer from difficulty sleeping. The video treatment, created by New York psychologist Dr. Robert Schachter, teaches problem sleepers how to settle down and get some sleep instead of tossing and turning for most of the night. It provides helpful hints to induce drowsiness, relaxation exercises, and peaceful scenes with soft, soothing music to set the mood for sleep.

According to Dr. Schachter, the video offers the same sort of help you would get at a treatment center for sleeping disorders. Perhaps the best thing about the video treatment is that it is drug-free. There are none of the problems that often develop with the use of sleeping pills.

The video treatment is designed for people who suffer from general, non- specific insomnia or sleeplessness which isn't caused by physical or psychological problems. People with such general sleeping disorders can often be cured by learning to relax at will and that's just what "The Sleep Tape" tries to teach insomniacs.

"The Sleep Tape" includes some helpful hints from Dr. Schachter on how insomniacs can reset their body's sleep clocks, resulting in new, healthier sleep habits. Here are a few of the tips contained on the video:

1) Stay away from heavy meals, alcohol, chocolate and caffeine late in the day.

2) Exercise can help you relax but not if it occurs too close to bed time. Try to workout at least several hours before you plan to retire for the evening.

3) For the best sleeping environment, set the temperature in your bedroom to cool.

4) Go to bed and get up every day at the same time. Never sleep late— not even on weekends.

5) Before you go to bed, try relaxing with a warm bath and soft music.

Almost 40 percent of insomniacs say that the inability to get a good night's sleep interferes with their work. Many automobile accidents and on-the-job accidents are caused by sleepiness. The Sleep Tape can cure sleep problems in about two weeks, if the "patient" is responsive.

The Sleep Tape consists of a set of two videos and an audio tape. The entire package sells for $24.95 plus $3.50 for shipping and handling, and can be ordered by calling (616) 621-2040 or writing to Rosebud, P.O. Box 8033, County Road 687, Hartford, Mi 49057.

Four Common Causes Of Back Pain

There are many different causes for back pain. However, in most cases, those people afflicted with back pain can trace it to one of four common causes:

1. Being out of shape— this is probably the most common cause of back pain. The muscles that support the spine include the abdominals, the back extensors, and the hip and thigh muscles. These muscles become weak and stiff without regular exercise, and pain in the lower back is usually a consequence.

2. Being overweight— carrying around excess weight can cause back pain because it increases the amount of pressure on the spinal disks, which provide cushioning between the vertebrae. Since most overweight people have flabby abdominal muscles which can not support excess weight, the back muscles become overburdened. This causes inordinate stress in the lower back, resulting in back pain.

3. Bad posture— when you walk with slumped shoulders you alter the natural curve of the back and cause stress for the muscles that serve as a girdle to support the spine. In order for the spine to receive proper support, your posture must be good, with your head and shoulders relaxed rather than thrown back and your buttocks should be tucked under slightly and your stomach held in firmly without straining.

4. Tension— anyone who experiences an excessive amount of stress is also susceptible to back pain. While most people can't eliminate all the stress from their lives, they can cut down on the risk with some simple relaxation techniques and by exercising.

How To Prevent Back Pain

Since most back disorders are caused by putting the muscles of the back under too much strain, paying attention to your posture, avoiding certain awkward movements, and exercising on a regular basis, can reduce the risk of straining and injuring your back. In effect, you should learn to lift, sit, stand, and sleep in ways that protect your back, and help you avoid back pain.

Here are several tips that may help you prevent back problems:

1) Begin, and stay with, a regular exercise program that emphasizes general fitness, aerobic, conditioning and strengthening of the muscles that support the spine.

2) Always warm up before and cool down after a workout.

3) Lift with your legs, hold objects close to your body, face your work and use lifting aids if at all possible.

4) Adjust table heights to a comfortable level.

5) Use back rests and lumbar supports when sitting.

6) Stop smoking.

The Best Chair To Sit In To Prevent Back Problems

The best chair to sit in is one that has a firm, upright back which enables you to press your lower and middle back against it, supporting the spine. The chair should also be of a size and height that will allow you to place your feet flat on the ground and to bend your knees comfortably at a right angle. Your chair should also support most of the back of your thighs.

The Best Sleeping Position To Alleviate Back Pain

Sleep on your side with your knees bent and with a pillow between them. This not only will relieve pressure on your back muscles, it will also prevent you from overstretching your hip muscles during the night. Other Back Pain Relief Tips:

It is important that you stand up straight with your head up, your shoulders back, and your weight resting equally on both feet. Always avoid standing in one position for longer than a few minutes. If you can't avoid standing in one position, try shifting your weight from foot to foot. This will prevent any single area from being subjected to excessive stress. You can also try putting one foot up on a stack of books or a stool to keep your back from arching. And always try to avoid wearing shoes that have high heels, because they can place unnecessary strain on your lower back.

When you pick something up, you should squat in front of the object, keeping your back straight while holding the object close to your body. You should then rise slowly by straightening your knees. This allows your legs to do most of the work.

When carrying something relatively heavy, such as luggage, always try to keep the load balanced with equal weight in each hand. You should never twist at the waist when carrying a heavy object— rather move your feet instead.

Easy Exercise Program To Prevent Back Pain

1) Lie on your stomach, with your hands on the floor directly beneath your shoulders. Slowly straighten your arms, while keeping your spine relaxed. Allow only your upper torso to move up from the floor.

2) Arch your back passively as your hip bones remain on the floor. Straighten your arms as much as is comfortable for your back. Slowly bend your arms so your upper torso returns to the floor. Repeat these movement about ten times.

Swimming is probably the best form of exercise to relieve chronic back pain. When you swim the breaststroke, you must be careful to put your face in the water every few strokes, otherwise you will be arching your lower back which is likely to aggravate your back pain.

Jogging is also a good form of exercise for people who suffer from back pain. Those people who experience chronic, or recurrent back pain, and who take up jogging as a form of exercise, should avoid all hard surfaces. They should also wear cushioned insoles to reduce the amount of jarring through the spine each time your feet hit the ground.

Strength exercises that require lifting weights can also be of benefit in relieving back pain. However, it is important that you take some precautions when doing strength exercises. Always use an exercise mat for any floor exercises that you do. You should also keep your knees bent during sit-ups in order to reduce the chances of aggravating existing problems in your lower back.

To ease back pain, you can try elevating your knees a foot or so. Place a pillow under your knees so they are elevated about 12 inches in order to keep your hips lightly flexed. The best pillow to use may be an inflatable pillow because foam pillows are likely to become compressed with use.

This Works Much Better Than Conventional Treatments To Ease Back Pain

While conventional treatments for lower back pain, such as surgery; traction; massage; bed rest; and acupuncture; are all helpful in bringing temporary relief, many experts believe that exercise can be an effective long-term solution.

Recent research has shown that people with chronic back pain who participate in some form of regular exercise are better able to manage the pain than those who remain inactive. But, before you decide to undertake any particular type of exercise, consult your doctor about the exact cause of your back pain. If you have problems with your vertebral discs, or if you have osteoporosis, it is essential that you have a doctor guide you in your exercise program.

New Technique To End Back Pain

A recently developed "external" technique that simulates spinal fusion can provide the sufferers of back pain with a preview of the results of back surgery.

Spinal fusion is a surgical procedure designed to alleviate painful movement by holding selected pieces of bone in place. The new preview technique was developed at Baylor College of Medicine in Houston and utilizes steel rods and screws which are held in place by a device originally designed to correct spinal fractures. The new technique allows doctors, who have a difficult task of determining which of the ten lumbar joints in the spine is creating the lower back pain, to fuse, temporarily, the joint suspected of being the culprit.

With the external device in place, a patient can go about his or her routine daily tasks and at the same time determine if the problem joints have been located. If the patient experiences complete relief, he or she is likely to get that same result from permanent spinal fusion. However, if the pain persists, the patient and doctor can examine other possible problem areas before proceeding with major surgery.

Five Things You Should Know Before Going To A Chiropractor

Simply put, chiropractic treatment relies on physical manipulation and adjustments of the spine for therapy, rather than on surgery or drugs. Before consulting a chiropractor about a lower back problem, there are several things you should know.

1) Since lower back pain can have many different causes, including kidney disease, bladder tumor and prostate cancer, it is essential to have the condition and its cause properly diagnosed. Since a chiropractor deals with manipulation and adjustments of the spine, some patients may require the treatment of another specialist. In other words, some lower back problems require treatment which is beyond the scope of a chiropractor.

2) While chiropractors are licensed health care practitioners, individual chiropractor's credentials may differ, which can have an effect on the type of therapy regimen prescribed. There are also varying state laws regarding credentials and certain kinds of treatment. Make sure you check out a chiropractor's credentials before undergoing any treatment.

3) Chiropractors generally diagnose like other doctors. Chiropractic treatment, however, does not involve the use of drugs or surgery as therapy— it involves adjustments and manipulation.

4) As a chiropractic patient, you should undergo a comprehensive consultation, which includes a review of your body systems and your medical history. You should also undergo a thorough physical examination in which the chiropractor looks for "subluxation" or the partial dislocation of a joint. The physical should also look for postural problems and/or problems caused by improper positioning or functioning of one bone in relationship to another.

5) A chiropractor should come highly recommended by former

and current patients. One way to find a good chiropractor is to talk with friends or associates who have had chiropractic treatment. Their positive recommendations should give you confidence in the chiropractor's ability.

Exciting Breakthrough For Headache Sufferers: These "Trigger Foods" Are Proven To Cause Headaches.

Extensive studies have revealed that 10% of chronic headaches are caused by certain foods, often referred to as "trigger" foods. Most often the headache is a reaction to a chemical in the food, which causes the blood vessels in the head to expand or contract, causing pain. Here are several of the foods that can cause headaches:

1) Aged cheese, liver, nuts, bananas, sour cream, yogurt and freshly baked bread— these foods all contain the chemical tyra mine which can also be found in pickled foods such as relish and beets.

2) Chocolate— contains the chemical phenylethylamine.

3) Cured meats such as bacon, ham, bologna, salami, and hot dogs— these foods all contain nitrates.

4) Some meat tenderizers and Chinese food— these can contain momosodium glutamate (MSG), a flavor enhancer (also found in some canned soups and TV dinners).

You can determine if your headaches are being caused by the food you eat by giving up all potential trigger foods. Once you do this, wait about 30 days and if you still experience the same type of headaches, your problem is not being caused by your choice of foods. However, if your headaches become less intense or they occur less often, food most likely does play a role. To find out if there is a specific food causing your headaches, reintroduce large quantities of one trigger food. If your headaches flare up, you've found a culprit. Continue this method until you've tested each food.

Aspirin May Lead To A 20% Reduction In TheOccurance Of Migraine Headaches

A five-year study has shown that minimal doses of aspirin—about 325 milligrams every other day—may lead to a 20% drop in the occurance of migraine headaches among acute migraine sufferers. This information does not mean that migraine sufferers should begin taking aspirin on their own, however. Even in low doses, aspirin is a powerful drug which can cause bleeding in the stomach and aggravate other conditions as well. However, with the guidance of a doctor, many migraine sufferers can try out this new way for alleviating headache pain.

What To Take For A Headache If You Take Aspirin For Arthritis

If you take aspirin for arthritis pain, you should take acetaminophen for headaches and other nonarthritis pain. If you take only aspirin for all those afflictions, you run the risk of overloading your system with anti- inflammatories.

Nasal Spray And Migraines

A new nasal-spray pain reliever, marketed by Mead Johnson Laboratories, offers relief for people who suffer from migraines and postsurgery pain. Stadol, the brand-name drug which has been available for about 15 years as an injectable pain reliever, is now available in a nasal inhaler. The new nasal spray can be administered at home by the patient.

According to Mead Johnson, the new nasal spray can be used when narcotics are not recommended. The drug Stadol is an analgesic and not a narcotic. It is not a federally controlled drug. Ask your doctor for more information about Stadol and the new nasal spray.

Sex And Headaches

The old joke "not tonight dear, I have a headache" isn't all that funny to the many people who suffer from sex-induced headaches. However, according to a new Danish study, such "post-orgasm" headaches may be just a temporary problem, so be patient.

While headache specialists have long been aware of benign coital headache, or orgasmic cephalgia, knot much is known about why orgasms trigger headaches or the likelihood of recurrences. But the study, which involved 26 people who suffered sex-related haedaches, suggests that the discomfort will eventually stop recurring as long as the person also does not suffer tension headaches or migraines.

Herbal Salt Substitutes

One good way to cut down or eliminate your intake of salt is to take advantage of several herbal combinations which can be placed in shakers and used as salt substitutes. Here are two basic herbal salt substitutes:

1) The most basic herbal salt substitute consists of garlic powder, basil, oregano and powdered lemon rind. Place 2 teaspoons of garlic powder and one teaspoon each of basil, oregano, and powdered lemon rind in a blender and mix thoroughly. Keep the mixture in a glass container with the addition of rice to ensure that it doesn't cake.

2) For a more spicy salt substitute, place 1 teaspoon each of cloves, pepper, and crushed coriander seed, 2 teaspoons of paprika, and 1 tablespoon of rosemary in a blender and mix well. Keep the mixture in an airtight container.

Should You Use Real Sugar
Or A Sweetener Substitute?

It's true that, except for supplying calories and energy, sugar has no nutritional value. However, it is not true that sugar prompts hyperactivity in children or causes diabetes, heart disease, and acne. And while sugar can contribute to obesity, it is much less a factor than fatty foods in causing a person to be overweight. The problem with using sugar is that many people don't know "when to say when". Consumed in small amounts, sugar actually provides some healthful benefits. Sugar can help relieve anxiety and stress, induce relaxation and sleep, act as an antidepressant, help heal wounds, and eliminate bacteria. New studies also suggest that small amounts of table sugar might even be safe for some people with diabetes.

On the negative side, sugar does promote cavities, and can cause sudden increases in insulin and blood glucose (although some vegetables, such as potatoes and carrots rank above sugar in ability to spur a quick rise in blood sugar). As mentioned earlier, sugar can promote weight gain if consumed in excess. It can also replace nutritional value when sugar-laden junk foods are a main part of one's diet.

Unless a medical condition dictates the use of artificial sweeteners rather than sugar, it's a matter of individual choice. If you do use sugar, do so moderately, and make sure you don't replace nutritional value for the sake of a "sweet tooth".

This Tastes Just Like Chocolate... Plus It's Healthy

You might not want to hear it, but chocolate is not especially good for you. Besides being fattening, it also contains a chemical—tyramine— which can trigger headaches. And since it is nearly all fat and contains caffeine, it should be avoided at all costs if you're suffering from heartburn.

There is some good news, however. For those people who love the taste of chocolate, many people have found that "chocolate" frozen yogurt actually tastes like real chocolate, and it's a healthier choice for dessert, or anytime. Try it!

Why You Must Eat Fiber-Rich Foods

Fiber consists of the indigestible matter in the diet. It can be divided into two types—soluble and unsoluble—depending on its ability to dissolve in water. An adequate supply of fiber in the diet increases the speed with which food passes through the intestines, helps to prevent constipation and reduces the risk of hemorrhoids, and may help reduce the risk of bowel cancer. A diet high in fiber will also slow down the absorption of sugar from the intestine, resulting in reduced blood sugar levels. And new research indicates that a high-fiber diet may cut down on the risk of breast cancer.

How To Add More Fiber To Your Diet

Current research indicates that the average American consumes 10 to 12 grams of fiber per day which, according to the National Cancer Institute, is not nearly enough. The NCI advises that you increase your daily consumption of fiber to 25 to 30 grams. This increase doesn't have to occur overnight— it can take place gradually. Experts at the NCI suggest that you first try to reach 20 grams per day, and then increase to the 25 to 30 gram level.

A gradual, but determined increase in the amount of fiber in your diet doesn't have to be an unpleasant experience. The best approach is to cut down on all the visible fat from the meat you consume, switch to low-fat dairy products, and increase your intake of whole-grains, fruits and vegetables. Such items as bran, apricots, prunes, cabbage, and celery, are all excellent sources of fiber you can add to your daily diet to help you attain the recommended 25 to 30 grams per day.

Best Fiber-Rich Foods To Lower Your Cholesterol

Soluble fiber dissolves in water and is present in peas, beans and oats. Research indicates that soluble fiber may help lower your cholesterol level. Insoluble fiber, which is found in whole grains, such as wheat bran and many vegetables, does not dissolve in water. This type of fiber helps hold water in the colon, and can also help prevent constipation.

Eating Too Much Fiber Can Cause Bowel Problems

Even though an inadequate amount of fiber in your diet can lead to serious health problems, you shouldn't become unduly alarmed and try to consume as much fiber as you possibly can. That's because, just like any other nutrient, too much fiber in your diet can also cause health problems. An excessive amount of fiber in your diet can bind important minerals in your intestine, not allowing your body to absorb them. This can cause abdominal cramps and lead to an irritation of your digestive tract. While it is not likely that you will take in too much fiber from food sources alone, there are limits to the amount of high-fiber foods you can comfortably consume. And you should be especially prudent if you consume products that are highly concentrated sources of fiber, such as processed bran or commercial fiber supplements. People who have a low mineral intake, such as the elderly, are especially vulnerable, and should try to avoid concentrated forms of fiber as much as possible.

The Truth About Milk

Nineteen Ninety Two has been an interesting year for cow's milk. First came the study linking cow's milk to juvenile diabetes. Then, the Physicians Committee For Responsible Medicine—a group of health and animal rights activists based in Washington—suggested that milk from cows may not be a healthy choice for children. Even Dr. Benjamin Spock, venerated child care guru and respected pediatrician at Johns Hopkins University, got into the fray with his questions about the benefits of cow's milk as food for children.

The diabetes research, reported in a study in the New England Journal of Medicine, suggested that drinking cow's milk in infancy might promote juvenile diabetes in people who are genetically predisposed to the disease. The researchers speculated that children who have certain genetic characteristics produce high levels of antibodies to a protein in cow's milk which is very similar to one found in the pancreas, which produces insulin. Researchers theorized that the children's antibodies then mistakenly go about destroying the cells which produce insulin, leading to diabetes. Other studies had indicated that there may be some link between milk and iron deficiency in infants as well as colic, allergies, and digestive problems.

The American Medical Association (AMA) has responded to the "attack" on cow's milk by denying that there is any "scientific proof" to back up conclusions of potential risks to children. Medical and nutritional experts point out that the research on diabetes is not conclusive and is therefore, not a "proven cause and effect study". However, most experts say that it is best not to give cow's milk to babies less than one year old. The American Academy of Pediatrics in Elk Grove Village, Ill., recommends that babies up to one year old should be breast-fed or given iron-enriched formula.

While the controversy continues, many respected medical experts say that for most people, drinking cow's milk is the only way they can get enough calcium in their diets. That's why such experts say that it isn't necessary or wise to give up on milk completely. It is estimated that 70 percent to 75 percent of the average American calcium intake comes from dairy products including milk. Therefore, for many people in this country, eliminating milk from their diets would cause nutritional deficiencies.

One noted dietician recommends that cow's milk not be eliminated from the diets of either children or adults, but that it be consumed in moderation as part of a varied diet. However, if you are determined to remove milk from the diet, you should check with a qualified dietician or pediatrician first.

How Kids Can Get Enough Calcium Without Milk

Here is a list of foods which will provide the RDA of 800 milligrams of calcium for children ages 1 through 10. (8 ounces of whole milk has approximately 291 milligrams of calcium; 8 ounces of skim milk has about 302).

1) 8 1/2 cups of frozen broccoli.

2) 4 1/2 cups of frozen kale. (90 milligrams of calcium in each cup.)

3) 14 ounces of canned salmon, with juice and bones.

4) 2 to 3 cans of sardines.

5) 16 oranges.

6) 4 1/2 cups of ice cream or 4 1/2 cups of frozen yogurt.

7) 5 to 6 slices of American cheese.

8) 5 cups of 2 percent cottage cheese.

Cooked kale or broccoli, tofu (soybean curd), dried or cooked beans, and canned sardines, with the bones, are all good nondairy sources of calcium.

Should You Take Mineral Supplements?

Most people get adequate amounts of minerals from their diets and have no need of supplements, which are available over-the-counter in liquid or tablet form.

Iron is the most commonly used mineral supplement. It is used to treat iron- deficiency anemia and is often needed by women who are pregnant or who are breast-feeding. You can boost your iron intake—without supplements—by eating such iron-rich foods as lima beans, spinach, whole-grain cereals, lean beef and clams.

Only one other type of mineral deficiency—magnesium—occurs with relative frequency. Magnesium deficiency usually occurs as a result of alcohol abuse, prolonged treatment with diuretic drugs, or a kidney disorder. Low levels of magnesium have been associated with high blood pressure. To increase your intake of magnesium without resorting to supplements, you should try eating more whole grains, green vegetables, dried beans, nuts, legumes, chocolate skim milk and yogurt.

In general, unless a deficiency exists, mineral supplements are not necessary, and should be used only after consultation with your doctor.

How To Choose The Best Supplement

In general, if you have your doctor's approval to take a supplement you should be sure to choose a multivitamin that contains a balanced mixture of the essential vitamins and minerals, rather than a single vitamin or mineral. It's important to remember that an excessive amount of any one nutrient may prevent the body from absorbing and using other nutrients. Therefore, the multivitamin you choose should be at 100 percent of the Food and Drug Administration's RDA for each nutrient. It isn't necessary to exceed those recommended levels.

You should also make sure the multivitamin has an expiration date. Most vitamins and minerals lose their potency after a time and anything over three years old is most likely no longer effective. Many supplements don't list any expiration date, making it impossible to tell how long they have been sitting on the shelf. If the bottle doesn't have an expiration date, don't buy the supplement.

The most important thing to remember when considering supplements is that you should not depend on them to make up for your own bad eating habits. The best way to get the nutrients you need is through a well-balanced diet.

Lower Breast Cancer Rates Linked To Diet

An ongoing study to determine why Hispanic and Black women have lower rates of breast cancer than whites, suggests that diet may play an important role. The study suggests that a diet rich in beans, fruits, and vegetables may be one factor and alcohol may be another. Although all three groups consumed similar amounts of fat and fiber, Hispanics appear to be more likely to eat beans and vegetables containing antitoxidants, substances with anti-cancer properties, and tend to eat the type of monosaturated fat found in olive oil. Whites also consume more alcohol, especially beer, than either Hispanics or blacks,

4 Proven Ways To Lower Nutrient Loss In Foods

1) When shopping for produce, always choose fresh fruits and vegetables with care. Regardless of the price, don't buy produce that has bruises or cuts or that simply doesn't look fresh.

2) Don't soak fresh fruits and vegetables in still water for any length of time or the nutrients may pass into the water. Instead, wash your fruits and vegetables under cold, running water. You can lso use a small amount of dishwashing liquid to help remove any residue of fat-soluble pesticides that may remain on the food. And be sure to rinse all of your produce thoroughly.

3) Whenever possible, make salads just before you eat them. Valuable vitamins are lost when fruits and vegetables are cut up in advance and left exposed to air.

4) You should cook food for the shortest time possible. Then, eat it as soon as you can and don't allow the food to stay hot for prolonged

periods. If you thaw frozen vegetables or fish before cooking, cook them immediately.

Three Health Hazards Of Microwave Cooking: What Not To Do

Recently, some British researchers found that the amount of salt or sugar in prepared foods may change the way foods absorb microwave energy. According to the research, a high salt or sugar content prevents food from reaching a high enough temperature to kill salmonella and other dangerous bacteria. Instead, microwaving such foods may only heat bacteria to a temperature that, rather than killing them, helps them grow.

When microwaving prepared foods, the best way to avoid food poisoning is to microwave them longer and at a lower temperature than the package recommends. Let the food sit for a few minutes—after microwaving—to be certain that dangerous bacteria are dead.

Another possible health hazard associated with microwave ovens is the adverse effect they can have on pacemakers. Modern pacemakers are relatively unaffected by interference, but in some cases they can be affected by powerful electromagnetic pulses and their ability to help regulate the heartbeat may become impaired.

You should also check the microwave door gasket regularly to make sure the seal is tight so that no stray radiation can leak out.

To get the best nutritional value out of fruit and vegetables, you should eat them raw. Without cooking, vegetables retain their essential vitamins intact and are more potent as health protectors. If you don't care for raw vegetables, the next best thing is to cook them as quickly as possible. When you microwave vegetables you will preserve nutrients such as vitamin C to a much greater extent than you do when you allow them to simmer in large amounts of water. And if not overcooked, microwaved vegetables will remain both crisp and brightly colored.

Tips To Buying
The Most Nutritious Fruits & Vegetables

When selecting fruits and vegetables for food preparation, bright is better. That means you should choose those fruits and vegetables with the most intense colors. For example, Dark-green lettuce leaves have more vitamins than lighter-colored ones. Carrots that are bright-orange have more beta-carotene than those that are pale. And sweet red peppers contain more nutritious vitamin C than is present in green peppers.

Thiamine Mistake That Many People Make

You should not wash rice or pasta—both high-thiamine foods—before cooking. Don't rinse these foods after cooking either, because you'll most likely wash away the nutritious thiamine.

Easy Way To Read Food Labels For Real Fat
And Calorie Content

Most people visit supermarkets between 2 and 3 times each week, and quite often those shopping trips are confusing because of a lack of information about product labeling. While many manufacturers are meeting the public's demand for healthful low-fat, nonfat, and low-salt foods, others have attempted to take advantage of consumer health concerns with deceptive labeling practices. For example, the word natural as it appears on some food labels can be quite misleading. Many consumers would expect the word natural to at least suggest that the food so labeled is low in calories. The fact is, a food may contain sugar in a different form, such as honey or molasses, and still be high in calories. In order to find and select truly healthful foods both parents and children should learn to read and understand the information on food labels.

When studying food labels, the key items to look for are size, grams of fat, and calories. While most serving sizes listed on labels are correct, some are unrealistically small, misleading some consumers into believing the fat content or calories contained in the product are low. You should be wary of products that list serving sizes that are smaller than is generally the custom.

While serving size is important, it can be confusing, so your ultimate decision may be better based on this easy to remember guideline: 3 grams of fat per 100 calories per serving. Remember, the total allowance of fat is recommended to be about 30% of your caloric intake. At 9 calories a gram, 3 grams would be about 27 calories, or 27 percent of the 100 calories, which falls within the recommendation for total fat. Keep in mind that those guidelines are for your entire diet and not each individual food. But a food containing more than 3 grams of fat per 100 calories will have to be offset by other low-calorie foods.

It is also important that you compare foods for ingredients, price, quality and nutritive value and then select the ones that best suit your needs. By law, all package labels must include the name of the foods; the weight of the contents; and the name and address of the manufacturer, packer or distributor.

Foods which are categorized by the U.S. Food and Drug Administration as standardized foods, such as mayonnaise, ketchup, margarine, and canned and frozen vegetables, do not require a list of ingredients. Many companies, however, provide such ingredient lists voluntarily. All other food which isn't standardized must have ingredients listed.

Many labels feature a Universal Product Code symbol for use with computerized checkout systems. The symbol registers the price of the food. It also updates the inventory of the stock.

Food labels may also contain other symbols. A "K" or "U" inside a circle means that the food was prepared in accordance with Kosher standards. When the Yiddish term "Pareve" appears on a food label, the consumer is being made aware that neither milk nor meat was used in the preparation of the food.

You should also look for markings that may appear on food labels, signifying the grade shield or quality of the product, such as Grade A for eggs and AA for butter and cheese. An inspection stamp indicates that the food was prepared for marketing under sanitary conditions.

Juice Label Confusion - How To Buy The Best

Even though you may learn how to decipher the information contained on product labels, you may still be misled by labels that do not "tell the whole story". For example, fruit juices come in a wide variety of choices, from drinks that are rich in vitamins and minerals to fruit-flavored sugar water, and it can be hard to tell the difference. Health-minded shoppers can make the right selections by following these suggestions:

1) Try to find fruit drinks that are labeled "100 Percent Fruit Juice", "100 Percent Fruit Juice Blends", "100 percent Juice From Concentrate", or "100 Percent Pure Juice".

2) Avoid juice drinks with labels such as "100 Percent Natural" or "100 Percent Real Juice". Such concotions are not guaranteed to contain 100 percent fruit juice.

3) Beware of juices labeled "juice cocktail", "fruit drink" or "juice beverage". Such drinks may contain only as little as 10 percent juice.

4) Pay close attention to the first ingredient listed on the label. Since ingredients on the label are listed in quantity, your best choice is usually a drink whose first ingredient is juice, not water.

How New Food Labeling Rules Will Help You

Thanks to new labeling regulations, consumers, for the first time, will be able to compare the nutritional value of every packaged food available in the supermarket.

The new federally required labels on all processed foods will have to list calories, total fat, saturated fat, cholesterol, carbohydrates and protein, and sodium content, and show them in the context of a daily diet featuring 2,000 calories and 65 grams of fat. The idea is to show the consumer how much of a day's total of each individual ingredient he or she is getting from a particular food. Also, designations such as "low-fat", "high-fiber" and "light" are to have federally imposed definitions under the new labeling regulations.

Here are the federal govenrment's definitions for some of the terms most commonly used to describe calories, sodium, sugar, fiber, fat, and cholesterol in food:

1) Free— fewer than 5 calories; less than 0.5 gram of sugar; less than 5 milligrams of sodium; less than 0.5 gram of fat; less than 2 milligrams of cholesterol, and 2 grams of saturated fat per serving.

2) Low— less than 140 milligrams of sodium; fewer than 40 calories; 3 grams or less of fat per serving size.

3) High— provides more than 20 percent of the amount recommended for daily consumption, as in "high_fiber".

4) Source of— provides 10 to 19 percent of the amount of a specific nutrient recommended to be consumed each day.

5) Reduced, or less— at least 25 percent less than the original product in sodium, calories, fat, saturated fat or cholesterol.

6) Light— if the product has more than 50 percent calories from fat, this designation means at least a 50 percent reduction in fat. However, if the product has less than 50 percent calories from fat, it can be either 50 percent reduced in fat or have 1/3 fewer calories.

7) Light in sodium— reduces the sodium content of the original product by 50 percent.

Until now, high-fat foods seldom carried nutrition information, and labels that did include such information based it on varied serving sizes, and words used to describe food had no uniform meaning. The new labeling requirements will not only supply the federally imposed definitions for such terms, they will also require that servings sizes be uniform.

Raw meat and poultry are not included in the new labeling rules but products containing meat and processed meat, such as bologna, are covered by the new guidelines. The labeling rules will also not apply to restaurant menus, but any restaurant posting a sign advertising a "low-fat" food must be sure the food complies with the federal government's definition.

According to nutrition experts, the point of the new labeling rules is to enable consumers to have better control of their diets. Such control would be protection against chronic diseases such as heart disease and some cancers.

While food companies are not required to have the new labels on their products until May 1994, many are expected to begin placing the new labels on their foods by the spring of 1993.

8 Keys To Cooking For Better Health

Healthful does not mean low on flavor. Here are some excellent methods of preparing tasty, healthful low-fat meals:

1) Bake, grill, roast, broil or braise meat, fish and poultry.

2) Baste meats and poultry with broth or stock and just a small amount of margarine or butter.

3) Use flavored vinegars, marinades of lemon juice, or fruit juices mixed with herbs when grilling or broiling. These items also make good tenderizers for lean cuts of meat.

4) Make your own sauces by combining stock or broth with pan juices. Thicken by boiling rapidly for a few minutes. Season your sauce with herbs and a small amount of wine.

5) Learn to stir-fry. Use a nonstick wok or saute pan and a minimum of oil.

6) Use your microwave to cook fish, vegetables, and poultry with a minimum of fat, and to reheat your leftovers.

7) Try extra lean ground beef or ground turkey in casseroles, spaghetti sauce, and chili.

8) Season meats, vegetables, stir-fry, and sauteed dishes with small amounts of flavorful oils, such as sesame, olive and chili oil. You can also season cooked vegetables with lemon juice, herbs, or stock.

Best Things To Eat And Drink, In The Morning To Feel Great All Day

There's usually no good excuse for skipping a meal as important as breakfast. Even a light breakfast helps us get into the day with more energy and the necessary nutrients. Good breakfast foods should be low in fat and cholesterol, high in calcium, contain some source of vitamin C and/or vitamin A, be high in fiber, and contain some protein.

Fresh fruits, such as berries, peaches, plums, melons, and kiwifruit, are excellent sources of both vitamins C and A, as well as fiber. Your favorite bread or a toasted English muffin can be topped with nonfat cottage cheese or a low-fat yogurt/raisin spread. You'll be adding protein to your meal as well as eliminating butter or jam. Add a glass of juice or 2 percent milk to the menu, and you have a quick, healthy, energizing, low-fat meal.

Here are some other breakfast suggestions you can work into your menu:

1) Have a bowl of hot or cold cereal with skim milk.

2) Sprinkle your favorite cereal or wheat germ on top of a bowl of plain or flavored nonfat yogurt.

3) If you add scrambled eggs to your breakfast menu, use only one yolk for every two whites, eliminating over 200 milligrams of cholesterol and 60 calories.

4) Try waffles with low-fat frozen yogurt or a fat-free frozen tofu-based dessert.

How To "Snack" Between Meals Without Gaining Weight

Eating between meals doesn't have to be bad for your health. In fact, if you choose the right foods, snacking between meals can actually be good for your health. The key is to choose snack foods that are lower in fat, cholesterol, sugar, and salt than the standard "junk food" items. If you can't bring yourself to do that, you'll need to make some adjustments for the extra fat, sugar and sodium you intake with a favorite snack by reducing the amount of those "offending" substances you consume during regular meals.

The Worst And Best Junk Foods

Most people already know some of the worst offenders in this group— candy bars, soda, and potato chips. All of those foods are either loaded with fat or sugar, and high in calories.

Candy bars are heavy with saturated fat and calories, but as long as you are also eating a well-balanced diet, they are not especially bad for your health. However, a more sensible and healthful alternative is low-fat or no-fat candies, such as jelly beans, gumdrops, marshmallows, and hard candies.

Sugar is the big culprit in soda. Drinking one can of soda is about the equivalent of eating 10 packets of sugar and washing it down with water. Soda will also make you thirstier than you were before you drank it, because your body will require more fluids to dilute that much sugar. As an alternative to soda, try a 16 ounce drink made from equal parts of your favorite fruit juice and flavored seltzer. This 16 oz. drink has only about 55 calories (1 12 oz. can of soda has about 128 calories) and the sugar will appease your appetite.

Even if the label states "no cholesterol", potato chips get as much as 60% of their calories from fat. In just one ounce of potato chips (10 or 12 chips) there are about 150 calories and 9.8 grams of fat. And most corn chips are just about as bad. Instead of chips, try snacking on baked tortilla chips. There are only about 110 calories and 1.4 grams of fat in an ounce of tortilla chips that are baked instead of fried.

These Taste Better Than Cola, And Are Good For You

To avoid consuming an excessive number of calories in the things you drink, try giving up cola. Most colas are overloaded with calories and have very little nutritional value. Instead of cola, try substituting more healthful drinks such as club soda, decafinated tea and coffee, fruit juices, and of course, water.

5 "Healthy Foods" That Are Bad For You

Sometimes we are misled into assuming certain snack foods are healthful when, in fact, they aren't. Here are several such foods that are usually, by reputation, thought to be healthy:

1) Peanuts— Although peanuts do contain protein, about 74% of their calories come from fat. A small bag of dry roasted peanuts (vending machine size) has 170 calories and 14 grams of fat— the same amount you would get from eating almost three pats of butter. Another little known "quality" of peanuts is that they are slow to be digested— that's why you can consume great quantities of them before you get a "full" feeling.

2) Granola— It's high in fat— frequently saturated fact such as coconut oil.

3) Cheese— On the positive side, cheese contains a lot of calcium and some protein. The bad thing about it is that cheese has one of the highest saturated fat contents of any food.

4) Muffins— Unless you make them yourself with low-fat ingredients, you'll most likely be eating an unhealthful food. Most of the muffins now sold in stores are 4 1/2 ounces to 6 ounces at about 100 calories per ounce. And they contain about as much fat as three pats of butter.

5) Sunflower seeds— While a package of roasted sunflower seeds contains some protein, it has about the same amount of fat as a bag of potato chips.

The 7 Best Snack Foods

1) Cereal— dry cereal, topped with skim milk and fruit, is both nutritious and easy to fix.

2) Bagels— while bagels contain 160 to 180 calories, they have almost no fat.

3) Pizza— as long as you get very little cheese and lots of peppers, onions, and mushrooms, pizza can be either a nutritious snack or

light meal. It's high in calcium and in vitamin A, B-complex, and C.

4) Fudgesicles— this is a good way to get the flavor of chocolate without the fat. A fudgesicle contains only about 100 calories (the diet version has about 35 calories), compared with as much as 300 calories in the average candy bar.

5) Hershey's chocolate syrup— this syrup is made with dry cocoa powder and has very little fat. You can make a low-calorie shake by mixing this chocolate syrup in a blender with skim milk and ice cubes. Or you can pour it over low- fat ice milk if you crave a sundae.

6) Popcorn— lightly salted, unbuttered, and air-popped.

7) Dried fruits— apricots, dates, figs, raisins, and prunes all make excellent, healthful snacks.

8) Soft Pretzels— you can find these in the frozen food sections of most supermarkets, and they contain very little fat.

8 Tips To Eat Healthier At Fast Food Restaurants

Today's busy lifestyles have led to an increased popularity of fast-food restaurants. We like fast food because it's quick and convenient. But, if you've made changes in your diet to avoid high-fat, cholesterol-rich and sodium-heavy food, can you still enjoy the fare at a fast-food restaurant? The answer to that question depends on the restaurant and what type of food they offer.

Most fast foods provide some of the nutrients you need, including some vitamins, minerals and protein. However, they don't often provide calcium, and vitamins A and C. They also have a tendency to be high in fat, sodium, and calorie content relative to the nutrients they provide. They can also be low in fiber. An order consisting of a cheeseburger, large fries and a shake can contain nearly 28 grams of saturated fat. In just one meal such as that, you've most likely come pretty close to your daily fat, cholesterol, sodium, and caloric allowance.

The good news is that many fast-food establishments are taking steps to accommodate people who are concerned about the nutritional value of their food. For example, many fast-food restaurants have switched from frying food in saturated beef tallow to polyunsaturated vegetable oil. Also grilled chicken and lower-fat beverages, such as 2% milk are now being offered by many outlets. Salads and reduced-calorie dressings have become standard items on most fast-food menus. And several of the biggest fast-food chains are now providing reduced-fat hamburgers, such as McDonald's McLean Deluxe, a hamburger with less than half the fat of their Quarter Pounder.

Here are eight tips on how you can enjoy many of your favorite fast foods, while cutting back on fat and sodium:

1) Avoid sauce. Have your hamburger, fish, or chicken sandwich without mayonnaise, tartar or other "special" sauces.

2) Eliminate cheese. The varieties of cheese commonly used by fast-food restaurants on burgers and chicken sandwiches, and breakfast muffins and biscuits are high in fat, cholesterol and calories.

3) Smaller is better. If a sandwich is your preference, avoid entrees called "big", "double", "jumbo", or "whopper" because they usually contain a "super load" of fat. By ordering the plain, small hamburgers you can cut the fat by as much as 70%.

4) Look for chicken, fish, or lean-meat entrees that are grilled, broiled or roasted.

5) Have your toast, english muffin, or pancakes be prepared and served without butter or margarine. Use jelly or jam instead.

6) To reduce the amount of sodium in a regular-size hamburger, eliminate condiments such as pickles and ketchup.

7) If you order breakfast, avoid the ham, bacon, or sausage, and trim the sodium content by more than 30%.

8) If you eat your fries plain, without adding salt and ketchup, the sodium content can be reduced by more than 60%.

Cereal— The best and the worst

Not all cereals are equal in nutritional value. Some are high in sugar, while others have none. Some are fortified with up to 15 nutrients, and others aren't fortified at all. Depending on which type you choose, cereal may not be your most healthful choice for breakfast. Here are some insider tips on choosing the best cereals from the worst:

1) The 6 to 8 grams of fiber in a one ounce serving of bran flakes with fresh fruit could make a good daily start on the National Cancer Institute's recommendation that American adults consume from 25 to 30 grams of dietary fiber a day.

2) Cereals that contain iron are also a good choice, especially for women. If you don't eat red meat or other iron-rich foods, the American Dietetic Association suggests that you choose a cereal that contains at least 45 percent of the U.S. Recommended Daily Allowance for iron. Also be sure to have orange juice or another vitamin C-rich drink with your cereal, otherwise the iron won't be well-absorbed.

3) Nutritionists agree that breakfast should make up about one quarter of your daily nutrient requirements. A fortified cereal, with 25 percent of the U.S. Recommended Daily Allowances can be helpful as long as you also eat a variety of healthful food throughout the day.

4) Select a cereal with no more than five grams of sugar. In general, the more sugar a cereal contains, the fewer complex carbohydrates and less dietary fiber it contains.

5) If you are primarily interested in insoluble fat—the kind that prevents constipation and may protect against colon cancer—select a cereal made with whole wheat. The best advice is to eat a multigrain cereal that will provide you with both soluble and insoluble fiber, or you can rotate among different types of cereals. Whatever you choose, it should have at least 2 grams of fiber per serving.

6) Try to avoid many of the hot cereals that are now available in single- serving packets. Hot cereal bought in large, economical boxes is not only as easy to cook on the stove or in the microwave, it's also much less expensive. While the instant varieties may seem convenient, they quite often contain a lot of unnecessary salt and sugar.

7) Many cold cereals are highly processed, while hot cereals are less tampered with. However, some hot cereals, such as farina and Cream of Wheat are processed so highly they become very smooth and creamy and loose a great deal of their fiber. You can fortify your own cereal with fiber, by adding fresh or dried fruit, and with calcium by using skim or low-fat milk.

Whatever brand of cereal you buy, be sure to read the label so you'll be certain it contains the nutrients you need.

How Fish Oil Can Lower Your Cholesterol

Fish oil contains a special type of unsaturated fat called omega-3. Research has shown that fish oil may be effective in counteracting a high-cholesterol diet by lowering blood levels of very-low-density cholesterol and triglycerides. There seems to be no disagreement that fish is good food, but most authorities, including The American Heart Association and The National Heart, Lung, and Blood Institute, strongly recommend that you get fish oil from fish rather than through the use of fish-oil capsules.

The latest research hasn't show how much fish oil you need to get the beneficial effects, but there are indications that certain doses of fish oil may be harmful. In any event, eating fish as much as three times a week may indeed be good for you, but since precise dosages are not known, it's best that you avoid fish-oil capsules, and get your oil strictly from the fish.

The Healthest Type Of Fish You Can Buy

Studies have shown that farm-raised fish are less contaminated by pollutants, such as mercury, PCBs and DDT than fish that are caught in open waters.

Little-Known Thing You Should Know About Oat Bran

In the late 1980s, oat bran developed the reputation of being a painless way of lowering blood cholesterol without having to endure major dietary changes. The demand for oat bran increased to such an extent that new products, such as oat bran potato chips and oat bran beer found their way onto supermarket shelves. Soon afterwards, oat bran was largly discredited as being ineffective.

Today, the best research indicates that oat bran can be effective in conjunction with a low-fat diet. Oat bran, by itself—or in high-fat products such as potato chips— does not appear to be the answer to lowering blood cholesterol. However, oat bran as part of a low-fat diet can help control blood cholesterol.

Oat bran is still available plain, in rolled oats, and in some oat-based cold cereals (those with 1 to 2 grams of fat per serving are best).

Nuts May Reduce Heart Disease Risk By 50%

Even though nuts are high in fat content, they may have some beneficial effect when it comes to preventing heart disease. The Archives of Internal Medicine reports that a study which kept track of 30,000 men and women indicates that nuts actually do help prevent heart disease.

In the study, a group of people who ate nuts at least five times a week had half as many heart attacks and other fatal heart diseases as did other groups who did not eat nuts nearly so often.

While researchers aren't sure how a food which is high in fat can be good for the heart, they do note that the most commonly consumed nuts—peanuts, walnuts and almonds—are high in monounsaturated fats and contain only small amounts of saturated fats.

The 10 Best Vegetables To Eat

Many fruits and vegetables are high in fiber, low in calories and contain vitamins A and C, which promote good health and even reduce the risk of some cancers. Recently, a California study ranked the top ten vegetables for overall content of major vitamins and minerals. Here is the top ten list:

1) Broccoli 2) Spinach 3) Brussels Sprouts 4) Lima Beans 5) Peas 6) Asparagus 7) Globe Artichokes 8) Cauliflower 9) Sweet Potatoes 10) Carrots

Many of these 10 highly nutritious vegetables are not widely used in the typical American diet. You can easily make your diet more healthful by including any or all of these top ten vegetables.

Cancer-Fighting Vegetables

Researchers at Johns Hopkins University in Baltimore say that the best way to take advantage of special cancer-fighting chemicals found in broccoli is to microwave or steam the vegetable. These two cooking methods leave the chemical intact, enabling you to get its full benefit.

For those people who don't like broccoli regardless of how it is prepared, the same cancer-fighting chemical is also found in high levels in other vegetables including cauliflower, kale, Brussels sprouts, carrots, and green onions.

How Many Fruits And Vegetables You Should Eat

A five-year nationwide program, "5 a day— For Better Health", which is being promoted by the produce industry and supermarket retailers is aimed at those people who don't eat enough fruits and vegetables. The National Cancer Institute and many health professionals are recommending and encouraging people to eat at least five servings of fruit and vegetables each day to help reduce the risk of certain cancers and other chronic diseases.

According to a recent survey, following the 5 a day program would mean a substantial increase in the average American's daily consumption of fruits and vegetables. The 1992 survey of 2,800 people showed that the median daily consumption of fruits and vegetables in the U.S. is only 3 1/2 servings. Just under 90 percent of the men and women who responded to the survey said they eat fewer than five servings a day. Only 8 percent of those surveyed were aware they should be eating at least five servings a day, and two-thirds of the respondents said they thought that two or fewer servings was enough.

The 5 A Day program itself is very flexible, allowing three vegetables plus two fruits one day, the opposite the next day, or any combination so long as the food choices meet the guidelines of the National

Cancer Institute, which include the following:

1) Eat from 5 to 9 servings of fruits and vegetables each day.

2) Eat at least one vitamin A-rich selection every day. Vegetables containing high levels of vitamin A include broccoli, carrots, kale, bok choy, turnip greens, beet and mustard greens, Swiss chard, spinach, romaine lettuce, sweet potatoes, winter squash, and tomatoes. Fruits include apricots, mangoes, cantaloupe, papaya, and watermelon.

3) Consume at least one vitamin C-rich food selection each day. Vegetables include asparagus, broccoli, bok choy, cabbage, Brussels sprouts, green peppers, cauliflower, and tomatoes. Fruits include oranges, grapefruit, kiwi fruit, honeydew melon, strawberries, raspberries, cantaloupe, papaya, and watermelon.

4) Eat at least one high-fiber food every day. Practically all fruits and vegetables are good sources of fiber.

5) Eat cruciferous (cabbage family) vegetables at least 3 times a week. Some studies suggest that cruciferous vegetables might have natural anti-cancer properties. These vegetables include broccoli; Brussels sprouts; bok choy; cabbage; cauliflower; mustard, turnip and beet greens; kale; and Swiss chard.

The National Cancer Institute has provided several mealtime tips on how to incorporate the 5 a day program into your diet.

Breakfast

A) Add fruit, such as strawberries or sliced bananas to cereal.

B) Have a bowl of fruit such as peaches or melons.

C) Top pancakes and waffles with fruit instead of syrup.

D) Drink a glass of fruit juice.

Lunch

A) Eat a salad or soup that has vegetables.

B) Put lettuce, sprouts and tomatoes on a sandwich.

C) Add carrot, celery, or zuchini sticks to your menu.

D) Have a piece of fruit— an apple, orange, etc.

Snack

A) Munch on grapes, raisins, apricots, prunes, figs, or cut raw vegetables.

B) Drink a glass of juice.

Dinner

A) Put raw vegetables or fruit in a green salad.

B) Add vegetables to main dishes, such as broccoli to pasta.

C) Order extra side dishes of vegetables when eating out.

D) Garnish main dishes with fruit.

Dessert

A) Add fresh fruit to a plain dessert.

B) Add pineapple or papaya to frozen yogurt.

C) Add chopped fruit or berries to cakes, cookies or muffins.

How Much Water You Should Drink

Nutrients are substances you need to get every day from what you eat and drink, and by that definition water is an essential nutrient. The recommended amount of water is 8 glasses (64 ounces) per day. That may seem excessive, but under average conditions—a moderate temperature, and only light exercise—the body loses 2 to 3 quarts (2 quarts equals 64 ounces) of fluid a day through sweating, breathing and waste products.

All that fluid must be replaced to maintain an adequate fluid balance in the body. Some of the fluid is replaced when you eat solid foods, such as fruits and vegetables—which contain a lot of water. Other liquids, such as juice, milk, soup, and soft drinks, also help replace lost fluids.

Plain water is best, however, because it is more efficiently absorbed than other fluids, especially those that are high in sugar. Coffee and caffeinated soft drinks are not good replacements either because caffeine acts as a diuretic and causes even more fluid to be lost. Alcohol has the same negative effect.

Suprise! Caffeine Can Get Rid Of A Headache - Or Give You One

In many cases the caffeine in coffee, cola, or several popular over-the-counter painkillers will ease the pain of a headache. The caffeine stops pain by constricting dilated blood vessels in the head and by speeding the absorption of other painkilling medications in the stomach. But all that doesn't mean that the more caffeine you intake the fewer headaches you'll get.

If your daily caffeine intake exceeds 500 milligrams—the equivalent of five cups of brewed coffee or eight cans of cola—you're likely to experience caffeine-rebound headaches. These caffeine headaches occur whenever the caffeine consumption schedule is disrupted—such as when a coffee drinker sleeps later than usual. Many people try to "treat" such headaches by having another cup of coffee. The most effective way of getting rid of these headaches is to avoid caffeine entirely.

The New News On Coffee Drinking. Is It Really Bad For You?

It may surprise you to find out that coffee, while it has some potential health hazards, can actually be good for you. Recent research reveals that coffee may provide several therapeutic benefits. Researchers say that, consumed in moderation, coffee can help improve mental performance, boost energy, relieve asthma and hay fever, prevent cavities, and elevate one's mood. Of course, moderation is the key word.

Heavy coffee consumption has been linked to heart disease, and pregnant women have been advised to cut out or cut down on caffeine, but most experts agree that moderate coffee drinking can provide health benefits.

The recommended "allotment" for coffee drinkers is two cups a day— one in the morning and one in late afternoon. This seems to be the best amount to help you stay alert and concentrated, help keep you in a good mood, and give you a boost of energy. Heavy coffee consumption— five cups or more a day—can lead to health problems, and you shouldn't drink coffee at night if you want to get a good night's sleep.

Decaffeinated Coffee May Be Harmful To These People

A recent study conducted by Swedish researchers revealed that decaffeinated coffee promotes the production of stomach acid which could be damaging to people who have ulcers. It was earlier thought that the caffeine in regular coffee was the source of the stomach acid stimulation, but the new research proves otherwise. While both decaffeinated and regular coffee stimulate gastric acids which could irritate existing stomach ulcers, neither appears to have any role in the actual development of gastric or duodenal ulcers.

The Type Of Person That Decaffeinated Coffee May Be Harmful To

While it is now known that there are several possible benefits from regular coffee, many people feel that decaffeinated brands of coffee are more healthful than caffeinated brands. While it is true that caffeine, consumed in excess, poses health problems, decaffeinated coffee can also be harmful in some instances. The best advice, whether you now drink regular or decaf, is to do so in moderation. You shouldn't consume more than two or three cups a day whether or not you are consuming caffeine.

If your current brand is regular coffee and you are concerned about the amount of caffeine you consume each day, you might make the switch to decaf. The switch should be made gradually, and you should allow yourself enough time to determine which type of coffee is best for you. If you find that caffeine tends to make you "edgy" or anxious, decaffeinated coffee may be a better choice.

Children, Milk And Lower Blood Pressure

New research suggests that an adequate calcium intake during childhood may prevent high blood pressure from occurring later in life. The Framingham Children's Study kept track of the calcium intake of 80 preschoolers from a total of 10 food diaries which were kept by their parents during the course of one full year. The researchers found that each 100 mg. increment in daily calcium intake was associated with a systolic blood pressure that was two points lower. The recommendation is that children between the ages of 1 and 10 should get 800 mg. of calcium per day. One 8 ounce glass of either whole or skim milk contains about 300 mg. of calcium

Get Rid Of Diarrhea With This Natural Drink

Fluids lost from the gastrointestinal tract during a bout of diarrhea contain vital minerals called elecytrolytes. These electrolytes include potassium, magnesium, chloride, sodium, and calcium. In order to speed your recovery from diarrhea, you should drink more than just water. Many sports beverages, such as Gatorade, now available contain the essential electrolytes that plain water cannot replace. Drinking these beverages helps you restore your nutrient balance more quickly.

Delicious Drink That Helps Get Rid Of Hangovers

A hangover can be relieved by drinking lots of nonalcoholic fluids lost by the diuretic effect of alcohol. Nonalcoholic beverages, such as apple juice, may also help relieve the unpleasant taste in the mouth many people experience after consuming a lot of alcohol. While there is no miracle cure for a hangover, apple juice and other nonalcoholic beverages can ease the misery to some extent. Of course, the best way to avoid a hangover is to drink in moderation, or not at all.

New Eating Plan Helps Alleviate Dizziness

According to recent studies many cases of dizziness may be caused by what we eat. Furthermore, the studies suggest that many people who suffer from dizziness don't properly absorb food, and that they can be helped by a simple change in their diets.

The diet to combat dizziness consists of large amounts of complex carbohydrates, such as spaghetti and rice, small amounts of lean meat, and only polyunsaturated fats. The exact amount of food and calories consumed should be based on your age, weight, height, and body frame. The main thing, however, is the breakdown of the calories.

It should be noted that some people, including most diabetics and hypoglycemics will not benefit from this diet because their dizziness is caused by other factors.

6 Foods That Actually Help You Think Better

Recent research by the USDA suggests that foods which contain the mineral boron—pears, grapes, apples, carrots, broccoli—may help your brain maintain its normal activity level. The research indicates that people may feel less alert when their diets are low in boron than when their boron level is adequate.

Researchers at MIT have also discovered that a diet which includes fish can result in a boost in mental-energy. Researchers are quick to point out that no food can actually make you smarter, but the protein found in fish can help raise your mental capacities to their fullest potential.

These Supermarket Foods Will Give You Almost "Instant Energy" That Lasts Up To Five Hours

Nutrition experts say that foods rich in vitamin B12 help to energize the body, especially when there is a B12 deficiency to begin with. New research suggests that B12 can also help energize otherwise healthy people who may be experiencing stress or stress-related fatigue.

There are several good dietary sources of B12, including fish, dairy products, organ meats (such as liver and kidney), eggs, beef, and pork.

Wine May Be The Healthiest Thing To Drink With Your Dinner

While you can never go wrong drinking water with your meals, some experts believe that wine is perhaps the healthiest choice. Studies indicate that wine has several possible healthful benefits including prevention of heart disease, increasing good HDL blood cholesterol, and killing bacteria and viruses. Wine has also been shown to contain chemicals which may prevent cancer in animals.

Some studies indicate that the people of France, who drink wine regularly with their meals (and consume foods high in fat) experience fewer instances of heart disease, and are generally healthier than the majority of Americans. While the studies are not conclusive proof that wine is the healthiest drink to have with your dinner, the evidence does suggest possible benefits.

Of course, there are potential dangers when consuming alcohol, so moderation is the key.

Two Foods That Will Help Boost Your Immune System To Fight Off Disease

1) Yogurt— studies in the United States, Switzerland and Japan, show that yogurt helps boost the immune system in both animal and human cells. Researchers say that yogurt also has several cancer-fighting properties and may help prevent colon cancer.

To make sure you get the best therapeutic value from yogurt, buy only those products which contain "active cultures".

2) Cabbage— recent studies suggest that cabbage can destroy bacteria and viruses and provide a significant boost to the immune system in its efforts to fight off disease. Experts recommend that you eat both raw and cooked cabbage.

Eat These Little-Known Grocery Store Foods If Your Hairline Is Receding

Foods that are rich in biotin, a water-soluble B vitamin, may help put a halt to a receding hairline. Studies show that a biotin deficiency can cause hair loss (as well as dry, flaky skin, and a facial rash). Many hair treatment products feature biotin as an ingredient to help produce healthy hair and prevent graying. The evidence also indicates that hair loss due to an extreme biotin deficiency is reversible with adequate biotin supplementation.

The best dietary sources of biotin include whole grain foods, nuts, organ meats, vegetables, and milk. Biotin is also available in supplement form.

Hearing Problems? This Wonder Food Will Help

Recent studies show that some instances of hearing loss may be a result of a vitamin A deficiency. According to researchers, an inadequate amount of vitamin A in the diet actually leads to an increased sensitivity to sound, which in turn increases the risk of hearing loss from noise damage.

If you experience hearing problems, such as a hearing loss,, good dietary sources, of vitamin A include liver, milk and dairy products, carrots, apricots, cantaloupes, and oranges.

Men: Increase Your Sexual Desire With This Natural Food

Some recent studies suggest that men who have zinc deficiencies are more prone to produce inadequate amounts of male hormone testosterone and sperm than those men with normal zinc levels. There is also evidence to indicate that a zinc deficiency can result in impotence.

One way to overcome a zinc deficiency is to take a zinc supplement. Another way to increase your intake of zinc is through dietary sources such as whole- grain products, brewer's yeast, and wheat bran and germ. Oysters, however, have a far richer concentration of zinc than any other food source. That may be why oysters have long had a reputation of being a "sexual food".

Foods That Cause Heartburn

Fatty foods and foods and beverages containing caffeine frequently cause heartburn. These foods can cause the sphincter muscles between the stomach and the esophagus to relax, which allows an irritating backup of stomach acids into the esophagus. Once your esophagus is irritated, consuming acidic or spicy foods can make the heartburn worse.

If you are prone to heartburn, here are some specific foods to cut down on or avoid altogether: coffee and tea (both regular and decaffeinated); cola; citrus fruits and juices; chocolate; mustard; peppermint; spearmint and alcoholic beverages.

You can also try eating several small meals a day, instead of fewer, larger meals. You should also wait several hours after you've eaten a big meal before you lie down.

Foods That Get Rid Of The Common Cold Faster

Eating spicy foods when you have a cold may bring you some needed relief. Spicy foods irritate nerve endings in your eyes, nose and throat, making your eyes and nose run, and helping to clear congestion. Some spices, such as cloves and hot peppers, also have an expectorant effect, making it easier to cough up mucus.

New Study On How To Avoid Eating "Bad" Foods When You Have A Craving

For many people, weight control is a battle against cravings for fats and sweets. The cravings may be difficult to deny because when sweets or fats are consumed the body produces "pleasure chemicals" called opioids. And while experts say that there is no cure for food cravings in the forseeable future, they may have taken a step toward just such a solution recently.

In a study at the University of Michigan, researchers injected nine women with the drug naloxone, which is also used to prevent heroin from being absorbed by the brain when people have taken overdoses. The drug, known as a "pleasure killer", stopped cravings for fats and sweets.

Researchers say naloxone worked in their test because it effectively blocks opioids from delivering their message of pleasure to the brain. Once the message of pleasure has been eliminated, the craving ceases to exist.

To confirm their initial findings, the researchers reversed the experiment. Another group of women were injected with "extra" pleasure chemicals with the drug butorphanol. The women injected with this drug reported an increase in pleasure when eating fats and sweets.

Even though naloxone was successful in blocking food cravings in the controlled study, it is not available to the public for that purpose. Scientists say its effects are only temporary and wouldn't make much of a difference. However, continuing research using the information uncovered in the University of Michigan study could lead to an eventual solution to food cravings and a significant victory for many people battling weight problems.

Free Chart On Chemical Additives In Food

The Center for Science in the Public Interest has available a color chart entitled "Chemical Cuisine" which provides a list of chemical additives commonly used in food. The chart also provides information about which additives appear to be safe, those to be viewed with caution due to poor testing or use in foods that people tend to eat in excessive amounts, and those to avoid as unsafe.

To get a copy of the chart, write to the Center for Science in the Public Interest, 1501 16th Street NW, Washington, DC 20036.

These Fruits And Vegetables May Contain Harmful Pesticides

Unless you know food has been organically grown, it has most likely been "treated" with some form of pesticide. The theory behind the use of pesticides is that they make crops much less vulnerable to a variety of harmful insects and other pests. This, in turn, helps to keep prices down.

According to the Food And Drug Administration (FDA), the pesticides used today by American farmers seldom "gets into food", and can be eliminated altogether by washing fruits and vegetables with water and wiping them off or peeling them. The FDA, which inspects thousands of domestic and imported foods every year, says that only "minute levels" of pesticide residues are found. The debate about pesticides on food, however, centers around whether or not the FDA's standards and frequency of testing are adequate.

If you are concerned about the use of pesticides on fruits and vegetables, you may want to consider starting your own organic garden. And look for abnormal spotting and coloring which could be cased by harmful pesticides.

Free Grocery Shopping Guidelines Advice Brochures

Free brochures offering grocery shopping advice and recommendations for a healthful diet are available by sending a legal-size self-addressed, stamped envelope to: Consumer Affairs Department (USAT), Food Marketing Institute, 1750 K Street N.W., Washington, DC 20006-2394.

Free Consumer Nutrition Hotline With Registered Dietitians

You can get accurate and timely nutrition information by calling the consumer nutrition hotline operated by the National Center for Nutrition and Dietetics. The center is the public education initiative of The American Dietetic Association and its Foundation.

Using a touch-tone phone, you can talk with a registered dietitian, choose one of three prerecorded messages on nutrition topics, and order free brochures. The recorded messages are available 24 hours a day. The dietitians are on duty Monday through Friday form 10 a.m. to 5 p.m. (Eastern Time). Call 1-800-366- 1655.

For more information about the National Center for Nutrition and Dietetics write to: National Center for Nutrition and Dietetics, 216 West Jackson Boulevard

"The Missing Ingredient"
- Why Your Diets Don't Work Or Last

The key to successful weight control is the ability to make changes in your diet that can be maintained on a long-term basis. In some instances, doctors believe that inconsistent weight management— losing and regaining weight repeatedly—may actually be more harmful than being overweight. In fact, dieters who don't maintain their initial weight-loss, often regain so much weight that they become heavier than they were before they went on a diet .

The safest and most effective way to diet is to go slowly, never losing more than two pounds a week. Losing more than two pounds in a week's time usually means the weight-loss is in fluids and muscle, and not in fat. Your diet should ideally consist of as wide a variety of foods as possible. In some instances, under medical supervision, you may be placed on a highly restricted diet. Such a diet will force you to pay closer attention to the composition of each meal.

The most recommended diet places special emphasis on veg- etables, fruit and complex carbohydrates, which are high in fiber and rich in vitamins and minerals. Such a diet contains fewer calories and less total fat, saturated fat, cholesterol, salt, alcohol, and slightly less protein. You don't have to eliminate any individual foods with this diet, but you will have to cut down on your intake of certain foods, while increasing your consumption of others.

Why "Crash Diets" Don't Work

Many people make the mistake of looking for a "quick-fix"— a way to lose excess weight in a hurry. This usually involves following a super low-calorie diet, without any kind of medical supervision. Crash dieting—sometimes called yo-yo dieting—can present many problems, especially if you get caught in the cycle of losing and then gaining weight.

Crash dieting is not an effective way to achieve long-term weight loss and maintenance. It may also be bad for your health. There is some evidence— although inconclusive— that the weight loss and gain cycle, which is typical of people who use crash diets, could promote heart trouble or even a stroke. This may be a possibility because crash dieting usually results in a shifting of weight from the hips and thighs to the stomach. Some research suggests that a heavy stomach can lead to increased risk of stroke in men as well as a high rate of heart failure in both men and women.

Another health risk associated with crash dieting involves the amount of stress that type of dieting places on the body. Such strain could increase the risk of sudden death from heart disease. Crash dieting is not a recommended course of action for anyone needing to lose weight. Not only is it ineffective, it can be quite dangerous as well.

A High-Fiber Diet Can Work For You

Diets that are high in fiber usually consist of foods such as pasta and cereals, whole-grain bread, beans and dried peas, fresh and dried fruits, and fresh vegetables, all of which contain plenty of fiber and complex carbohydrates. Such high-fiber foods are good for weight loss because they are more filling and contain fewer calories per gram than high-fat foods. As long as this diet contains a wide variety of low-calorie foods, it can be a safe and effective way to lose weight.

The only disadvantage of a high-fiber diet is that it may cause some initial indigestion and gas. These problems normally disappear in a relatively short time. They can also be effectively avoided in most cases by adding fiber to the diet gradually, and by not consuming an excessive amount of fiber.

A Low-calorie Diet
That Works Without Feeling Hungry

This type of diet consists of calorie-controlled meals which are made up of a wide variety of low-fat foods. In order for a low-calorie diet to be effective it must provide at least 1,000 calories per day. It should also include a variety of nutrient-rich foods. It's also essential that good eating habits continue after the initial weight-loss, otherwise the new weight will not be maintained. A low-calorie diet that meets all of the above requirements is highly recommended as a safe and effective means of proper weight control.

Many people think of low-calorie diets as bland and boring and because of that, fall back into old eating habits. Actually, a successful low-calorie diet doesn't have to be unappetizing or extremely low in calories. The important thing is that you lose weight on the type of diet you will continue to follow, even after you reach your desired weight.

Several ways you can reduce your caloric intake and still enjoy mealtime:

1) Cut down on the serving sizes of (or eliminate altogether) these foods:

Meats, including all meat with visible fat, bacon, sausage, salami, and lunch meat.

Dairy products, including butter, whole milk, cream, most cheeses, and ice cream.

Other foods, such as fried foods, potato chips, gravies or sauces, sweetened cereals, pastry, candy, chocolate, and beverages with added sugar. You should also limit your daily intake of alcohol to the equivalent of one ounce of 80- proof whisky—12 ounces of beer or 4 ounces of wine— or none at all.

2) Replace the above foods with small portions of the following:

Meat— lean beef, lamb and pork, skinless poultry (except duck or goose) and liver.

Fish—oily fish such as mackerel, sardines, herring, and salmon or tuna canned in oil. Also nonoily fish, such as cod, haddock and shellfish.

Vegetables— legumes, such as beans (lima, pinto, kidney, navy and soy), and all other vegetables, including potatoes.

Dairy products— eggs, 2% or skim milk, plain low-fat yogurt, and low-fat cheese.

Other foods—Crackers, nuts, dried fruit, bread, unsweetened cereals, pasta, rice, and polyunsaturated soft margarine and vegetable oils.

If you fail to lose weight following the above menu suggestions, then try cutting down on the foods in the above group and increasing your intake of the following:

Meat— all poultry (except duck and goose) with skin removed, and liver.

Fish— nonoily fish such as tuna and salmon soaked in water, shellfish, haddock, and cod.

Vegetables— all vegetables

Dairy products— skim milk and plain low-fat yogurt.

Fruit— fresh fruit and unsweetened fruit juices.

Other foods— bran and whole-grain, pasta, cereals and bread.

Before you modify your menu to accommodate a low-calorie diet such as suggested above, consult your doctor for his or her recommendations.

Low-Fat Diet Tips

Here are some tips from the American Heart Association to help simplify a low-fat eating plan:

1) Limit your intake of lean meat, seafood and poultry (with no visible fat trimmed or drained) to no more than 6 ounces a day.

2) Substitute meatless main dishes as entrees, or combine with small portions of meat.

3) Use no more than 5 to 8 teaspoons of fat and oils a day for cooking, baking, spreads and salads.

4) Cut back on egg-yolk consumption to three or four per week. (Egg whites are all right).

5) Eat five or more servings of fruits and vegetables a day.

6) Eat at least six servings of cereals and grains a day.

7) Use skim or 1% milk and other low-fat dairy products.

8) Limit your consumption of organ meats, such as kidney, liver, heart, and gizzards.

How To Eat Many High Fat Foods
And Still Lose Weight

Many people are under the mistaken impression that in order to lose weight you have to suffer through meals featuring bland foods that are fat-free. Experts agree that the most efficient way to lose weight is to eat less and exercise more. Generally, to lose weight, people should eat 500 to 1,000 calories a day less than their energy requirements. Cutting out fat and eliminating your favorite foods to lose weight is simply not necessary.

It is neither practical nor recommended that you eliminate high-fat foods from your diet altogether. The key is to eliminate only excess fat. Most experts say that your total intake of fat should not exceeed 30 percent of your daily caloric intake. As long as you stick to a total fat intake within the recommended guidelines, you can still enjoy such high-fat foods as porkchops, hamburger, french fries, cheese, dairy products, high-fat dressings such as hollandaise, mayonnaise, veal, and so on.

Obviously you should not eat such high-fat foods three times a day. You must be aware of your total fat intake. If it exceeds the number of grams per day of fat that's right for you, you won't lose weight. If, on the other hand, you exercise discipline and willpower and keep your total fat intake within or under the recommended limits, you can still enjoy high-fat foods and lose weight.

You can use the following formula to calculate the number of grams of fat that's right for you:

1) Multiply your ideal (desirable) weight by 15 if you are moderately active, or 20 if you are very active. Then subtract 100 if you are 35 to 44 years old; 200 if you are 45 to 54; 300 if you are 55 to 64; or 400 if you are 65 or older. The number you get is your "ideal daily caloric consumption".

2) To determine your daily limit of calories from fat, multiply your ideal caloric intake (see above) by 0.30.

3) Divide the above number by 9, as each gram of fat contains nine calories. The result is the maximum number of grams of fat you should eat daily.

To determine your daily limit of saturated fatty acids (recommended at less than 10 percent of total caloric intake), use the above formula you used for fat grams, substituting 0.10 for 0.30. Or, even simpler, you can divide the number of grams of total fat by 3.

The Truth About Liquid Diets

Liquid protein diets—also known as "fasts" and "Very Low Calorie Diets" (VCLDs)— are liquid formulas which contain a relatively high proportion of protein. This type of diet takes in no solid food for up to 16 weeks, just several flavored protein drinks per day. The diet supplies a total of 400 to 800 calories per day. Weight loss with a VCLD can be rapid and dramatic—four to ten pounds can be lost within the first week, with up to five pounds each week thereafter.

Proponents of VCLDs claim the new liquid diets are nutritionally complete and vastly improved from the dangerous liquid diets that were available a decade ago. The new liquid diets are much safer than the old formulas because they contain essential nutrients, including an abundance of high-quality protein, carbohydrate, fatty acids, the recommended amounts of the major vitamins and minerals, and micronutrients. These new, "improved" liquid diets are also administered under medical guidance—many as part of hospital-based programs that monitor each patient at least twice a month to ensure their safety.

Another new feature of the current liquid diets is that "fasters" also attend regular support meetings, and start a controlled "refeeding" after finishing the fast. They are also encouraged to join follow-up programs in order to learn more about proper nutrition, exercise and behavior modification. The people who stay with a follow-up support group for at least a year appear to have a good chance of controlling their weight. Other people have a tendency to fall victim to "yo-yo dieting" and return to their old eating habits and life- styles and regain all the weight they lost while "fasting".

While the new liquid diets are greatly improved from the old formulas, which were associated with several deaths, they still have some significant disadvantages. One disadvantage is the cost. Since these diets should be taken only under medical supervision they can be quite expensive. There is an initial charge of up to $300 for a complete physical examination, nutritional and psychological evaluation and lab tests. You may also pay at least $100 per week for 12 to 16 weeks. That fee is for all medical screening, monitoring, group meetings and the protein product itself. Your insurance will usually cover the medical tests and all doctor's fees, but not the cost of the protein product or the group meetings.

Another distinct disadvantage to liquid diets is side effects, including headaches, dizziness, constipation, fatigue, dry skin, chills, and hair loss. Some of the side effects disappear within the first few weeks and all of them vanish once you start eating again. Most serious complications, however, are extremely rare with the new liquid diets.

The important thing to remember is that these liquid diets are designed for and acceptable for only the one in fifteen Americans who are at least 30 percent overweight. In fact, the average person accepted by a VCLD program has between 50 and 60 pounds to lose, along with serious weight-related health disorders, such as hypertension, high fat levels in the blood, and diabetes. Most people who desire to lose weight only want to lose 10 to 15 pounds. Those people should choose a more moderate diet plan and avoid liquid diets.

How Safe Are Those TV-Advertised Weight-Loss Shakes?

The most important thing to remember is that no diet product is safe if it does not provide the essential nutrients a healthful diet requires. Most TV- advertised weight-loss shakes are safe if taken properly and all nutritional requirements are met. However, many people who are trying to lose weight want to do so quickly, and turn to weight-loss products that promise such a weight loss. As a result, these people may be taking a product that provides a severely restricted caloric intake. Although there may be rapid weight-loss in the beginning, most of these products do not work over a long term and the lost weight is usually regained.

As a rule, any type of diet or diet product that provides less than 1,000 calories per day should be undertaken only with medical supervision. It is also considered "unsafe" to lose weight too fast. Experts recommend that you lose no more than 1 1/2 to 2 pounds a week.

While some TV-advertised weight-loss shakes can help you lose weight fast, you should consult your doctor for his or her advice and recommendations before you start using one.

Fasting May Not Be Faster

The latest research on fasting—400 to 800 calorie-per day diets that prohibit eating anything except scientifically devised liquid supplements— shows that it actually may not help you lose weight any faster. The research was conducted by weight-loss experts at Syracuse University and at the University of Pennsylvania over a period of six months. A total of 76 obese women were separated into 3 groups and placed on on 420, 660, and 800 calorie- per-day diets. All of the women lost weight—an average of 45 pounds— but there was very little difference in the amount of weight lost on any of the diets.

It is interesting to note that losing 45 pounds in six months actually averages out to about 2 pounds a week, which is the rate of loss that most doctors recommend. And that type of weight loss can be accomplished by carefully maintaining a low-fat diet, coupled with adequate exercise. No fasting is necessary.

Why Low-Carbohydrate, High-Protein Diets Don't Work

This type of diet features a limited amount of high-protein foods, such as red meat, eggs and cheese, with little or no carbohydrates being consumed. There are no restrictions on caloric intake with this type of diet.

A diet that is essentially high in protein and low in carbohydrates will ordinarily bring about a rapid weight loss due to a loss of fluid and lean body tissue. And since the amount of calories consumed is not restricted, little or no body fat is lost. This type of diet is not nutritionally well-balanced, and is very high in fat content. It can also lead to such problems as diarrhea and fluid imbalance.

How To Lose Weight Without Rigid And Restrictive Planned Meals— Even If You Have A "Sweet Tooth"

A recent innovation in diet planning and weight control is custom-tailored, computerized diets. These computerized diets allow you to enjoy all of your favorite foods and still lose a desired amount of weight— even if you like chocolate candy and pastry. One such customized diet is the Woman's Day "Have- It-Your-Weigh" Diet, which is available from WOMAN'S DAY magazine for about $20.00. You supply the information that goes into your computerized diet by filling out a questionaire.

The "Have-It-Your-Weigh" diet features six weeks of customized menus for breakfast, lunch, and dinner. You'll also get two alternate menus for each regular menu—one for splurging when the mood strikes, and another to make up for splurging. The diet also provides a list of food substitutions in case you can't find some of your favorite foods on the questionaire. You'll also get a small cookbook featuring recipes for a variety of foods.

The computerized diet also features a guide for "eating out". The guide explains what kinds of food to avoid, what to order and how your food should be prepared in just about any kind of restaurant imaginable, from fancy to fast-food. The "Have-It-Your-Weigh" computer will also automatically give you the correct balance of proteins, carbohydrates and fats, including saturated fats, in your diet.

Your custom-tailored diet will be based on the information you provide about how much you exercise, your favorite foods and your lifestyle.

You can find out more about the Woman's Day "Have-It-Your-Weigh" computerized diet by calling 1-800-553-8599 (this toll-free number will be answered "A.D.A." and is in operation Monday through Friday from 8:30 a.m. to 5:00 p.m. EST. The number is not available in Canada), or write to: The Woman's Day Have-It-Your-Weigh Diet, A.D.A./Dept. B 32, Box 17007, Hauppauge, NY 11788.

Fruit Juice Diet Makes You Eat Fewer Calories

Researchers have found that fructose—the kind of sugar found in fruits—mixed with water can be an effective appetite suppressant. According to the research, you'll get the best results if you drink a glass of orange juice— rich in fructose—about a half hour to one hour prior to a meal. By doing so, you'll most likely consume fewer calories at mealtime. Even though a fructose-laden fruit juice drink contains about 200 calories, the net calorie suppression averages about 100 to 225 calories per meal.

While fructose mixed with water works as an appetite suppressant, and doesn't require eliminating any specific foods from your diet, or doesn't produce a rapid weight loss, a doctor's opinion should be considered before you attempt to lose weight in this manner. Even a moderate reduction diet should have a doctor's consent before beginning.

4 Tips To Prevent Overeating

1) Eat three small meals a day instead of two large meals. If you still feel hungry, you can fill up on whole-grain bread and fluids, such as water and fruit juice.

2) Choose a smaller plate than usual to prevent taking "extra-large" portions, eat slowly, and don't go back for seconds.

3) Don't eat a large meal just before bedtime.

4) Monitor your weight. If your weight increases, cut down on the amount of food you are eating and get more exercise.

Lose Weight Faster And Easier With These "Wonder Foods"

Breakfast— unsweetened cereal with low-fat or skim milk, citrus fruit, and whole-grain bread with a minimum of low-fat spread and preserves.

Lunch— sandwich with lean meat, onion, lettuce and tomato, and soup or a salad of mixed greens and fresh vegetables topped with a low-calorie dressing.

Dinner— broiled fish dressed with parsley, thyme and lemon juice, broccoli and rice, a fresh fruit salad served with yogurt.

Why Most Oriental People Are So Skinny

Most nutritionists recommend a reduction in daily fat intake as a means of maintaining a more healthful diet. Weight-watchers are advised to cut down on the amount of fat they consume each day as a way to reach and maintain their ideal weights. Does fat really make that much difference?

Perhaps the answer to that question can be found in the difference between the typical American and typical Oriental diet and the much higher prevalence of obesity in the U.S. than among Oriental people, such as the Japanese. A typical Japanese diet contains approximately 2,300 kilocalories per day. Fifteen to twenty percent of those calories come from fat, Another thirteen to fifteen percent come from protein, and from sixty-five to seventy percent from carbohydrates (less than 10% from refined sugar).

In America, the typical diet also provides about 2,300 kilocalories per day, but from thirty-eight to forty percent of those calories come from fat. Protein is responsible for twelve to fifteen percent, and the remainder—less than fifty percent—comes from carbohydrates (about 15% from refined sugar).

Besides a diet much lower in fat and sugar, some nutritionists believe that Oriental people get more exercise than most Americans, which could also contribute to their lower incidence of obesity.

Apples And Weight Loss

We've all heard that "an apple a day keeps the doctor away", and now it appears that apples might also help keep excess weight away. Whole apples keep glucose levels up for a while and they also help provide you with a "full" feeling. That means, apples make great snack food, especially if you are dieting. While apple juice is good for you in many different ways, whole apples are much better for weight-loss. Apple juice acts much quicker in prompting a rush of insulin and a drop in blood sugar, which tends to make you hungry.

How To Avoid Sweets In Food

Excessive sugar intake is a problem for many people who are trying to control their weight. While an occasional "sweet binge" will not disrupt a serious weight management program, a regular high intake of sweets can be self- defeating. Here are several ways to cut down on, or avoid altogether, sweets in foods:

1) If you must have dessert, develop the habit of serving fruit. Fresh fruit is best, but if you must rely on canned and/or frozen fruit, purchase brands that are packaged in water rather than sweetened syrup.

2) Always read food labels to get an idea of the sugar content. One good clue as to sugar content is if the words sugar, sucrose, glucose, maltose, dextrose, lactose, fructose, or syrup appears first on the label, then the product most likely contains more sugar than any other ingredients.

3) Choose plain, unsweetened cereals and add sliced fruit or raisins instead of sugar. While raisins contain some sugar, they also supply vitamins, minerals and fiber.

4) Make your own cookies, pies or cakes and cut the sugar in the recipe by a third or even as much as a half.

Easy, Little-Known Ways To Stick To Your Diet When You Are At A Restaurant

You can be "true" to a low-fat diet even when you eat out by following these tips:

1) Choose a restaurant which features a good salad bar, or one that is known for its delicious, healthful salads.

2) Lime or lemon juice is a good low-fat salad dressing substitute available at most salad bars. Seafood coctail sauce is another excellent low-fat substitute dressing.

3) Ask the waitor, or the chef to prepare your vegetables without butter, sour cream, or cheese sauces.

4) Order chicken broiled instead of fried.

5) Try a low-fat entree, such as cooked chopped broccoli, on your potato.

6) Don't give in to temptation. Most chefs will prepare your food exactly as you request.

News About Nutrasweet

The artificial sweetener Nutrasweet, found in many diet soft drinks, begins losing sweetness after about three months. To avoid getting "sweetless" diet soda, look at the code on the bottom of the can or bottle. Many diet sodas containing nutrasweet have codes which usually begin with a number that corresponds to the last number in the current year. For example, 2 for the year 1992. That number is followed by three digits that signify the day of the year. For example, a drink canned on January 1 (the first day of the year), 1992 would be stamped with the code 2001— and may taste watery before the end of April.

4 "Diet Foods"
That Make It Harder To Lose Weight

1) 2% low-fat milk— one cup of 2% milk contains 125 calories, about 35% of which come from fat. That is really not much different from whole milk, which has 150 calories per cup, almost half of which come from fat. A better way to lower your fat intake is to use 1% or, even better, skim milk.

2) Cottage Cheese— 40% of the calories in cottage cheese come from fat. Also, you would have to eat almost 2 cups of regular cottage cheese (about 470 calories) to get the same amount of calcium you get from one cup of skim milk (90 calories). Regular cottage cheese can also contain almost 1,000 milligrams of sodium per cup. People who are concerned with their intake of fat are better off to limit themselves to cottage cheese which is labeled 1% or 2% fat.

3) Soy-Based Frozen Desserts— these desserts usually contain 19 grams of fat and 330 calories in just a 3/4 cup serving. That's not much difference from the same size portion of ice cream, which contains about 24 grams of fat and 395 calories (depending on the flavor).

4) Lean Ground Beef— ground beef doesn't have to adhere to the same standards for "lean" as do unground cuts of meat. That means that lean ground beef may not actually be all that lean. To be assured of getting truly "lean" ground beef, you should ask a butcher to trim fat off a piece of bottom round steak and then grind it.

How To Quit Smoking Without Gaining Weight

According to a recent government survey, people who stop smoking are likely to gain weight, but the average increase is relatively small—under ten pounds. It is believed that ex-smokers gain weight for two reasons— they burn about 100 fewer calories per day and they consume an extra 200 to 300 calories a day (mainly in carbohydrate snacks). Although it isn't known exactly why ex- smokers eat more, it may be because that in the absence of nicotine, the brain releases a smaller amount of the chemical serotonin, which influences both appetite and mood.

Some recent studies suggest that serotonin-enhancing drugs, may cut down on weight gain in ex-smokers. The studies are, however, not conclusive, and more research is needed. For now, the best recommendations for people who stop smoking are as follows:

1) Get more exercise to counter the slow-down in metabolism which occurs after giving up nicotine.

2) Cut calorie intake by trimming fat from your diet.

3) When you have a craving for sweets, try eating hard candy or chewing gum.

4) Sip cold water to suppress your appetite. Spicy Foods And Weight Control

One of the keys to maintaining a desirable weight is the ability to control the urge to eat too often, and too much. New research suggests that consuming spicy foods, such as Szechuan, Mexican, Thai, or Indian, may help satisfy your appetite before you've eaten too much. Such spicy foods appear to satiate the appetite better than does less spicy foods . It is almost impossible for most people to overeat when dining on spicy foods, possibly because the flavors are so intense they don't need to eat as much.

Experts Say Chew Your Food Slowly To Eat Less At Mealtimes

One way to ensure that you eat less at mealtime is to eat slowly. By eating slower you provide extra time which lets your body know when it has received enough fuel and doesn't require any more. One of the most natural and healthful ways to slow down eating is to consume more fiber. Fiber is not only satisfying but it provides mouthfuls that must be chewed thoroughly. In other words, when eating fiber, you must take your time. The end result is that you'll eat less food than you would if you hurried through your meal. Fiber also requires a lot of room in the stomach, which reduces the appetite and makes you feel full longer.

Water And Your Appetite

One of your best weapons in the "battle of the bulge" is water. Many times we think we are hungry when we are actually thirsty. Sipping water throughout the day—especially when you feel a craving for food— may satisfy your hunger and help you avoid unnecessary eating.

Exercise Is A Must To Lose Weight

Any weight control program must include regular exercise. It doesn't necessarily have to be vigorous exercise like aerobics, jogging, or swimming. A brisk 20 to 30 minute walk can be very helpful as well as increasing the rate that excess calories are burned off. Here are some common exercises and the number of calories that are expended practicing each one for an hour at a time:

1) Brisk Walking (4 mph)— 440 calories expended in one hour.

2) Jogging (5 mph)— 740 calories expended in one hour.

3) Bicycling (6 mph)— 240 calories expended in one hour.

4) Running in place— 650 calories expended in one hour.

5) Jumping Rope— 750 calories expended in one hour.

6) Swimming (25 yards per minute)— 275 calories expended in one hour.

7) Tennis (singles)— 400 calories expended in one hour.

Recent research indicates that aerobic exercise may reduce fat first and quickest in the stomach. A study conducted at the University of Washington monitored a group of men participating in an intensive six-month aerobic program. The men lost 20 percent of their abdomen fat— practically twice the amount of fat reduction in their arms and legs.

9 Popular Exercises To Help You Lose Weight

1) Cross-country skiing— this form of exercise is more strenuous than running, but it is an excellent way to burn off a great deal of fat without a lot of discomfort. There is also a relatively low risk of injury with cross-country skiing because the movements involve gliding rather than bouncing. Cross-country skiing is recommended for people who are already in good condition, because it requires skill, balance, and good arm and leg coordination. The starting cost is relatively low, and you can rent equipment.

2) Running— this exercise offers excellent long-term fat-burning potential. The injury risk with running is considered moderate for less than 35 miles per week and very high for more than 35 miles a week. The only equipment needed to start running is a pair of good running shoes.

3) Cycling— the long-term fat-burning potential from cycling is moderate. The injury risk from the exercise itself is low, but can be high if you cycle in areas of high traffic. Since it uses fewer muscles than running, and because it is not weight-bearing, you have to cycle about 40 minutes to equal 20 minutes of running or jogging.

4) Walking— if the total walking time is 30 minutes or less, or if the walking speed is less than 15 minutes a mile, the long-term fat-burning potential is moderate to low. If the walking time is more than 30 minutes, or the walking speed is more than 15 minutes a mile, the long-term fat-burning potential is moderate. The risk of injury with walking is low.

In order to get maximum fat-burning benefits from walking you should try to set a brisk pace of at least 100 steps a minute and less than 20 minutes a mile. About 45 minutes of brisk walking is equal to 20 minutes of jogging.

5) Swimming— both the long-term fat-burning potential and injury risk are low. Swimming is actually the most injury-free sport and it provides excellent benefits for the cardiovascular system. It also tones practically all muscles. However, if you are overweight, swimming should not be your only exercise. Of all the people tested for body fat, swimmers usually carry more fat than either runners or cyclists.

While swimming will help keep you lean and fit, you will not lose fat as fast as you would with land sports. Even with that drawback, swimming is a good starting program for overweight people who aren't used to exercise.

6) Rowing— the long-term fat burning potential of rowing is high, and the injury risk is low. Either indoors or outdoors, rowing is an excellent fat- consuming exercise. It exercises most of the large muscle groups without placing stress on joints and it also helps develop the muscles of the upper body. It should also be noted that rowing causes back problems in some people.

7) Stair-climbing— while the long-term fat-burning potential with this exercise is high, the risk of injury is moderately low. While you are not really simulating stair-climbing, this exercise does require as much energy as running. But it places only about the same amount of stress on the joints as walking.

8) Treadmill— depending on the incline and speed, the long-term fat-burning potential is moderate to high. The injury risk is low. Treadmills require a good deal of balance and involvement, which enhances the exerciser's motivation. The best pace on a treadmill is a fast walk or a slow jog.

9) Stationary Bicycling— like its counterpart outdoor cycling, the long-term fat-burning potential is moderate, and the injury risk is low with stationary bicycling. Stationary bikes are are both stable and easy to use. This type of exercising has become popular because you can do two things at one time— exercise, and read a book or watch television.

5 Tips To Help You Stick With Your Exercise Program

Obviously the best exercise tip is to— just do it. But that can be pretty difficult. Especially if you've been inactive for a long time and are just beginning a regular exercise routine as part of your weight-loss program. Many times, it seems easier to just "skip-it". Since exercise is such an essential part of weight-control, you really can't afford to skip-it on a regular basis. Here are some tips on how you can enhance your exercise routine, and keep yourself from becoming "lazy":

1) Fix specific times for your workout and then stick to your plan as closely as possible. Self-discipline is an important part of maintaining a regular program of exercise.

2) Invite a friend. Many people find exercise to be quite boring, no matter what type of workout they're doing. Getting a friend to join you in working out may help alleviate your feelings of boredom. It will also enable you to get and give support.

3) Make a tape of your favorite music. The music you most enjoy will trigger a good mood, making your workouts more fun. Of course, your exercise music should have a strong beat which is conducive to repetitive movement.

4) Go at you own pace. Many people push themselves too hard and soon become discouraged or injured. You should work hard, but not beyond your capacity. Increase the physical challenges a little at a time, when your body is ready for them.

5) View Exercise Videos. There are scores of good video instructors—Jane Fonda, Kathy Smith, Denise Austin, and so on— who have valuable information on form and technique that will be of benefit to you. Rent some videos and "pretend" you are part of the group in the video.

The Best Time Of Day To Exercise To Burn Off Fat

One of the keys to maintaining an exercise regimen is to pick a time of day that is best for you. Our bodies have certain rhythms that have subtle effects on our athletic ability which in turn may influence how we feel about exercising at certain times of the day. Knowing what works for you is an essential factor in getting the greatest benefit from exercise designed to help you maintain a desirable weight.

Morning— research has shown that exercising in the morning is best for people who have a hard time sticking with a regular exercise program. That may be because it's easier to find excuses to skip exercising as the day progresses.

Midday— this is a very good time for dieters. Prelunch workouts provide two important benefits—they not only burn off calories, they also help suppress the appetite.

Late afternoon— this is the time of day many people trying to reduce stress find most beneficial. An end-of-the-work-day workout helps these people relax.

Evening— moderate activity right after dinner shouldn't cause any problems, but you should wait at least an hour before doing anything strenuous. Also keep in mind, that exercise will invigorate you and may keep you awake if you do it just before bedtime. Secret: Try each time - one will allow you to burn fat faster and easier.

The Truth About Weight-Loss Centers

Joining an established and reputable weight-loss center may be beneficial for those people who find it very difficult to lose weight. Weight-loss centers provide structure and the discipline of a regular weigh-in, serving as both motivation and inspiration. They also offer the companionship of people who are experiencing a shared problem, and a shared goal.

Before joining a weight-loss center, it is essential that you check out the center's credentials. Make sure the center has a professional staff, backed up by a good reputation. One way to find out about a particular weight-loss center is to talk with past and present members. Their recommendations, or lack of same, should help you find a center that's right for you.

The best weight-loss centers are those that follow a balanced, low-fat diet and employ behavior modification. However, This book can do the same for you as any weight loss center - without having to spend hundreds of dollar!

How To "Think Thin" And Lose Weight

The state of your mind has a lot to do with the state of your body. Since thoughts influence feelings and behavior, it is quite possible to "think thin" and succeed in losing a desired amount of weight, and maintain a desirable weight. Many weight-loss experts are convinced that the mind can be a powerful diet tool in treating problems of excess weight. These experts recommend a balanced diet and exercise program, along with newly developed techniques that emphasize mind over body in weight loss. Here are some mind over body techniques:

1) Learn About Yourself— this involves the personal discovery and understanding of the feelings and circumstances that lead you into overeating. You could be using food simply as a response to boredom or stress, or some other situation that you could change. Think about your eating habits and when you are most likely to overeat. Does your overeating occur at a certain time of day, or in a certain place? Do you eat a lot of junk foods between meals? Do you eat a lot while you're watching TV? Write down what you find out about yourself, and you are likely to find a pattern to your overeating.

Once you've established the feelings and situations associated with your overeating pattern, you can begin to make the necessary changes. If you find that you are eating as a response to boredom, you can try breaking that habit by doing something else you enjoy, instead of eating. The important thing is to understand why you are overeating and then make a determined effort to create the emotional and situational changes necessary to help eliminate the problem.

2) Pay Attention To What You Eat— many of us are too busy or too tired to actually notice and fully appreciate the food we eat. In effect, we don't take the time to really enjoy our food. Strangely enough, this sort of inattention often results in eating more than we want or need. At your next meal, try this simple exercise: close your eyes and take a few moments to enjoy the aroma of the food you are about to eat; run a bite-size portion of the food lightly along your lips to get a feel of its texture; take a small bite and chew slowly, noticing the flavor and the juices; then, very slowly, enjoying each bite, eat the rest of your food.

It may seem rather silly at first, but the point is to take your time and appreciate all the food you eat. By eating this way, you'll find that you are not only more satisfied, but that you are also eating smaller portions.

3) Self-Motivation— your intentions may be good, but if you don't take the time to motivate yourself, you are not apt to have much success losing weight and keeping it off. In order to motivate yourself, you need to have a clear idea of why you want to lose weight. Health is certainly a pri-

mary factor in many decisions to lose weight, but there may also be other reasons, such as simply wanting to feel better about yourself. Whatever your reasons, write them down and use them diligently as your self-motivation. Your success or failure depends largely on how well you motivate yourself.

4) Don't Set Your Goals Too High— if you set a goal of losing 4 to 5 pounds a week, you're not thinking in realistic or healthy terms. Most experts agree that a healthy weight-loss should be no more than two pounds a week. You should set a realistic goal of one half to one pound a week. That will allow you to establish a realistic ultimate weight goal. For example, if you want to lose ten pounds, give yourself at least ten weeks. That way you have a desirable weight goal within a realistic time frame.

5) Choose The Right Foods— selecting and preparing a healthful low-fat diet shouldn't be a boring or unpleasant task. Think about the healthful foods you like and put extra time and thought into their preparation. Be creative with your diet and de-emphasize the high-fat foods that you are cutting down on, and you'll begin to look forward to mealtime.

6) Choose The Right Exercise— regular physical activity is the best way to help you take off excess weight and maintain the loss permanently. But choose an exercise you will enjoy doing. Don't just choose an aerobic exercise, such as walking or biking simply to have an exercise program. Think about what you like to do and will continue to do. Otherwise, you'll find it very difficult to continue.

7) Don't Give Up— once you've made the decision to reach your desirable weight, adopted a positive attitude, and changed your eating behavior, don't become discouraged if you "backslide". You don't have to be inflexible to succeed. Allow yourself room for occasional lapses, and realize that such occurrences don't mean you are a failure. Instead of seeing your diet and/or exercise lapses as a lack of willpower, think of them as learning experiences. Learn to identify the events that preceded the lapse(s) and how to avoid them in the future. In short, learn to forgive yourself, and keep trying. If you keep telling yourself "I can do it", you're more than likely headed for success.

11 Low Calorie, Fast Meals That Help You Drop Pounds

Breakfast

Oat Breakfast

1 bowel of oatmeal, prepared as directed on package 1-2 cups of lowfat milk 1-2 slices whole wheat toast 1 grapefruit or orange

Fruit Breakfast

Two generous servings of fruit (orange, grapefruit, mixed, or dried fruit) 1-2 cups low-fat milk 1-2 slices of whole wheat toast

Hearty Breakfast

1 boiled egg 1 bowel shredded wheat 1-2 cups of low-fat milk 1 glass of juice or serving of fruit 1-2 whole wheat muffins or corn muffins

Lunch or Dinner

Fajita Rice Meal

1 1/2 cups Minute Instant Brown Rice, 3/4lb flank steak, cut into thin strips, 1 medium onion sliced, 1 each green and red pepper sliced, 1 1/2 tea. garlic powder, 1 Tbls. oil, 1/2 cup water, 1/4 cup lime juice, 1 teas. hot pepper sauce, 1/4 teas. black pepper.

Prepare rice as directed on package, omitting margarine and salt. Cook and stir meat, vegetables and garlic powder in hot oil in large skillet until browned. Add remaining ingredients, bring to boil. Reduce heat and simmer 5 minutes. Serve over rice. Makes 4 servings.

Salad Lunch

One large salad — lettuce, spinach, tomatoes, carrots, celery. 1 small serving of pasta 1 slice of whole wheat bread 1 glass iced peppermint tea

Fish Lunch

1 baked fish 1 cooked vegetable (green beans, corn, etc.) 1 generous helping of raw vegetables (carrots, celery) 1 small baked potato small glass of milk or iced pepermint tea to drink

15-Minute Meals Of 600 Calories Or Less

Beans And Rice

1/2 cup of canned black beans on a bed of 1 cup of quick-cooking brown rice; with chopped, raw onions; 1/2 ounce of reduced-fat cheddar cheese; and a dash of Tabasco.

1 slice of bread with a half teaspoon of margarine. 1 orange 2 low-fat cookies

Pasta

1 cup of vermicelli, topped with 1/2 cup of commercial spaghetti sauce 1 cup of frozen Italian vegetables 2 tablespoons of Parmesan cheese 1 sourdough roll 1 12 ounce packet of dried fruit

Turkey

4 ounces of medium-sliced turkey, 1/2 ounce of Swiss cheese, lettuce, tomato, and sprouts in a whole-wheat pita pocket

broccoli florets (raw) with low-fat salad dressing

an apple

Tuna

water-packed tuna low-fat mayonnaise chopped celery lettuce 1 slice of 7-grain bread 1 can of vegetable soup 8 ounce glass of skim milk tangerine 2 low-fat cookies (ginger snaps or low-fat oatmeal cookies)

Potato

1 large, microwaved potato (baked) topped with 1/2 cup of

canned chili and 1/2 ounce of reduced-fat cheddar cheese

1 fresh pear 2 ounces of whole-wheat pretzels

Recommendations

Drink few if any caffinated bevereages and replace them with juice drinks or herbal teas.

Eat less meat and fat-containing products and less high sugar foods. Replace with more fruits and vegetables.

New U.S.D.A. Food Recommendations

The US Department of Agriculture has recently revised its rec-ommended daily food intake. These new recommendations include more fruits and vegetables. Here are these new recommendations.

1. Bread, Cereal, Rice, and Pasta— 6-11 servings

2. Fruit Group — 2-4 servings

3. Vegetable Group — 3-5 servings

4. Milk, Yogurt, and Cheese — 2-3 servings

5. Meat, Poultry, Fish, Dry Beans, Eggs, and Nuts Group — 2-3 servings

6. Fats, Oils, and Sweets — Use sparingly

New Breakthrough: Little Known Mineral May Help Weight Loss

Mention chromium and many people think of chrome plating on automobiles. But to researchers at the University of Texas at San Antonio, chromium is an essential trace mineral which may help people lose weight without requiring a significant reduction in caloric intake. Recently the researchers found that increasing the intake of chromium can help an individual lose up to 2 pounds a month without the necessity of following a strict low-calorie diet.

The mineral is found naturally in some fruits, vegetables, meats, whole grains, and shellfish. However, most Americans fail to consume the RDA of chromium which is 50 to 200 micrograms. According to researchers, 200 mcg per day is enough to aid in weight control.

In order to increase chromium intake, weight conscious individuals may consider taking chromium picolinate. This supplement combines the mineral with picolinic acid which is a natural substance produced from an amino acid. The picolinic acid transports minerals such as chromium rapidly and efficiently to areas in the body where they will be of most benefit.

The researchers say that the chromium picolinate supplement may help keep your insulin levels within a normal range, thereby playing a key role in weight control. High insulin levels can lead to overeating. The supplement also seems to help burn stored fat by reducing the body's metabolic rate.

The Natural Healing Power
Of Vitamin A And Beta-Carotene

While vitamin A may be far from being a world-wide panacea, it is high on the list of vital nutrients. In recent years numerous medical research studies have revealed that certain fruits and vegetables rich in beta-carotene can help prevent cancer; cataracts; fight heart disease; strengthen the immune system; protect your skin from wrinkles; maintain good vision and prevent certain eye disorders such as night blindness; speed up the effective healing of wounds; eliminate acne and boils; and much more. While the research continues, there is no doubt that the natural wonders of Vitamin A, especially in the form of beta-carotene, is essential to the maintenance of good health.

There are two forms of Vitamin A—preformed Vitamin A or retinol is found only in foods of animal origin and provitamin A or carotene is found in foods of both plant and animal origin. It's important to know the difference because preformed vitamin A can be toxic in large enough amounts over a long period of time. It builds up in the liver and can not be excreted from the body in any significant amount. Toxicity can result from prolonged daily doses that exceed 50,000 IU in adults and children. The symptoms of a vitamin A overdose include nausea, diarrhea, headache, dizziness, loss of hair, dry itching skin, and drowsiness. The toxicity will clear up in a few days if the excessive intake is halted. Overdoses of Vitamin A (retinol) can be caused by eating an excessive amount of animal liver over an extended period of time, but is more commonly due to high doses of vitamin supplements.

Here are several ways you can avoid an overdose of vitamin A:

1) To supplement your body's store of vitamin A, take carotene supplements instead of vitamin A supplements. Consult with your physician for his or her advice.

2) If you take a vitamin supplement, be sure you never exceed the RDA for vitamin A (see chapter 2) unless you have your doctor's permission.

3) Don't take vitamin A supplements if you are currently taking fish oil or cod liver oil supplements. Both of these contain large amounts of vitamin A, and the result could be an overdose. Because of their high level of vitamin A, you should use cod liver oil and other fish oil supplements only under a doctor's supervision.

4) Don't take vitamin A supplements if you are using birth control pills, unless you have your doctor's permission. Some studies indicate that women taling birth control pills sometimes experience an increase in their levels of vitamin A.

5) You shouldn't take vitamin A supplements if you are currently taking prescription drugs that are made from vitamin A. There are two drugs in use today which are derived from vitamin A— Accutane for acne and Tigason for psoriasis. Retin A is a vitamin A ointment which is used for smoothing out wrinkles in skin which has been damaged by prolonged exposure to the sun and aging.

Beta-Carotene

Carotene is actually a precurser of vitamin A, and is a substance that is changed in the body to vitamin A. The transformation takes place in the wall of the small intestine. Depending on the type of food we eat and the form in which it is eaten, the amount of carotene that changes into vitamin A varies between 30 and 70 percent. Carotene itself is not active in the body and is not toxic. An "overdose" of carotene may cause the skin to turn slightly yellow, but nothing more serious. The main sources of Provitamin A, or carotene, are red, orange, yellow and green vegetables and fruits, such as carrots, sweet potatoes, winter squash, yellow corn, tomatoes, broccoli, spinach, chard, turnip greens, kale, apricots, peaches, oranges, cantaloupe, and watermelon.

4 Safe Ways To Add Vitamin A To Your Diet

1) Eat 1 to 2 daily servings of red and/or orange vegetables. For example, one carrot will provide you with about 7,950 IUs of beta-carotene and one medium tomato provides 820 IUs of beta-carotene.

2) Eat at least two green leafy vegetables per day. Two ounces of spinach will provide about 4,600 IUs of beta-carotene.

3) Eat at least one piece of fruit—with colored flesh—every day.

4) Take a beta-carotene supplement. While the best source of any vitamin is food, it may sometimes be necessary to take a supplement. And while there is no conclusive evidence that daily supplements of pre-formed vitamin A, with up to 15,000 IUs, poses any serious health risk, many experts advise taking a beta-carotene supplement instead.

The recent advent of inexpensive and readily available beta-carotene supplements, along with mounting evidence suggesting that beta-carotene can provide many of the same benefits (and possibly more) as preformed vitamin A, make taking a daily supplement of 5,000 to 25,000 IUs of beta-carotene the way to go if you need a supplement. But again, you should consult your doctor before using any supplement.

Warning: Don't Mix Beta-Carotene And Alcohol

Even though carotene is not considered toxic, new evidence indicates that it's not a good idea to mix beta-carotene with alcohol. A recent study at Mount Sinai School of Medicine in New York suggests that heavy drinkers who take beta-carotene supplements could develop liver problems.

According to the study, levels of beta-carotene normally considered safe or non-toxic can in fact become toxic when combined with alcohol. That's because alcohol tends to inhibit the body's usual ability to remove beta-carotene from the blood. The beta-carotene may then heighten whatever damage alcohol causes to the liver.

Beta-Carotene May Help Prevent Emphysema

No one would dispute the fact that the harsh chemicals and tar in cigarette smoke can injure and destroy lung tissue. Ultimately, the lungs lose their elasticity and their ability to bring in oxygen from the air. The result is emphysema. Now, some new research suggests that beta-carotene may help prevent emphysema. That's encouraging news for active smokers, and passive smokers as well. (According to some studies, the levels of harmful chemicals in the blood of people who live in larger cities where the air isn't very clean and who do not smoke—passive smokers—can amount to that of a one-pack-a-day active smoker).

While the research into the potential of beta-carotene as a way to prevent emphysema continues, many experts are recommending that anyone who smokes or who lives in an environment that is heavy with smoke and fumes should get ample amounts of beta-carotene.

Natural Help For Skin Disorders

Clinical tests suggest that while beta-carotene supplements can alleviate many skin disorders, such as acne and psoriasis, vitamin A derivative drugs may do a much better job. The tests seem to indicate that Accutane is effective against cystic acne, while Tretinoin (the active ingredient in Retin A) works well as a treatment for acne vulgaris, which is the most common form of acne. There have been some good results using Tigason (etretinate) in the treatment of psoriasis. Tests have shown that etretinate may be as much as 80 percent effective when taken for 3 to 4 months. Researchers say that is a much higher rate of effectiveness than is found with any other drug currently being used to treat psoriasis.

It is important to note that women of childbearing age who are not using birth control pills, and pregnant women should not take Accutane or etretinate because they have been linked to certain birth defects. And everyone—both women and men—should consult with a physician before using these vitamin A derivative drugs.

Another vitamin A derivative, Retin A, which was initially developed as a treatment for acne, is now proving to be a fairly effective treatment for sun- damaged skin. According to recent studies, the overall improvement provided by Retin A to skin which has been damaged by exposure to the sun is, in most cases, modest.

Natural Way To Improve Your Eyesight. And Night Driving, Too

You can prevent night blindness by eating an adequate amount of vegetables high in vitamin A—especially in carotene form. Yellow vegetables such as carrots are high in vitamin A, which is required for the maintenance of good vision. An early sign of a deficiency in vitamin A levels is the loss of vision in near darkness or night blindness. By regularly eating vegetables that are rich in vitamin A, you can prevent night blindness, and you may actually improve your night vision.

Reduce Your Risk Of Cataracts By 37%

A study of nearly 1,400 men and women over age 40 suggests that vitamins in food may help prevent cataracts, the most common cause of blindness. Researchers at the State University of New York at Stony Brook, found that subjects whose diets were high in foods containing vitamins A, C and E had fewer cataracts than people with a low intake of those vitamins. It may be that vitamins A, C and E help neutralize certain electrically charged compounds known as free radicals, which can damage eye tissue.

The study also found that people who had taken multivitamin tablets at least once or more a week for one year had 37 percent fewer cataracts than those who hadn't. But the experts also warn against increasing vitamin dosage as a means of enhancing natural benefits. Consult your doctor before using any multivitamin tablet.

In a related study, researchers at the Social Insurance Institute in Helsinki say that people with low levels of vitamins A and E are almost twice as likely to need cataract surgery as are people who have high levels of both vitamins.

The Finnish study, which measured the levels of nutrients in the blood, appears to support the theory that free radicals, which are formed naturally in the body, cause the growth of cataracts. Both vitamins A and E help to neutralize free radicals. Researchers say the new findings show a strong link between low nutrient levels and the eventual need to have cataract surgery.

According to the researchers, the study, published in the British Medical Journal, is not conclusive, and further investigation is required to prove that eating foods rich in vitamins A and E can actually reduce the likelihood of getting cataracts.

Natural Compound In Fruit May Help Prevent Cancer

Recent research suggests that some natural chemical compounds found in fruit may help prevent certain types of cancer. The compounds are known as limonoids and were tested on rats. The results showed that limonoids caused an increase in the secretion of an anti-cancer enzyme in the rats' stomachs, providing them with added protection against stomach tumors and stomach cancers. Limonoids are the natural compounds that create the slightly bitter taste in some fruits, including oranges, lemons, limes, and grapefruit.

Many Nuts And Berries May Help Prevent Cancer

According to results from a study conducted at the Medical College of Ohio in Toledo, elegic acid—a substance found in many nuts and berries—may help your body fend off cell damage caused by certain cancer-causing chemicals or carcinogens. Researchers discovered that elegic acid neutralizes carcinogens which have invaded the bloodstream.

The researchers note that the substance only seems to work if it is introduced into the body's system immediately before or during the time the body is exposed to the cancer-causing carcinogens.

Because the body has difficulty absorbing elegic acid in a concentrated form, supplements of the substance aren't very effective. The researchers indicate that elegic acid in its natural form—in nuts and berries, such as Brazil nuts and strawberries—is more easily absorbed by the human body.

Natural Insect Repellent

According to a study conducted at Lake Superior State College in Michigan, vitamin B1 supplements (thiamine) may provide a helpful natural bug repellent. As part of the study, volunteers were placed in two groups—those who took thiamine supplements and those who took a placebo or phony supplement. All of the volunteers were sent out into the woods immediately after taking the real thiamine supplements and the placebos. Once outdoors, the volunteers kept track of the number of mosquito bites they received. The results showed that the volunteers who took the thiamine supplement experienced the fewer number of bites.

The study at Lake Superior State College involved only a few volunteers. New research is underway, involving more people, in an attempt to confirm the earlier indication that thiamine supplements may provide an effective natural insect repellent.

Vitamin C Protects Sperm Cell DNA
- Prevent Birth Defects

Researchers have found strong evidence indicating that men with inadequate levels of vitamin C may be more likely to have DNA (the basic molecule for transmitting hereditary traits) damage in their sperm. This could lead to an increase in their chances of fathering children who have birth defects. The research also indicates that smokers appear to be at the greatest risk. Medical experts recommend, for all men, a diet that features fruits and vegetables which are high in vitamin C content. In some cases, daily supplements are recommended— especially for smokers.

Vitamin E And Parkinson's Disease

Preliminary research has found that vitamin E, or a combination of vitamins E and C may delay the appearance of tremors, rigidity and loss of balance, which are all associated with Parkinson's disease. The significance of the discovery is that vitamin E (and possibly C) may make it possible to postpone the need for therapy with levodopa. Researchers are hoping that a larger, ongoing study will be able to shed more light on the matter. As of now, nothing conclusive has been established.

Vitamin E can be found in such foods as green leafy vegetables, fish, vegetable oils, dried beans, whole-grain cereals, and eggs.

Foods That Prevent Cancer And Birth Defects

Scientists studying an apparent link between HPV (human papillomavirus) and cervical cancer now think that folic acid (a B vitamin) may help protect some women. The study, conducted at the University of Alabama at Birmingham, discovered that of the 464 women subjects, those with medium to low levels of folic acid and who also had HPV, were more likely to develop the abnormal cervical cells (dysplasia) that can lead to cancer than those with high levels of folic acid in their blood.

Scientist who participated in the study, recommend that women get at least the Recommended Daily Allowance of folic acid (400 mcg a day). Those women who smoke or take birth control pills are likely to have an even greater deficiency of folic acid.

New research also suggests that all women of childbearing age should consume the RDA of folic acid in order to reduce the risk of brain and spinal defects in children. The evidence indicates that folic acid deficiencies may contribute to neural tube birth defects such as spina bifida and anencephaly. Spina bifida is a deformation of the spine that leaves the spinal cord exposed. Anencephaly is a condition in which all or part of the brain never forms.

According to the Centers for Disease Control, in order to reduce the chances of spina bifida and anencephaly, folic acid must be in the woman's system at conception because the defects are caused during the first month of pregnancy.

Folic acid is found in many fruits, dark green leafy vegetables, yeast, bread, beans, and fortified cereals. It is also available in over-the-counter vitamin pills.

Little-Known, Natural Ways
To Easier Pregnancy And Delivery

Giving birth is the greatest responsibility that any woman will ever face. It is essential that a mother-to-be take every step possible to provide her unborn child and herself the best possible chance for a life of good health and a healthy environment. Here are several natural ways a mother-to-be can improve her chances of having an easier, healthier pregnancy and delivery:

1) Nutrition is one of the most important factors contributing to the health of a mother and her baby. Even before pregnancy you should maintain a healthy, balanced diet with lots of fresh fruit, vegetables and fiber. You should also get plenty of fluids and adequate amounts of protein. This type of balanced diet should be maintained throughtout your entire pregnancy to provide proper nutrition for you and your unborn child.

2) Weight control is also an important factor for expectant mothers. A woman who is underweight or overweight during pregnancy risks possible harm to herself and her baby. It is important that you exercise and practice proper weight maintenance with a well-balanced diet.

3) If you smoke, quit. If you don't smoke, don't start. You should also avoid second-hand smoke as much as possible. Smoking can cause serious problems for you and your unborn child. Second-hand smoke can also be harmful.

4) Most doctors recommend that you eliminate smoking and alcohol during pregnancy. Alcohol consumption during pregnancy can have an adverse effect on you and the fetus. Avoid drugs as well.

5) Make sure you have been immunized against rubella (German measles). Contracting rubella during pregnancy could harm your unborn child.

6) If you are taking any medications, check with your doctor to make sure they are safe to take during pregnancy.

7) Get plenty of sleep.

8) Choose an obstetrician you can trust. You can get recommendations from friends, relatives and associates. It is important that you have a good relationship with your doctor, and that he or she has your complete confidence.

The 100% "Natural High" Without Drugs Or Alcohol

Although it may be hard to believe, there are substances in your brain which, when released, can provide you with a natural high— without drugs or alcohol. Back in the 1970s, scientists discovered that molecules similar to morphine were produced in the brain. The substances, called endorphins, are released during vigorous physical exercise. They also help relieve pain. This may explain why some athletes, injured during a contest, can continue playing without pain. These natural substances also help control responses to stress and can even improve mood. Many athletes experience a sense of well-being after a strenuous physical workout— a "natural high" brought about by the release of endorphins in the brain.

Cranberry Juice Can Fight Mild Urinary-Tract Infection

While scientists continue to debate the benefits of cranberry juice as a natural remedy for mild urinary-tract infection, the evidence continues to mount in favor of the berry juice. Several recent clinical studies show that cranberry juice and it's botanical cousin, blueberry juice, contain a compound that—at least in the test tube— prevents Escherichia coli bacteria from clinging to bladder cells and causing infection in the urinary tract. No other juices which were tested displayed the ability to combat the Escherichia coli bacteria.

In one clinical study, over 50 people with urinary-tract infections drank a pint of cranberry juice every day for three weeks. None of the subjects took any special medication. More than half of the individuals showed marked improvement. Twenty percent showed slight improvement and about 30 percent showed no improvement at all. An interesting footnote to this study is that about six weeks after all the subjects stopped drinking cranberry juice, more than half of those who had showed some improvement came down with another urinary-tract infection.

This Natural Grocery Store Food
Can Actually Help Ease Depression

Some recent medical studies suggest that nutrition plays a vital role in your overall state of mind. Researchers say that a deficiency in B vitamins and certain amino acids may result in depression. Some cases of depression, resulting from low levels of the B vitamin, folic acid, have been successfully treated with folic acid supplements. While the link between vitamin B deficiency and depression is not conclusive, the evidence suggests that proper levels of folic acid can help ease mild depression in some people. If you think you may have a vitamin B deficiency, consult your doctor.

Good dietary sources of folic acid include lima beans, liver, whole-grain products, asparagus, oranges, and green, leafy vegetables.

The Natural Wonder Of Water

Many people constantly underestimate the value of water to overall health. The truth is that water is of benefit to your body in many ways. It helps prevent kidney stones, protects the body against disease, regulates body temperature, and is necessary for regular bowel movements. But that's not all— water also helps prevent urinary-tract infections by keeping the bladder well-flushed, and it's the best "diet" drink you'll find (see chapter 4).

As a matter of fact, water is your body's most vital nutrient— you can't survive for more than about 5 days without it. Generally, doctors recommend that you drink eight 8-ounce glasses of water each day. You may need to drink even more water if you live in a hot climate, if you do heavy, physically demanding work or if you exercise regularly.

Is Tap Water Best?

Sometimes the methods used in treating water, so that it is free from harmful bacteria, also leave chlorine and chlorinated hydrocarbons in the water. This can present a health danger because of the association between chlorinated water and the rate of certain cancers. It is also possible to have your water contaminated between the water treatment facility and your home. You can remove the contaminants, along with the chemical residue from treatment, by using an activated charcoal filter which attaches to your water tap. One good way to avoid contamination is to drink only high-quality certified-pure spring water.

If you choose bottled over tap water, make sure what you are buying is pure. To help ease the confusion over the water you get from your tap, versus the water you buy, here's a look at the most popular bottled water sources:

1) Bulk water— this is usually sold in gallon jugs or large containers, known as carboys. Some bulk water is actually processed tap water, while others come from springs and wells.

2) Spring water— this comes from underground. Pure, or "Natural" spring water has not been processed. It is also much less likely to be contaminated than ground water.

3) Mineral water— compared with tap water, mineral water contains significant, but highly variable, quantities of mineral. Some advertising claims are misleading in that the minerals in bottled water are no more easily absorbed than other minerals.

4) Distilled water— this is purified by evaporation. Since distilled water contains no minerals, it tastes rather flat. It may also contain some of the organic chemicals you sought to avoid by buying bottled water.

5) Soda or Sparkling Water— this includes seltzer, club soda and

many soft drinks that have added ingredients, such as caffeine and fla-vorings. Most straight soda water contains high amounts of sodium.

Algae May Make Good Sunscreen

Researchers at the Australian Institute of Marine Sciences in Townsville, Queensland, have reported the discovery of an amino acid that apparently absorbs ultraviolet radiation. The amino acid was discov-ered in algae growing inside coral on the Great Barrier Reef. The scien-tists say that without the protection provided by the amino acid in the algae the complex structure of the coral and the reefs would be impaired.

The amino acid has been produced in synthetic form, and while it has not yet been tested on humans, early lab results indicate that the substance successfully blocks even the dangerous UVB rays which can cause sunburn and trigger cancer. More potential good news from the research is that the algae lotion may be less likely than conventional products to cause allergic reactions which prevent many people from using sunscreens.

The Amazing Vegetables That Help Prevent Cancer

Even though one American president publicly admitted he didn't like it, many scientific studies suggest that eating broccoli, as well as Brussels sprouts and other yellow and green vegetables, may lower the the risk of colon and other cancers. Although scientists are not certain why, recent evidence indicates that several substances in these foods, such as fiber, beta carotene and vitamin C, all have a part in protecting the body from carcinogens. And recent research at Johns Hopkins University may have uncovered another vital substance in these foods.

The substance, called sulforaphane, is present in significant amounts in broccoli. It appears to promote increased production of spe-cial enzymes in the body's cells. The enzymes in turn neutralize cancer-causing agents. More testing needs to be done to determine sul-foraphane's true potential for certain kinds of cancer prevention, but the latest evidence is encouraging.

The Best Natural Ways To Cure And Prevent Heartburn And Indigestion

According to some recently released statistics, about 10 percent of adult Americans get heartburn everyday. New research may offer these people an effective and natural way to ease their discomfort.

People get heartburn when stomach acid backs up from the stomach, irritating the lining of the esophagus. Normally, the esophageal sphincter muscle forces itself shut, preventing stomach acid from coming upward. But foods that are high in fat can instigate heartburn, and lying down on the "wrong side" may only make matters worse.

Recent studies suggest that lying down after eating a big meal makes many people susceptible to heartburn. The studies also indicate that which side you lie on may make a significant difference in the amount of discomfort you experience. Lying on the right side may allow the esophagus to open where it enters the stomach, making it easier for stomach acid to enter. Here are some suggestions to help you combat heartburn, naturally:

1) Try to wait at least three hours after eating before you lie down. If you can't wait that long, lie on your left side.

2) If your heartburn continues, prop up your head at least six inches. This should help keep stomach acid from surging upward.

3) Don't eat fatty foods, chocolate, drink alcoholic beverages, or smoke cigarettes. All of these tend to relax the esophageal sphincter, and lead to heartburn.

4) Try some gingeroot. Many people have found relief from heartburn with this herbal remedy. Some medical experts say that gingerroot seems to work by absorbing acid and by helping to calm the nerves. It's best to take it in capsule form just after you eat.

5) Apple cider vinegar is another natural remedy that works well for some people who experience heartburn. The recommended "dosage" is 1 teaspoon of apple cider vinegar in 1/2 glass of water. The concoction should be taken during a meal.

If your heartburn persists you should see your doctor.

A Banana A Day Keeps The Doctor Away
And Reduce Stroke Risk By 40%

Researchers have discovered that potassium deficiency may contribute to high blood pressure. The results of a recent study involving several healthy men who ate either a low-potassium diet or a normal potassium diet for one to two months showed that those on the low-potassium diet had considerably higher blood pressure levels after eight weeks than did the men on normal potassium diets.

The best way to add more potassium to your diet is to consume plenty of fruits and vegetables such as bananas, beans, and potatoes. While there is no Recommended Daily Allowance for potassium, most medical experts suggest a daily intake of from 2 to 3.5 grams. Your doctor can tell you more specifically how much your potassium intake should be each day. This is especially important if you are on medication or have some type of illness or disease.

The potassium in such fruits as bananas may also help ease the discomfort and pain of indigestion. Recently, researchers in India conducted a test involving 40 people who had all suffered stomach pain and nausea for several months. Half of the subjects were given a natural treatment consisting of capsules which contained banana powder. These people took eight capsules a day for about 2 months. The other 20 subjects in the test were given nothing for their pain and nausea. And all 40 subjects avoided such things as antacids and/ or ulcer medication.

The results of this test showed that half of the subjects who took the banana capsules gained complete relief. Most of the other people in this group reported at least some level of relief from their almost constant discomfort. Eighty percent of the people in the other group—those who were given nothing for their indigestion—reported no relief at all.

Other research suggests that potassium-rich foods, such as bananas and potatoes, may also help to reduce your chances for having a stroke. A 12-year study conducted by the Department of Community and Family Medicine at the University of California in San Diego has provided strong evidence in support of that theory. The study, involving over 850 men and women, showed that the people with the lowest intake of potassium had the highest number of stroke- associated deaths. The people who consumed high levels of potassium seemed to be relatively "stroke-free". Also, according to the study, an increase in daily potassium intake by 400 milligrams showed an almost 40 percent reduction in the risk of having a stroke.

The Anti-Cancer Power Of The Pawpaw Tree

Recent research has led to the isolation of a potentially powerful anti-cancer drug and a safe, natural pesticide, both contained in substances found in the pawpaw tree. Researchers say the cancer drug, which has been tested only in animals, appears to be significantly more potent than some widely used cancer drugs. While more research needs to be done—the National Cancer Institute has begun its own tests—researchers are encouraged by early testing.

The pawpaw tree, which grows throughout the eastern United States, is a shrublike tree, bearing edible fruit shaped like bananas. The two substances isolated by researchers were found throughout the tree, but mostly in twigs and small branches. Researchers were able to identify the two substances thanks to a new screening test which was devised to rapidly identify potentially useful drugs and pesticides in plants.

The new screening test is based on the fact that most drugs, given in high enough doses, will kill. Researchers expose tiny brine shrimp to plant extracts. According to the researchers, if the shrimp die, the plants contain drugs. If the shrimp live, the plants don't contain drugs. If the results from step one of the screening test warrant it, potentially useful plant extracts are then placed on tumors which are growing in the laboratory. If the tumors die, the extracts are then tested further for potential anti-cancer potential.

Apparently, the pawpaw drug acts on cancer cells in a new way, opening up the eventual possibility of an entire new class of anti-cancer drugs. While the research so far is promising, more testing needs to be done .

Natural Way To Prevent Clogged Arteries

Balloon angioplasty—surgery to open blocked arteries—is performed on over 280,000 Americans each year. While the operation, which brings about unrestricted blood flow by expanding the arteries, is highly successful, it may also damage the vessel walls. And, if the body tries to repair the injury, cells at the site multiply, often creating a new blockage. Recent research at the University of Washington School of Medicine may have discovered a way to prevent the new blockages from developing.

Earlier studies have suggested that a natural substance, platelet-derived growth factor (PGDF), plays an important role in the development of new blockages in angioplasty-repaired arteries. In order to put that theory to a test, researchers first had to find an antibody to PGDF. They obtained the antibody by injecting goats with PGDF taken from humans. The goats' immune systems then produced antibodies against PGDF.

Armed with the PGDF antibody, scientists then performed angio-plasty surgery on about 40 rats. The balloon was inflated in an artery, causing damage to the vessel walls—the same thing that happens in human angioplasty. Researchers then injected half of the rats with the goat-produced PGDF antibody. The other rats were injected with a differ-ent goat-produced antibody. The results showed a 41 percent reduction in arterial thickening at the angioplasty site in all the rats who had received the PGDF antibody. There was no such reduction in any of the rats who were injected with a different antibody.

Scientists believe that if the PGDF antibody can eventually be successfully applied to humans, they will be making a great step forward in preventing some cases of clogged arteries.

This Natural Cure For Muscle Aches Works Better Than Medicine

While medication can relieve the pain and discomfort of assorted muscle aches and pains, a natural remedy—massage—often works bet-ter. Massage can increase the circulation of blood and relieve the pain by reducing muscle spasms and loosening cramps.

To massage a muscle cramp, you'll need to work on the entire area, and not just that part that has a cramp. For example, if the cramp is in your foot, you should massage the entire leg. Using your hands, stretch the area of the muscle cramp. For best results, use gliding and then kneading strokes until you feel the cramp begin to loosen. You can end your "self-massage" with some chopping strokes to help the blood supply in the cramp area.

5 Natural Ways To Get Rid Of A Headache Fast

Some studies indicate that as many as 70 million Americans may suffer from frequent and chronic headaches. And many of those people take medication to chase away the pain. While medication can certainly help combat headaches it can also cause unwanted side effects. That's why some experts are now recommending natural, nonmedical treatments instead of drugs. These natural treatments, while not guaranteed headache-pain relievers, sometimes work as effectively as drugs, but without the negative side effects.

Here are 5 ways you can get rid of headache pain fast, naturally, without drugs:

1) Give your eyes a rest. Eyestrain headaches can be prevented by avoiding the circumstances that cause the condition. Reading in dim light, staring at a computer screen, using corrective lenses that are not right for you, or not using lenses when you need them, are among the leading causes of eyestrain. Under such circumstances, the muscles around the eyes contract in an attempt to help you "see" better. The contraction instigates headaches and triggers muscles in the face and scalp to contract as well—all making for a pretty powerful eyestrain headache.

You can prevent eyestrain headaches when you are reading or working at a computer terminal by taking periodic breaks and re-focusing your eyes on some distant object. If you feel eyestrain coming on, remove your glasses or contacts (if you wear them) and dim the lights. Then, keeping your eyes open, cup the palms of your hands over your eyes to create total darkness. Stare into this darkness for about 30 seconds. Then, close your eyes and lower your hands. Slowly open your eyes.

2) Give your muscles a rest. If your work requires that you maintain a fixed position—sitting or standing—for long periods of time and/or if you have poor posture, your muscles, including those in the head, face and neck, are likely to tighten up and in effect "freeze". This can in turn trigger or aggravate the misery of tension headaches.

To prevent muscle freeze, you should try to vary your position as much as possible. You should also take five-minute breaks at a minimum of every two hours. This will help you release both the physical and psychological tension that could lead to a headache. If you are standing for a long period of time, try to pace a little, tilt your pelvis forward and back, and rotate your shoulders. People who are in a sitting position for long periods of time should occasionally straighten and stretch their spines. Good posture can also help to further reduce the strain of maintaining one position for hours at a time—especially when sitting. You should sit with your shoulders square and your back straight against the back of your chair. Also keep your feet flat on the floor and your knees at hip level.

3) Try hot and cold treatments. While some people have discovered that applying cold helps to ease their headache pain, others prefer heat. You should try both treatments and find out which one works better for you.

To give your headache a cold treatment, wrap ice cubes in plastic and then in a damp towel. Apply the wrapped ice directly on the area that is generating the pain. You can also try applying cold to the back of your neck, the base of the skull and the top of your head. Cold may also be applied by using a damp washcloth which has been in a freezer for at least 10 minutes, or a frozen gel pack which you can find at most drug stores and some supermarkets.

Heat can be applied with a hot-water bottle, a heating pad, or with a hot, wet towel draped across the back of the neck. Another method of applying heat is to sit under a hot shower, with your arms resting on your bent knees, and your forehead resting on your arms. The hot water beating down on the back of your neck and shoulders should help ease your headache pain.

4) Learn to breathe deeply. You stand a good chance of calming yourself and avoiding a tension headache if you learn to breathe slowly and deeply whenever you begin to feel stress. Most experts recommend breathing through the nose because it carries oxygen more directly to the brain. You should take a deep breath, filling your lungs completely as you inhale to a slow count of four. Hold the breath through a slow count of four, and then exhale to a slow count of four. If you do it properly, you should feel your stomach puff out slightly.

5) Perhaps the best natural way to prevent headache pain is to exercise. Regular physical activity helps keep your blood circulating through your body, delivering more oxygen and removing metabolic waste more efficiently.

Natural Methods Of Preventing Heart Disease

Many recent medical research studies indicate that certain natural methods for treating and/or reducing the risk of developing coronary heart disease or coronary artery disease can be very effective. Here are two such highly recommended methods:

1) Switch to a low-fat diet. It is especially important that you cut down on your intake of saturated fats, most commonly found in meat and dairy products. Basically, a healthful low-fat diet requires that you consume less meat, eggs, dairy products and other sources of saturated fats and cholesterol. You should consume more starches and low-fat sources of protein.

2) Replace red meat and dairy products with fish. Studies have shown that the omega-3 oil found in many saltwater fish and some freshwater fish can help raise HDL levels in the blood. The new studies indicate that people who eat lots of cold water fish, such as salmon, trout or cod, tend to have lower rates of coronary heart disease than do other people. This seems to be true even if the amount of fat in the diet stays about the same.

11 Natural Remedies For Common Health Problems: Arthritis, Constipation, Dental, Diabetes, Diarrhea, Emphysema, Hemorrhoids, Hypertension, Insomnia, Skin Disorders And Toothaches.

Hundreds of scientific studies have shown the following natural treatments for various diseases, illnesses and conditions to have a relatively high degree of effectiveness. Even so, you should have regular professional medical checkups, and seek your doctor's advice before trying any treatment— natural or otherwise.

1) Rheumatoid Arthritis— omega-3 fatty acids found in fish, such as lake trout, salmon, mackerel, and sardines, may help prevent or alleviate a good deal of arthritic pain and swelling.

2) Constipation— wheat bran is the most effective natural laxative. Other good natural laxatives include prunes, dried beans and most

high fiber fruits and vegetables.

3) Dental Problems— if you want an effective cavity-fighting natural mouthwash, try some tea. Other natural cavity-fighters include grape juice, black-cherry juice, and cheese.

4) Diabetes— foods such as peanuts, soybeans, lentils, kidney beans, black- eyed peas, chick-peas, and apples all produce a desired slow, steady increase in blood sugar levels rather than a more dangerous rapid rise.

5) Diarrhea— yogurt, with live cultures, can be very effective, especially if the diarrhea is caused by prescription antibiotics. It is also important that you replace the fluids your body is losing by drinking lots of liquids, such as fruit drinks, chicken broth without fat, and Gatorade.

6) Emphysema and Chronic Bronchitis— hot, spicy foods, such as onions, mustard, horseradish, chili-peppers, and garlic will help keep mucus flowing and the bronchial tubes open.

7) Hemorrhoids— wheat bran and other high fiber fruits and vegetables will help produce a soft, bulky stool and reduce the strain in bowel movements.

8) Hypertension— eating mackerel a couple of times a week can help lower your blood pressure. Other foods, such as oat bran, and high fiber fruits and vegetables can also help.

9) Insomnia— sugar or honey can be effective sleep aids. Either leads to an increased level of serotonin—a chemical which helps calm down brain activity —in the brain, bringing about relaxation and sleep.

10) Skin Disorders— salmon, herring, sardines, mackerel, and all other seafood containing high levels of omega-3 fatty acids may bring relief from psoriasis. And certain skin inflammations can be treated with oatmeal packs.

11) Toothache— oil of cloves has proved to be effective in providing temporary relief.

How To Start Your Own Organic Garden
For Fun, Health And Money Savings

For many people, planning a garden is a source of great enjoyment. How and when a garden is planted is the key to getting the most food savings, as well as to the quality and quantity of the harvest. So the prime objective should be a well-planned, well-planted, well-cared-for garden that produces a good yield.

Many beginners make the mistake of planning "too big". They plant a large plot of land, only to find that it takes too much time and work. The result is a poorly tended garden that produces a low yield. A small plot of land will require less work and enable the beginning gardener to get the most vegetables possible out of the least amount of space. It's both efficient and profitable.

The first phase of the planning process should take place during the winter months when you get as many seed catalogs as you can find. Browsing through seed catalogs will give you a good idea of what each company has to offer. You'll learn who specializes in what vegetables—disease resistant varieties, short season varieties—and who offers the best selection of each vegetable you are interested in planting.

Before you actually order your seeds, you should make a list of what foods you and your family like to eat. Make sure you order only those foods you want. Also be sure to include all those foods you like but seldom get to enjoy because of their high prices in the store. That way your garden will also provide some extra treats at very little cost.

The next step in the planning process is determining how big a garden you can take care of realistically. As already noted, a small plot of land can produce both quantity and quality if properly cared for. The best thing to do is to start small, and then expand as your needs dictate. Of course, the size of your garden also depends on how much land you have available. But the main thing you want to avoid is putting out more garden than you can take care of properly.

Once you have decided on what seeds to order and a general idea of how big your garden should be, you'll need to decide on exactly what type of garden you want to have. Here are three basic organic garden plans to consider:

1) The largest of the three garden possibilities is a garden that will furnish all your vegetables year-round. This type of garden takes extra work to prepare and maintain, but if you give it your best effort, you should harvest enough vegetables from it to last you through the year, with both fresh foods and foods to store and use over the winter months.

This type of garden will certainly demand a lot of time and work. And unless you have lots of mulch and/or several hours a day to work in this type of garden, you'll probably need to utilize mechanical cultivation.

The "year-round" garden also requires that you grow enough fresh foods to get you through the early and late growing seasons. Remember, the longer you eat fresh foods from your garden, the less you will have to store for use during the winter months.

2) The second type of organic garden to consider is one to produce selected vegetables for storage and the rest for fresh foods. As with the "year-round" garden, you should keep this type of fresh garden going as long into autumn as possible. It is also a good idea to try to be somewhat selective with this garden, planting vegetables that will accommodate your available storage areas. For example, if you have a freezer, plant vegetables that freeze well— if you have a root cellar, plant that type of crop. If you don't plan to pressure can any vegetables, then don't plant more than you can eat fresh and/or frozen.

3) The third possibility is a fresh food garden or a salad garden. This type of garden requires that you plant something every couple of weeks all season long in order to maintain top-quality fresh vegetables.

This type of garden allows you to experiment with small plantings of exotic vegetables you have never tried before, and it can be incorporated into either of the two other types of gardens.

Planning Tips

1) Location— ideally, you should try to have the garden near enough to the house so that it is almost like a "fresh food cupboard". That way you can get fresh produce any time you need it and put off harvesting vegetables for a meal until the last minute, keeping all their nutrients and flavor intact.

Having your garden close to the house also promotes better care by you and your family. You'll know what's going on in the garden nearly all the time and be able to avert many problems before they become serious.

2) Soil— most gardeners aren't fortunate enough to have perfect garden soil. Instead, they have to make do with whatever soil they have. This means you must usually keep on adding organic matter to your garden because the vast majority of soils require it and plants keep using it up. But you should not get discouraged by poor soil, because you can add natural matter to improve its quality.

3) Water— adequate water is another essential thing your garden will need. It isn't wise to depend on rain as the sole source of water for your garden— mulching will provide some help, but your garden should get, as a general rule, about 1 inch of rain per week.

One way to insure adequate water for your garden is to use a sprinkler system. Depending on the size of your garden, one or two strategically placed sprinklers should give it adequate coverage and water.

You can also try trench irrigation. This is done by digging trenches, about 6 inches deep, on a slight slant in a gridiron pattern between rows. This system doesn't work especially well in sandy soil and doesn't provide the freedom to change the pattern of the garden on short notice if such changes are needed.

4) Tools— for basic organic gardening, you will need very few tools. If you haven't gardened before, it is a good idea to try getting along with just the essentials to begin. Here are the basic tools you'll need for starting your organic garden: a spade; a fork; a trowel; a knife; a 3-pronged, hand-held cultivator (can be a short-handle for small gardens or on the end of a long handle for larger gardens); a rake; a hoe; and a file to keep the edges of your tools sharp and effective.

Planting Tips

1) All perennial crops, such as strawberries, asparagus and rhubarb, should be located at one side of the garden.

2) To avoid shading, tall-growing crops, such as corn, must not be planted near small crops like carrots or beets.

3) Space for spring crops which are harvested early may be used again for later crops. For example, tomatoes after radishes, and cucumbers after spinach.

4) Crops, such as lettuce, radishes, onions, early cabbage, etc., which are planted early, fast-growing and quick to mature, should all be grouped together.

5) In hilly areas, rows should follow across the slope.

6) If possible, rows should run north and south to keep plants from shading one another.

7) Spacing between rows should be designed for the method of cultivation you plan to use— hand or mechanical.

What Vegetables Should You Grow

The purpose of organic gardening is to grow food naturally, without pesticides and artificial fertilizers. It is an effort to utilize natural resources to provide various foods. You can have any type of vegetable you want in your organic garden. Here is a list of some of the foods which have been proven to contain natural substances that are both healthful and healing, and which can be organically grown for fun and money-savings:

1) Early spring planting— onions, lettuce, peas, spinach and radishes.

2) Mid-spring planting— carrots, beets, parsnips, chard, broccoli, cauliflower, and early potatoes.

3) Late spring planting— tomatoes, bush beans, summer squash, winter squash, and sweet corn.

4) Early summer planting— Brussels sprouts and snap beans.

5) Mid-summer planting— turnips, rutabagas, and kohlrabi.

Many of the above vegetables can be planted in more than one planting group.

Other healthful foods you can grow in your organic garden include, beans of all types; celery; eggplant; endive; garlic; artichokes; kale; sweet potatoes; parsley; okra; melons; peppers; and Chinese cabbage. Of course this is just a partial list. With your own organic garden, you can grow any type food you want. The results are good for both your health and your budget.

New Study Confirms The Amazing Effects Of Thinking On How You Feel

A recent study, conducted by researchers at Yale University, gives more strength to the theory that if you believe that you are healthy, you'll have a longer, healthier life. The results of the Yale University study showed that emotions, such as happiness at work, are better predictors of illness than medical history in people of all ages. Unhappy people usually dwell on the negative, while positive thinking people appear to be both happier and healthier. For example, the researchers say that being unhappy as a homemaker can pose an especially high risk of health problems.

An ever-increasing amount of scientific evidence supports the theory that the mind and emotions ahve a significant effect on the body's overall state of health. how we think and feel apperars to have a significant affect on the body's main defense mechanism for fighting off illness and disease, the immune system.

Many studies have shown that positive feelings such as love, sucurity and faith help to strengthen the immune response, giving the body a better chance of preventing and fighting of illness and disease. At the same time, negative feelings, such as tension, worry, and depression seem to undermine the immune response, making our bodies feel sluggish and worn-out. That's when we appear to be virtually defenseless, and prone to aches, pains, illness, and disease. Many suchj negative emotional states have been linked to diseases such as cancer, coronary heart and artery diseases, kidney malfunctions, lung ailments, diabetes, migraine headaches, and many other afflictions.

What this means is that you are far more in control of your life than you may realize. without being aware of it, you play a major role in creating your own state of health every day. Everything you eat, think, feel, and believe has a great effect on your overall health and happiness. Just as we've seen previouly a healthful diet and regular exercise can help improve and maintain our general state of health, a positive, optimistic outlook can also work wonders. It is possible, with a positive mental outlook, to learn to be the master of your inner resposes, and in so doing strengthen your body's immunity against illness and disease.

How To Fight Off Chronic Fatigue And Stress

Some experts estimate that as many as 10 million Americans are afflicted with chronic fatigue (CF). According to research, chronic fatigue is a stress- related illness which can be caused by long, frustrating hours at work, family pressures, and even by allergies brought on by industrial pollution. Most people who suffer from CF report a persistent, run-down feeling. In order to overcome chronic fatigue, medical experts recommend rest, proper diet, and stress management.

This Cure Works If You Feel Run-Down, Fatigued Or Stressed Out

1) As soon as you are fully awake, get out of bed and get into action. You'll soon discover that you have more energy when you don't lie around in bed.

2) Have a good breakfast. It is important that you eat an energizing breakfast, such as whole grain cereal, skim milk, wheat toast, and a piece of fresh fruit.

3) Take a daily vitamin-mineral pill. This should include the RDAs of all major vitamins and minerals. Ask your doctor for his or her recommendation.

4) Get regular exercise. Even moderate exercise,such as walking, will give you more energy.

5) Maintain your ideal weight. Having excess weight may cause

you to expend more energy than you should.

6) Reduce your consumption of alcohol. Drinking alcohol at night can interfere with your ability to get a good night's sleep.

7) Avoid caffeine. Since caffeine is a stimulant, it too can keep you from getting a good night's rest. Try decaffeinated drinks instead.

8) Get some time alone. You can reduce stress by taking 30 minutes each day to do something that you enjoy doing by yourself. Do some reading or work on a hobby. Explain to your family that you need some private time.

If you follow those suggestions properly and you still feel extremely fatigued, you may be suffering from a more serious problem known as chronic fatigue syndrome— also known as "yuppie flu". Some evidence indicates that a virus may cause CFS, but no one is really certain.

The Centers For Disease Control in Atlanta recently released a list of symptoms to help people know whether they have CFS. According to the list, you may have CFS if you have experienced chronic fatigue for at least six months and have been treated by a doctor who has ruled out any other problem that might be similar to CFS, such as an acute nonviral infection, depression, hormonal disorder, drug abuse, or poisoning.

Consult your doctor if you suspect that you have CFS. He or she may be able to diagnose your condition and provide treatment by prescribing low doses of an anti-depressant drug, such as Sinequan.

Hidden Psychological Distress May Lead To Heart Disease

A recent study suggests that cardiac overreaction to stress may increase the risk of heart disease in some people. The study revealed that people who were hiding psychological troubles—even from themselves—showed an abnormal jump in heartbeat and blood pressure when performing stressful tasks.

Earlier studies have linked such cardiac overreaction to heart disease, which often leads to heart attacks. Researchers say that while it is already known that being constantly anxious or constantly depressed is unhealthy, the new study suggests that suppressing such distress may be even more harmful.

In a related study, conducted at the University of Michigan, 58 people with an average age of just under 22 years and no known history of heart disease, were analyzed and tested in relation to their responses to stress. The participants filled out assessments of their psychological health as well as a test which dealt with their earliest memories. The tests of the subjects' early memories were used by a psychologist to uncover signs of emotional distress.

The subjects' responses to stress were analyzed while they performed assigned stressful tasks, such as timed mental arithmetic, making up stories about ambiguous drawings and saying the first thing that came to mind upon hearing certain phrases. According to researchers, the drawings and phrases used were designed to raise themes that many people find "psychologically threatening". A measure that combined elevations in blood pressure and pulse rate was used to analyze the subjects' responses to stress.

The results of the test showed that, of the people participating, those with hidden distress were twice as reactive to stress as genuinely healthy people. The participants with hidden stress were also more reactive than people who admitted that they were distressed.

While neither study provides conclusive proof linking heart disease and cardiac overreaction to stress, many scientists consider the evidence convincing. And, according to the researchers, the studies serve to emphasize the need to deal with anxiety and tension in an open and healthy manner.

Stress, Anger And Heart Attacks

Two recent scientific studies have uncovered evidence showing how stress and anger may cause heart attacks.

In one study, at Brigham and Women's Hospital and Harvard Medical School in Boston, 26 people with coronary artery disease were asked to perform certain "stress tasks", such as counting backwards by sevens while under the pressure of being timed. As the subjects counted, researchers monitored their coronary arteries.

The researchers focused on two randomly chosen artery segments for the participants. The segments were classified as "healthy", "mildly diseased" and "severely blocked". The results of the test showed that stress had no harmful effect on the healthy segments, but that it further constricted segments already constricted by coronary heart disease— almost 9 percent more constricted for segments which were mildly diseased and 24 percent for those that were severely blocked. And while blood flow in healthy arteries increased by about 10 percent, it decreased 27 percent in those that were diseased.

In another study, conducted at the Veterans Affairs Medical Center in Palo Alto, California, researchers studied the responses of 27 men in relation to anger and possible heart attacks. The subjects included 18 men with mild heart disease and 9 healthy men. All of the men were asked to talk about a recent event that had made them very angry. Researchers measured changes in the left ventricles of each subject.

Describing the disturbing incident had no ill effect on healthy ventricles, but in men with heart disease it reduced the pumping efficiency by up to 4 percent. The small reduction, although significant, caused no chest pain or other warning sign.

Researchers speculate that in the "real world" more intense, spontaneous anger may have a far more damaging effect on the heart's pumping capabilities. These experts think that anger may send diseased coronary arteries into spasm, thereby cutting off necessary oxygen to the left ventricle. When that happens the risk of a serious heart attack is likely to increase.

Is Stress Contagious? How To Protect Yourself

Many medical experts say that person under stress can easily "pass on" their tension and anxiety to people around them— especially to those people who tend to get caught up in the problems of others. Although being sensitive to another person's anxiety and tension is not a weakness, it can make us vulnerable to unnecessary stress which could then lead to serious health problems.

Since we all have our own fair share of stress to cope with every day, it is important that we know how to avoid "catching" stress from other people. Here are several expert tips on how to protect yourself from "contagious stress":

1) While it may seem harsh or unfeeling, you should, if at all possible, try to avoid people who seem to exude tension and anxiety. For example, if you seem to be coming into contact with such a person at the same time and place —at lunch or on the bus—rearrange your schedule so you are not constantly meeting him or her. After all, avoiding potentially unhealthy situations is an important part of proper health maintenance.

2) If you can't avoid "stress carriers", distract yourself so that you don't get caught up in their problems. Try to remind yourself that their problems are not yours. It's o.k. to sympathize, and even offer a few words of encouragement as long as you don't allow yourself to be swept away in their misery.

Try to distract yourself by thinking of peaceful images when you are in the presence of a stressed-out person. Visualize the most relaxing setting you can imagine—a sunny beach or a picnic in a lush, green meadow. This type of distraction should serve as a protective barrier against intrusive tension and anxiety.

3) A sense of humor may be one of your best defenses against contagious stress. Try to make yourself laugh as soon as possible after an encounter with a stressful person. Seek out a friend who can always make you laugh, or go see a funny movie. Research has proven that laughter can be a potent antidote to stress.

4) Another proven method of reducing stress is exercise. If possible, do some exercise—walking or running—after dealing with a stressful person. Exercise will be helpful, even if you simply walk around the block once or twice at lunchtime.

5) Keep your personal and professional environment as "stress-resistant" as possible with flowers, plants, posters, or pictures of relaxing scenes. In other words, try to surround yourself with proven "stress-busters".

Try This Natural Way To Eliminate Stress In Your Life

Having a good sense of humor may be one key to living a stress-free life. That's the indication from a recent study of 300 people at the University of Alabama. The study, concentrating on family life, suggests that funny remarks, playful attitudes and family jokes are characteristic of strong families, while those qualities seem to be lacking in weaker families.

According to the research, good-natured humor promotes a positive outlook, reduces tension and alleviates anxiety. In effect, people who can share laughter and who can laugh at themselves are more open and at ease. People who can laugh with others and at themselves are better able to put things in their proper perspective and not take their own problems too seriously. The most healthful, healing type of humor is that which makes people feel good.

Here are some insider's tips on how you can add more laughter to your family life:

1) Share jokes and favorite TV comedy shows and/ or comic strips.

2) Play games which encourage spontaneous, creative reactions.

3) Read funny stories aloud.

4) Participate in outside activities that you enjoy doing together.

7 Self-Help Techniques For Controlling Stress

1) Relax. Make time everyday for periods of relaxation— even if only for a few minutes.

2) Talk about your problems with someone you trust, or the people who may be the source of a problem.

3) Avoid making too many major life changes at one time. Whenever you can, plan for the future so that such changes won't occur at the same time.

4) Get regular exercise. Besides being good for your physical well-being, regular exercise will help take your mind off your troubles.

5) Set your priorities. Consistent planning of your daily priorities will enable you to gain control of your work load and help prevent frustration.

6) Establish reachable goals. You can avoid a lot of frustration if you don't set unrealistic goals. It's o.k. to be ambitious, but you must also be practical about what you can reasonably accomplish.

7) Take a break. Regular short breaks after periods of concentrated effort, or whenever you are frustrated with a project or a certain troubling situation, will help clear your mind.

If the stress in your life seems to be more than you can handle, consult your doctor immediately. He can evaluate you for the possibility of other effective stress fighting methods.

Amazing Two-Minute "Instant Relaxation Technique"

The most important part of any effective plan to control stress is learning how to relax. The following technique was designed by medical experts to promote deep muscle relaxation. With regular practice, the technique can provide you with such muscle relaxation in as little time as two minutes. For best results, it is recommended that you practice this technique once or twice a day before meals, or at least one hour after you have eaten.

1) The first step is to find a quiet, peaceful place where there are no distractions. Be sure to wear comfortable, loose-fitting clothes. You should take off your shoes, and undo any belts or tight buttons.

2) Lie down on your back with your feet about 18 inches apart. Your hands should rest on the floor, palms upward and about a half foot from your sides.

3) Once you have settled into position, begin tensing and then relaxing each part of your body. Start with your feet, then proceed with your legs, buttocks, abdomen, back, chest, shoulders, arms and hands,

head, and face. You should tense each part in its turn as hard as you can, then let it relax.

Quick Self Massage Gets Rid Of
Neck And Shoulder Tension In Seconds

For most people, anxiety and stress create discomforting muscle tension. To relieve such tension, it is necessary to "zero in" on the tense muscles— usually in the back of the neck and upper back—and massage them until you feel them relax. Here's an easy self-massage technique that, properly done, can relieve upper body tension:

1) Breathe slowly and deeply. Let your head drop forward, then cup the back of your neck with your hands. Press gently, so you will stretch your neck muscles without straining them.

2) Using thumbs and fingers, massage the back of your neck from the base of your skull down to your upper back.

3) As your muscles begin to relax, massage up from your shoulders to the back of your head, then around both sides of your head to your temples and back down again. Continue until your muscles are completely relaxed.

Self-Help Techniques That Work Fast
To Help Breathing Problems

Many people who develop breathing problems do so as the result of anxiety. The most common anxiety-induced breathing problem is hyperventilation, which is rapid and shallow or abnormally deep breathing. Some people, when frightened or worried, begin breathing rapidly and deeply which causes an abnormal loss of carbon dioxide, which in turn causes the blood to become alkaline. In such instances, a person who is hyperventilating may have a feeling of tightness in the chest, numbness in the fingers and around the mouth, muscle spasms, and dizziness.

Hyperventilation is not necessarily a one-time experience. In fact, it is not uncommon for such episodes to recur when you are anticipating anxiety-creating situations. However, there are several proven, self-help techniques that can help stop and/or prevent hyperventilation.

1) Breathe into a paper bag. Supposedly, breathing into and out of a paper bag helps to replace the carbon dioxide which has been lost while hyperventilating. While this technique can be effective, it should be used only if you are certain the hyperventilation is in fact caused by anxiety and not by a serious medical condition. If you have any doubt as to the cause of the hyperventilation, seek medical help immediately.

2) Relax. You can stop hyperventilation if you remain calm and slow your breathing. If you relax, your breathing will become slower naturally. As long as you remain tense, your breathing will be rapid.

3) Avoid stimulants. Since caffeine is a stimulant, it is a potential trigger for an episode of hyperventilation. Therefore, you should cut down on or eliminate such things as coffee, tea, colas, and chocolate which contain caffeine. Nicotine is also a stimulant, so smoking can also lead to hyperventilation.

4) Exercise. Regular exercise helps to decrease anxiety, therefore it can help cut down on the risk of hyperventilation.

5) Think of something else. After you have had your first experience with hyperventilation, don't become obsessed with the fear that you'll have another one. It is self-defeating to spend all your time thinking about your breathing and the possibility of hyperventilating again.

It should be noted that although hyperventilation is usually caused by anxiety, it may also occur as a result of uncontrolled diabetes, kidney failure, and some lung disorders. Such occurrences are, however, uncommon. If you should experience your first attack of hyperventilation, you should see a doctor and get a diagnosis.

How To Overcome Non-Medical Depression - Naturally

According to a recent report by the American Psychological Association's task force on women and depression, one of the best ways to cope with low moods is to increase one's energy level. Instead of basking in passivity and negative thinking, both men and women should "get into action" to help chase away the blues. The report recommends activities such as tennis and running, or simply doing something you enjoy. Once you feel less emotionally drained, you'll be better prepared to deal with the problems that brought on the low mood.

How To Use Hypnosis To Cure
A Medical Or Emotional Problem

Hypnotherapy and self-hypnosis are becoming increasingly popular methods of treatment for many stress-or fear-related conditions, such as eating disorders, insomnia and agoraphobia. Hypnosis has also been used to help people stop or modify unwanted habits such as smoking and excessive drinking. It has also been used to treat a wide range of physical ailments, including asthma, high blood pressure, skin problems, migraines, and certain digestive disorders.

While there is no conclusive scientific evidence as to the overall effectiveness of hypnosis, some doctors who have had success with this type of treatment say that most disorders respond within 1 to 12 sessions. The actual duration of the treatment varies according to each specific individual and problem.

The use of self-hypnosis usually follows treatment by a hypnotherapist, as it requires some initial professional guidance. The hypnotherapist will use various methods to help you develop a therapeutic trance (hypnotic state) in which you relax and focus your attention. For example, you may move into a hypnotic state by concentrating on the hypnotherapist's voice or by focusing on a specific object. Once you are "under" or in a hypnotic state— characterized by heightened mental awareness, deep relaxation and suggestibility—the hypnotherapist will communicate suggestions to your subconscious.

Being in a hypnotic state does not mean that you are asleep. Scientists who have studied EEG recordings of hypnotized subjects' brain waves,have discovered that the waveforms match those found in people who are awake but relaxed, with their eyes closed. Therefore, at the end of the session you will simply open your eyes and will be fully aware of everything that occurred.

Once a hypnotherapist has helped you to develop a therapeutic trance, you can use the same or similar techniques on your own to help fight physical or emotional problems. Many people are using self-hypnosis as a means of learning how to relax, to control emotionally based problems or habits and to reduce pain and other physical problems.

If you would like to get a referral to a licensed psychologist or doctor who practices hypnotherapy, write to the American Society of Clinical Hypnosis, 2200 E. Devon Ave., Suite 291, Des Plains, IL 60018-4534. Include a self- addressed, stamped envelope.

New Studies Reveal How Your Religion Affects Your Health

Several studies have confirmed the power of prayer in relieving tension and stress. The results from these scientific studies into the effect of prayer on stress reduction show that prayer is an effective means of evoking the relaxation response, which is the key to relieving tension and/or stress.

In one study, subjects were taught a basic relaxation technique—to make themselves comfortable, sit quietly and mentally repeat a word or phrase. Even though the subjects were offered a choice of relaxing words, eight out of ten chose a word or phrase indicative of their personal faith. These people also stayed with the program longer and enjoyed better results in terms of improved health than did those people who used words not related to religion or faith.

The results suggest that, while any technique which evokes the relaxation response will help reduce stress, the most effective technique may be one that conforms to your faith or religious beliefs—something you have conviction in and are comfortable with. For many people, that technique seems to be prayer.

In another related study—conducted at Purdue University—researchers recently discovered that people who practice their religious faith consistently, tend to be healthier than people who do not or people who do not claim a religious affiliation.

The study, involving almost 1,500 people, revealed that those who practiced their faith regularly—church attendance, prayer, readings—were in better general health than those people who were not actively involved in regular religious worship or who had no religious affiliations.

A Bath A Day May Help Keep Stress At Bay

While the most effective long-term way to deal with stress is to uncover and treat its cause(s), experts say it is also helpful to simply treat the symptoms. Being able to alleviate the symptoms of stress can allow you to improve your chances of relaxing long enough to understand and deal with its cause(s). One effective way of soothing stress-produced symptoms is taking an "antistress bath".

The most common antistress bath is the evening bath. Soaking in a tub of warm water helps to relax the muscles. It may also work by heating the brain slightly, which can have a calming effect. Experts say that only water that is comfortably warm to the touch (100 degrees to 102 degrees F.) is effective in easing symptoms of stress—water that is too hot or too cold can shock the system. It is recommended that you soak for no longer than 15 minutes.

Steam baths and saunas can also work as "antistress tools" for some people. However, you should check with your doctor before trying either a steam bath or sauna because they can both create a significant strain on the cardiovascular system.

Some people find flotation tanks to be an effective method of combatting stress. Such tanks are filled with water and a large quantity of Epsom salts to ensure buoyancy. They are made secure in a sealed, soundproof container. According to researchers, the warm water, plus complete silence and the elimination of virtually all outside distractions make flotation tanks a popular choice for many people who want to alleviate the symptoms of stress.

You can find out more about flotation tanks by writing to the Flotation Tank Association, P.O. Box 1396, Grass Valley, CA 95945. To find out if such a facility is available in your local area, check your local Yellow Pages.

How To Use Yoga Or Meditation To Relieve Tension, Relieve Pain, And Feel Better

For some people, the ancient practice of yoga is the ideal way to induce the relaxation rsponse. In fact, many doctors recommend the practice of yoga for pain control and stress reduction. As practiced in the West, yoga consists mainly of a combination of breathing, stretching and relaxation exercises which may be of great benefit in relieving tension and stress.

While there is no hard scientific evidence that yoga can be of benefit to overall health, there are indications that it may help in the cure and prevention of a wide range of disorders as well as in improving posture, strengthening certain muscles and enhancing flexibility.

The best way to perform yoga correctly is to attend classes led by an experienced instructor. Even though yoga exercises are performed slowly and are safer than many other types of exercise, improperly performed they can cause injury.

To perform yoga exercises, you should wear loose clothing and no shoes. You should also find a room with few distractions and utilize a mat or a blanket. When exercising, hold a position only as long as it is comfortable and breathe normally through your nose. Stretch slowly and focus on relaxing a tight muscle. You should not attempt an extreme yoga position without proper instruction.

Basic Yoga Breathing Exercises

1) Lie on your back and relax. Inhale slowly, to the count of four, pushing out your diaphragm, bulging your stomach and distending your ribs. Then, exhale to the count of four. Your stomach will flatten and your ribs retract. This breathing exercise can also be performed while you are walking or sitting.

2) Sit with your hips touching the back of a chair and your feet flat on the floor. Make sure your knees are comfortably apart, and then take a deep breath through your nose as you raise both arms over your head. Lean forward slightly and exhale slowly. Keep breathing through your

nose as you bend over until your chest rests lightly against your knees. Allow your head to hang between your knees and your arms to dangle by your sides as you press out all air. Hold this position for a count of 8 after exhaling. Begin breathing in as you lift your arms and return to a sitting position. Maintain the sitting position, with your arms overhead for a count of 8, then relax. Repeat the entire exercise a total of 3 times.

Basic Yoga Relaxation Exercise

Lie on your back, with your arms by your sides, palms up. Your legs should be slightly apart. Close your eyes and imagine that you are floating. Unflex your neck muscles— very slowly roll your head from left to right 10 times. Relax the other parts of your body, beginning with your feet, your ankles, your lower legs, and continue upward toward your head. Concentrate on each part of your body until it feels free of tension and you are completely relaxed.

Basic Yoga Stretching Exercises

1) Stand straight, with your feet well apart— your left foot pointing to the left and your right foot turned slightly inward. Stretch your arms out to your sides, palms down. Inhale, then bend to the left and slightly forward as you exhale. Slide your left hand down your leg and grasp the lowest part possible. Bring your right arm up vertically. Turn your head so you can look upward at your right hand. After a few full breaths, release the position and repeat the exercise on your right side.

2) While sitting up straight in a chair, bend your legs at right angles and plant your feet firmly on the floor. Put your right hand on your left knee and your left arm over the back of the chair. Look straight ahead and breathe in through your nose. Exhale slowly as you turn to the left. Pull easily with both hands in order to twist your spine gently. Maintain this position for a count of 3, and then go back to the starting position. Rest for a few moments, and then reverse the placement of your hands and perform the previous exercise. Repeat the exercise twice each way.

3) While sitting with your back against the back of a chair, stretch your arms straight out and parallel to the floor. Flex your hands so your palms are facing away from you. Begin a slow rotation of your arms— the

circles you make should be so large, your arms almost touch when they reach the front. Do from 3 to 5 repetitions, breathing deeply through your nose throughout the entire exercise. Repeat the exercise in reverse. You may also try making smaller, faster circles.

Meditation

Recent medical research indicates that daily meditation may help lower blood pressure, reduce stress and promote a general feeling of well-being. With meditation, the mind is released from the constant barrage of external stimuli, as well as from its own steady stream of consciousness. The result is a state or condition unlike either ordinary wakefulness or sleep.

While advanced meditation techniques may require rigorous training, the basic meditation technique can be learned by almost anyone. Here is a simple, effective, basic meditation technique which should be performed daily, preferably at the same time and in the same place.

1) Find a quiet place free of all distraction.

2) Sit in a comfortable, upright position.

3) Close your eyes.

4) Relax your entire body, from your feet to the top of your head.

5) Visualize a quiet, peaceful setting, or concentrate on a word or phrase of your own choosing, repeating it to yourself over and over.

At first, distracting thoughts, feelings and sensations may intrude on your meditation. Have patience. Renew your effort to concentrate on your image or chosen word. The more you practice, the easier it will become for you to reject distractions.

Try this technique for about 15 or 20 minutes, then open your eyes and sit quietly for a minute or two, then return to your regular daily routine.

10 Self-Help Techniques For Improving Your Memory

Memory experts say that what many people consider "having a poor memory" is really just forgetfulness, and it happens to everyone. Forgetfulness can strike at anytime— you can't remember what you did with your car keys, or you can't remember someone's name, or you can't seem to remember what you came into the kitchen to get—and can be most irritating and frustrating. Such forgetfulness affects the short-term memory, resulting in a brief memory lapse.

The good news is that forgetfulness can be overcome by utilizing some simple devices we all have at our command. Techniques, from mnemonics to tying a string around your finger are all proven methods of memory enhancement. All it takes is a little extra effort and patience, and forgetfulness can be just a memory.

Here are ten expert self-help techniques for memory improvement:

1) Positive thinking— one of the most potent memory boosters comes from developing a sense of confidence that you can, in fact, remember. If you assume you have a poor memory because of past memory lapses, you are only undermining your true memory capability. If, on the other hand, you assume a positive attitude, you will develop the self-assurance needed to relax and be totally aware of what is going on around you. Having a positive attitude and confidence in your mental capacity is the first step toward memory improvement.

2) Repetition—the foundation of an efficient memory is repetition. Whenever you repeat something—a phone number, a name, a date, an address—you fix the information in your memory. While practice may not always make you perfect, it will bring about improvement. If you get into the habit of repeating information you need to remember, you'll soon develop an effective retrieval system.

3) Mnemonic devices— at one time or another, most people use this artificial memory system without even being aware of it. Mnemonic devices are those that associate unknown information with familiar things. For example, in order to remember how many days are in a certain month we might recite a little poem we learned when we were children— "Thirty days hath September...". Another well-known verbal mnemonic is "Every

Good Boy Does Fine", for recalling the positions of notes in the treble cleff.

Mnemonic devices can also be visual as well. One effective type of visual mnemonic device associates items on a list with images in a visual scene.

4) Listen— much of what we attribute to a poor memory is actually a failure to concentrate on what we are   hearing. The way to correct this is to learn to listen actively, rather than passively. Don't expect to sit and listen passively and then have automatic recall of everything you heard. You must think along with the speaker, ask questions, and actually be involved. In order to listen actively, you'll need to eliminate distractions and give your undivided attention to what others are saying. Once you have learned to do that, you'll notice a marked improvement in your memory.

5) Write it down— the act of writing out information you want to remember is an excellent way to improve your short-term memory. It serves to reinforce your ability to recall specific information. Whenever possible, jot down on paper what you need to remember.

6) Improve your vocabulary— if you have trouble remembering words, it's probably because you aren't using them. Studies have shown that a good command of the language enhances memory. The best way to improve your language ability is to read as much as you can.

7) Relax— that old nemesis, stress, which contributes to so many problems, can also be a culprit in forgetfulness. Your short-term memory can be impaired if you are preoccupied with stressful problems and situations. Learn to relax with relaxation techniques, and try to clear your mind.

8) Associate names with faces— many people have a great deal of trouble remembering the names of people they've just met. This sort of memory lapse can be overcome by making some sort of instant and permanent association between the name and the person's face. For example, you may observe that Bob bobs his head while he is talking, or that Rose has rosy cheeks.

9) Use your imagination— if you need to remember something,

you can devise your own memory aids. For example, if there's something you need to take with you when you leave the house in the morning, set the item in front of the door before you go to bed for the night. It's a sure bet you'll remember to take the item with you when you leave.

10) Memory joggers— do something unusual that will serve to jog your memory. For example, wear your watch on the other wrist or call your answering service to leave messages for yourself.

Behavioral Training Can Help Incontinence

According to medical research estimates, urinary incontinence affects 10 million Americans, mostly women over the age of 55. Most of these people can be made better or cured with a simple program of behavioral training that can be implemented at home. The program, when properly followed, has proven to be most effective as a cure, or in alleviating many cases of urinary incontinence.

The training consists of patient education and a strict schedule for urination. The patients are taught relaxation techniques and how to distract the mind from the urgency to urinate. Under a doctor's supervision, the program can be implemented in the patients' homes.

More information about this program is available from a national nonprofit advocacy organization, Help For Incontinent People. Call 1-800-BLADDER or write to: Bladder Retaining, Box 554RD, Union, S.C. 29379. Include a self- addressed, stamped envelope.

The Best, Easiest Way To Stop Smoking

We've all heard it before—especially those people who use tobacco regularly— cigarettes and other forms of tobacco are addictive. We even know that nicotine is the drug in tobacco which causes addiction, and that all tobacco products contain substantial amounts of nicotine. The nicotine is absorbed quickly in the lungs from tobacco smoke and in the nose and mouth from smokeless tobacco, such as snuff and chewing tobacco. Even knowing all of this, millions of people continue to use tobacco, many of them, perhaps, because the addiction is so powerful.

How powerful is nicotine? Here are some facts, according to the 1988 Report of the Surgeon General on the Health Consequences of Smoking:

1) Used regularly, levels of nicotine accumulate in the body both day and night. In other words, daily tobacco users are exposed to the effects of nicotine 24 hours a day.

2) The more and longer you smoke, the more your body builds up a tolerance to nicotine, meaning the more nicotine you get, the more you need in order to produce the same feelings. That's the reason that certain unpleasant symptoms, such as headaches and dizziness, which usually accompany beginning smoking disappear once tobacco is used regularly.

3) Nearly every component of the body's endocrine and nonendocrine system is affected by nicotine and smoking.

4) Most patterns of tobacco use are regular and compulsive, and any attempt to give it up usually results in a withdrawal syndrome.

Whenever someone who uses substances that contain nicotine—cigarettes, cigars, pipes, snuff, chewing tobacco—attempts to quit, he or she usually experiences varying levels of the following withdrawal symptoms:

1) A craving for nicotine.

2) Frustration, irritability, anger.

3) Anxiety and tension.

4) Decreased heartrate.

5) Increased appetite.

6) Lack of concentration.

Most withdrawal symptoms seem to reach their zenith within the first 24 hours after quitting tobacco use and then decline gradually after that over several days or a few weeks.

Scientific research suggests that medicines can help reduce certain withdrawal symptoms as well as the likelihood of starting tobacco use again, but they seem to be more effective when used with behavioral intervention, such as relaxation methods and hypnosis.

Local offices of the American Cancer Society, the American Heart Association, and the American Lung Association can provide pamphlets on how to stop smoking and information on low-cost cessation programs. For those people who find quitting smoking "cold turkey" too difficult, the information supplied by these organizations can be very helpful. Look in your local telephone directory to find the office in your area or write to:

American Cancer Society
159 Clifton Road NE Atlanta, GA 30329

American Heart Association
7320 Greenville Avenue Dallas, TX 75231

American Lung Association
1740 Broadway New York, NY 10019

How To Disease-Proof Your Body
For A Longer, Healther Life

Diseases can be put into two main catagories — (1) Infectious diseases or (2) Noninfectious diseases.

Infectious diseases can be caused by exposure, by bacteria, or viruses. The tiny organisms can invade the body and infect it with a disease. A good example is the AIDS virus. You cannot get AIDS unless you are exposed to the AIDS virus. However, just because you are exposed to a particular infectious disease — that doesn't mean that you will get the disease.

You can lessen your chances of getting an infectious disease by (1) Taking steps to avoid exposure to that disease, (2) Keeping your body healthy so that it can fight bacteria or viruses, (3) Recognizing the symptoms of a disease so that you can get early treatment.

How To Avoid Getting AIDS. The Five Key Things To Do

(1) Abstain from sexual activities.

(2) Maintain a monogomous relationship with an uninfected person.

(3) Avoid drug use and possible infected needles.

(4) Do not share razors or any other skin-piercing instruments which could be contaminated with blood.

(5) Avoid hair salon treatments when worner's are cut - the blood can give you AIDS.

Using protective measures — such as condoms can lessen, but not eliminate, the chance of HIV infection.

Doctors are searching for a cure to AIDS. A new drug called AZT can help (but not cure) AIDS sufferers. While several drug companies are working on an AIDS vaccine — most experts feel that they are many years away from success.

If You Have Additional Question, Call The AIDS Hotline At (800) 342-AIDS.

Also Do These Things So You Don't Get Sexually Transmitted Diseases

1) Avoid sex that may damage a condom or tear the sensitive and delicate tissue which lines the vagina.

2) Use spermicidal jellies which contain nonoxynol 9.

3) Use water-based lubricants— oil-based lubricants can damage condoms.

4) Abstain from sexual activity if your partner has symptoms of a sexually transmitted disease, or is being treated for such a disease.

5) Avoid having multiple sexual partners. Maintain a monogomous sexual relationship.

7 Keys To Arthritis Relief

1) Ginger

An article in Medical Tribune (30,18,16) reports that ginger provides some relief from arthritis pain. Patients took 5 grams per day of fresh ginger root or 1 gram/day of ginger powder. They reported less swelling and less stiffness.

2) Fish Oil

Stanford Univerisity's Dr. Harris reports that some people gain benefits from using fish oil. Doctors recommend that you get the fish oil by eating cold water fish. A report in Arthritis and Rheumatism states that a daily dose of Omega-3 fatty acids (from fish oil) helped arthritis sufferers.

3) Exciting News For People With Arthritis

Biological response modifiers can ease a type of arthritis that is caused when a person's immune system goes out of whack. Dr. A. Gragzel states that these new drugs could soon be very important for fighting inflammatory arthritis. These drugs include: Interlukin-1, CD4, CD5, and IL-2. They are nearing FDA approval. Other new drugs include modified forms of old drugs: Azalfidine and Sandimmuade.

4) Lose Weight

One simple way to help ease arthritis suffering is to lose weight if you are overweight. Excess weight puts added pressure on your joints. This increases stress on your cartilage and bone, and can lead to more inflammation and swelling.

5) Floating

Some studies have shown that floating in a specially designed tank filled with warm water, can relieve arthritic pain. The water is heated to 93.5 degrees F and floating time is about 1 hour. There are over 200 tank centers in the USA. Here is a contact that can tell you the nearest flotation center to your home: Flotation Tank Association, Box 1396, Grass Valley CA 95945.

6) Exercise

Dr. Mollen recommends that people who suffer from arthritis should undertake aerobic exercise. He recommends walking, bicycling, or swimming. Dr. Mollen states that exercising in water is also excellent. The water reduces the pain that you may normally experience while exercising.

7) Vitamins

There is some evidence that increasing your vitamin C intake can help rheumatoid arthritis. One of the best sources for vitamin C is citrus fruit.

Prevent Getting Alzheimer's Diesease

The exact cause for Alzheimer's disease is not known. This disease effects the portions of the brain that are responsible for memory, thinking, and physical functions. It usually affects older people and is fatal in a period of a few months to 5 years.

What Many People Don't Know About Alzheimer's Disease:

Aluminum

Many autopsy studies have revealed high amounts of the metallic element aluminum in the damaged brain areas of Alzheimer's patients. This could mean that these people have too much aluminum in their diet or that they are unable to metabolize it properly.

Another study revealed that young patients who received abnormally high doses of aluminum begin to show signs of senility! A report in The Lancet shows increased Alzheimer rates among people who drink water with high concentrations of aluminum.

Some doctors warned that cooking with aluminum pots and uten-sils can be dangerous. Aluminum cooking pots when mixed with fluori-dated water could increase the amount of aluminum in your food. It does this by increasing the solubility of aluminum in the water used to cook the food.

Some natural occurring waters or treated waters contain large amounts of aluminum. This could result in increased aluminum in your body. Therefore, it could pay you to have your water tested.

Some doctors are convinced that there is an increased risk for Alzheimer's if you have high amounts of aluminum in your body.

Smoking

A recent study reveals that cigarette smokers have four times the risk of gettting Alzheimer's disease. The reason for this is not known. The best advice is to quit smoking entirely. You could lessen your chances of get Alzheimer's as well as many other ailments.

Diagnosis

A London University study reported that many doctors gave wrong diagnoses of Alzheimer's disease in about half of their cases. Other diseases can cause similar symptoms. Alzheimer's disease can only be correctly diagnosed by a doctor who is thoroughly experienced with the disease.

Alzheimer's Information Service

You can obtain information about Alzheimer's disease by calling the Alzheimer's Disease and Related Disorders Association at 800-621-0379.

Cancer - Cause And Prevention

Cancer is one of the most frightening words in the English lan-guage. This disease comes in many forms and is one of the deadliest afflictions of mankind. Cancer frightens people because it is very deadly, there are no sure cures, it can be very painful, and many people contact this disease.

Doctors cannot pinpoint any one single cause of cancer. But recent medical research has shown that a number of enviromental and diet factors can increase the risk of contacting cancer.

Cancer Facts

About 500,000 people die from cancer each year in the U.S.A.

Cancer treatment costs can run into the many thousands of dollars per week.

Lung cancer kills more Americans than any other type of cancer.

As deadly as cancer is doctors now have an increasing cure rate for many kinds of cancer. Also, there is much medical evidence which indicates that certain lifestyles can reduce your risk of getting cancer. In other words, cancer is not as mysterious or as deadly as it used to be. If you contact cancer you now have a greater chance for survival. Currently, about 5 million Americans alive today have had cancer and about 3 million of these are considered cured.

Cancer Causes

Many recent medical studies have shown strong links between certain environmental and diet factors, and an increased risk of getting cancer. Being aware of these possible cancer causing factors can help you avoid them. These could result in a lower cancer risk for you.

Last year colon cancer killed over 60,000 Americans, making it the second deadliest form of cancer. A recent study in the Journal of the National Cancer Institute (82,11:915) identifies two possible causes of colon cancer. These are (1) high saturated fat diets and (2) a low exercise lifestyle.

A Nutrition and Cancer study (13,4:271) indicates that a diet that is high in vegetable fiber may help to protect against colon and rectal cancer.

Numerous studies have shown a strong link between smoking

and lung cancer. The facts are very clear — people who smoke have a much greater risk of developing lung cancer than nonsmokers.

Recent evidence indicates that several types of cancer are mostly diet related. These include (1) Stomach, colon, and rectum cancer — 90% diet related. (2) Gallbladder, Pancreas, and Breast cancer — 50% diet related.

One recent study shows the risk of obtaining esophageal cancer for people who smoke and drink in various amounts. People who smoke and drink in moderate to heavy range have increased risks of 35 to 150 times greater than other people. This study shows that people who smoke and drink heavily are at enormously increased risk of getting esophageal cancer. Other studies have shown that smokers and drinkers also have increased risks of obtaining other types of cancers.

Environmental exposure to chemicals can also increase cancer risks. Americans are exposed to many chemicals in their workplaces and in large cities. Some known cancer-causing substances are: Asbestos, certain amines, and chlorine containing organic compounds.

Mouthwash Warning: This Mouthwash May Increase Your Chance Of Mouth And Throat Cancer

A recent study by the National Cancer Institute indicates that some mouthwashes may contribute to mouth and throat cancer. These brands of mouthwashes contain as much as 25% alcohol. So check the label on your mouthwash!

8 Ways To Help You Avoid Getting Cancer

The 1988 Surgeon General's Report on Health recommends a diet that would help to reduce the number of cancer cases. Here are the guidelines:

(1) Reduce fat intake to less than 30% of your total calories. The easiest way to do this is to eat less red meat and leaner cuts of other types of meats

(2) Increase the fiber in your diet to 20 to 30 grams each day. This

can easily be accomplished by eating plenty of vegetables and whole grain products.

(3) Include a wide variety of vegetables and fruits in your diet. You should have 4 to 6 servings of vegetables and 2 to 3 servings of fruit.

(4) Avoid being overweight. This increases your tendency toward many diseases by weakening your entire system.

(5) Limit your consumption of heavily spiced, salt cured, smoked, and pickled foods.

(6) Reduce alcohol consumption.

(7) Exercise on a regular weekly schedule.

(8) Don't Smoke

Reduce Your Breast Cancer And Colon Cancer! Risk By 50%

Dr. Leonard Cohen of the American Health Foundation states " You might reduce your risk of getting breast cancer by 50% — just by following the right diet."

Several studies suggest that diets high in saturated fats (from red meat & diary products) could increase your risk of breast cancer. This type of dietary fat increases a woman's estrogen levels and this could increase breast tumors.

Thus a suggested diet to reduce the risk of breast cancer would include:

(1) Only small amounts of saturated fats.

(2) Plenty of vegetables such as broccoli, brussel sprouts, corn, beans, lentils, kale, spinach, and sweet potatoes.

(3) 2 -3 servings of fruit each day.

(4) Use whole grain breads and pasta.

Some researchers have claimed that taking large daily doses of certain vitamin mixtures can cure or prevent cancer. However, most medical experts agree that megadoses of vitamins have not been proven to be a cureall.

In fact too much of certain vitamins can be very harmful to your body. At this time the best advice is not to overdo it when it comes to taking vitamins.

A number of studies have shown that physically fit people have a lower chance of getting cancer. One study revealed differs between women college classmates. Women who were active in sports and exercise had lower breast cancer rates than those who exercised little if any. Walking is one of the best forms of exercise.

Another study indicated that people who have some form of weekly exercise have 50% less chance of getting colon cancer. This indicates that you should at least get some form of mild weekly exercise.

Numerous studies have shown much greater cancer risks for smokers. Therefore, you can easily reduce this risk by not smoking. This increased risk is not just for lung cancer but also for many other types of cancer as well as other diseases. Many of the chemicals produced by burning are known to be strong irritants or cancer producing agents.

What Every Person With Light Skin Needs To Know

Fair skin people should avoid excessive exposure to sunlight. If you sunbathe use a sunscreen that blocks UV rays. Excessive sunlight is now beleived to be the primary cause of skin cancer.

Prostate Cancer Tips To Prevent And Treat

A new medication called Proscar (see chapter 11) can shrink some enlarged prostate glands. This could help you to avoid prostate surgery. If discovered early enough prostate cancer is almost 100% curable.

(1) So you should have annual prostate checks starting at age 50.

(2) Eat a low-fat diet.

(3) Don't ignore trouble signs such as: difficulty in urinating or frequent urination at night.

Cervical Cancer - Foods That Help Prevent It

The B-vitamin Folate seems to help prevent a virus that causes genital warts from turning into cervical cancer. This vitamin can be found in green leafy vegetables, citrus fruits, and beans.

Cut Your Colon Cancer Risk 60% To 70% With This New Test

A widely available test can cut your risk of dying from colon cancer. The test is called flexible sigmoidoscopy and costs $100 to $200. The American Cancer Society suggests that the test be done every 5 years after the age of 50. This could result in an early diagnosis of any colon problems. And with cancer an early diagnosis means you have a much better chance at curing the disease.

4 Skin Cancer Prevention Tips

Skin Cancer is spreading faster than any other type of cancer. Here are some tips for protecting yourself.

(1) Use plenty of sunscreen lotion — one ounce per treatment. Reapply every 2-3 hours.

(2) Wear a wide brimmed hat— 80% of all skin cancers are on the head, neck, or hands.

(3) Keep infants out of direct sunlight.

(4) Avoid exposure to direct sunlight from the hours of 11 A.M. till 1 P.M. This is the time when UV rays are the strongest.

Fish And Cancer Risk - The Untold Story

The Environmental Protection Agency (EPA) warns that eating fish from any of America's 46 polluted waterways could result in a slight increase in a person's risk of getting cancer.

Consumers shouldn't worry about the warning because grocery stores, fish markets and restaurants do not carry fish from the polluted waterways. The EPA says the chief danger is to sports fishermen and poor people who fish to provide food for their families.

The potential danger is all the more insidious because the pollution doesn't produce any physical signs of contamination on the bass, walleye, catfish, trout, pike, sunfish, and other freshwater fish affected. However, the EPA stresses that the risk of getting cancer from eating such contaminated fish is relatively small.

While the EPA has not discovered the cause of the pollution, it is known that most of the contamination came from a pesticide, called dieldrin; and polychlorinated biphenyls, or PCBs, widely used in electrical transformers.

The National Cancer Institute (NCI) says that even though there is only a small risk of getting cancer by eating contaminated fish, it does add to the overall risk of contracting the disease. NCI records indicate that as many as 2 out of every 10 Americans are diagnosed with cancer by age 70.

New Test Warns Of Cancer Cell Growth

A new test developed by researchers at Children's Hospital in Boston may enable doctors to gauge exactly when a cancer patient's tumor begins to grow.

The new test, which is still considered experimental, works by detecting a hormone-like growth factor which shows up in urine. The test has already been used in more than 1,000 cancer patients in Boston, and according to researchers, it seems to identify those people who are at the highest risk of relapse.

Most of the initial experimentation with the new urine test has been in breast cancer patients, but the researchers say it may also detect rapid tumor growth in patients with cancer of the prostate, lung, kidney, ovary, testicle, bladder, skin, colon and brain.

The success of the new test depends on the detection of an obscure protein, known as growth factor bFGF, in the patient's urine and blood once a tumor begins accelerated growth. If the new test identifies the presence of the growth factor, doctors know the tumor is growing.

Further tests are needed to determine the test's reliability, but researchers are hopeful that it may one day win government approval and become available to the public.

Free Cancer Test Booklet

A free booklet titled, "Cancer Tests You Should Know About", for people 65 and older is now available upon request. The booklet is published by the National Cancer Institute and describes various tests. It also includes foldout checklists to track screenings. To get a copy of the booklet call 800-422- 6237.

12 Ways To Heal Diabetes

Diabetes is a wide-spread disease that effects more than 11 million Americans. Diabetes comes in two forms — both with a major symptom of excessive urination. Diabetes Mellitus is by far the most common form and about 1/2 of all sufferers do not know that they are diabetic.

A diabetic person cannot make normal use of sugar. The kidneys discharge some of the excess sugar into the urine. Severe cases of diabetes also cause problems with the use of fats and proteins.

Diabetes cannot be cured. The serious form (Type I) requires that the patient take insulin. About 80% of diabetic cases are of Type II, these cases can often be controlled by diet alone. Diabetes can lead to blindness, kidney failure, nerve troubles, and circulatory problems.

Recent research has shown several ways for Type II diabetics to help control this disease and its effects. There are 3 major aspects for controlling diabetes: nutrition, exercise, and weight control. Some diabetics have eliminated many symptoms by following a careful plan worked out with their doctor.

The American Diabetes Association has determined what the best diet is for diabetics. Of course each person's diet must be tailored to his or her particular lifestyle. No diet should be undertaken without consulting a doctor.

(1) The ADA recommends that a Type II person's diet provide 50 to 60 percent of his or her calories from carbohydrates.

(2) Cut your fat intake. Try to use foods with polyunsaturated fats.

(3) Limit your intake of protein to 15-20 percent of your total calories.

(4) Eat high fiber food. These include vegetables, barley, oats, whole wheat products, fruit, and legumes.

(5) Cut your cholesterol by limiting your meat intake.

A diabetic should not make any drastic diet changes except under the supervision of a doctor. Make gradual changes, sudden changes could upset your body's chemistry and cause major problems.

(6) Exercise

Exercise is extremely important for a diabetic person. It helps to improve your circulation, control blood sugar, control your weight, strengthen the heart, and reduce cholesterol. The best type of exercises included: Walking, jogging, swimming, or bicycling. Three times per week with 20-30 minute sessions are best. Do not do heavy exercises like weight lifting.

(7) Reduce Stress

Increased stress can cause additional problems for diabetics. Therefore, you should take steps to relax, remain calm, and reduce the amount of stress in your life.

(8) Dental Care

Some diabetic people are very susceptible to infection. Therefore, leading dentists like Roger Levin D.D.S. recommends that you pay particular attention to the care of your mouth. You should brush and floss frequently, and have regular checkups.

(9) Your Feet

A diabetic must pay close attention to their feet. A diabetic's feet can become easily damaged and infected. This can often lead to amputation. Here is how to protect those feet:

(A) If you are overweight, then reduce your weight to take pressure off of your feet.

(B) Wash your feet well everyday.

(C) Keep your feet warm on cold days — A nice foot bath can help.

(D) Inspect your feet for bruises, cuts, swelling, and other damage — everyday.

(E) Wear confortable — well fitting shoes.

(10) Magnesium for Type-II diabetics

The mineral magnesium seems to help Type-II diabetic sufferers. This can help by lowering high blood pressure. One of the best ways to get extra magnesium (and fiber) is by eating fresh green vegetables and salads. You should never take a magnesium pill supplement except under the advice of a doctor.

(11) Peas

A medical study in Denmark showed that the kind of fiber found in peas could help diabetics. This fiber helped by smoothing out the sharp rise in blood sugar after a meal.

(12) Your Lifestyle

A person with diabetics must pay close attention to diet, exercise, weight control, stress, and injuries. This can greatly reduce the many complications that can develop in a diabetic person. By taking all these factors into account, making gradual changes, and listening to your doctor you could greatly reduce diabetic complications.

Diabetes Breakthrough: New Procedure
May Lead To Earlier And Better Treatment

There is a new blood test that will soon allow mass screenings of patients who are likely to develop diabetes. According to the American Diabetics Associaton this new test can identify potential diabetics several years earlier. This could allow for earlier treatment and result in less diabetes-related complications. The new test was developed by Allergy Immuno Technologies in Newport Beach, California.

Researchers have made some dramatic progress in the actual treatment of diabetes. With the new blood test and earlier detection, new methods of treatment of diabetes, including self-monitoring of blood sugar; new insulin delivery systems; improved oral medications; laser therapy to prevent blindness caused by diabetes; and a better understanding of the dietary needs of people with diabetes, can all be even more effective.

Brain Chemical
May Cause Complications For Diabetics

Many diabetics are plagued with an almost insatiable appetite and subsequent obesity. Now, researchers say they have found a chemical in the brain which is likely to be responsible for those complications of diabetes.

In a study reported in the December 1992 edition of Endocrinology, researchers tested laboratory rats, focusing on abnormal levels of neuropeptide Y, called NPY. According to a leader of the research team, "overproduction" of NPY in many diabetics may lead to a heightened appetite and a propensity for obesity, as well as high blood pressure and "impaired reproductive function".

What Causes Heart Disease?

Your heart is the hardest working organ in your body. This muscle must continually pump blood to every cell. If it stops for as little as 4 minutes death or permanent brain damage will result.

Heart disease accounts for about 1/3 of all adult deaths. Unfortunately many of these deaths are premature. And worse yet most of these premature deaths are preventable. You can greatly lower your risk of premature heart failure by following a few easy steps.

Most premature heart deaths are caused by coronary heart disease. This is a condition in which fatty deposits develop in the arteries that supply blood to the heart muscles. This leads to atherosclerosis (narrowing) and eventually can block off the arteries or cause a blood clot. This can result in many heart problems or sudden attacks.

Doctors have discovered an unusual pattern in world wide heart disease. The more developed countries (U.S.A., Great Britain, Northern Europe, Australia,) have a much higher rate of heart disease than the less developed countries. There are some strong potential reasons for this higher rate in the more developed countries, including a diet high in saturated fats, a lifestyle with little exercise, overweight, and eating more refined food. Of course these reasons also suggest some solutions for lowering your risk of heart attacks.

Many studies have shown that several factors increase the risk of heart attack. You have control over most of those factors and to a large extent determine the amount of risk you take.

Four High-Risk Factors For Having A Heart Attack

(1) Diet— foods that are high in saturated fats and cholesterol (mainly from animal fats) increase the risk of heart attacks.

(2) People who eat large amounts of salty food have a higher risk of high blood pressure and heart attacks.

(3) People who live sedetary lives (little or no exercise) have a higher risk of heart failure.

(4) People who are under a lot of tension, worry, and are "too busy" increase their risk of heart attacks.

Of course there are other causes of heart disease such as genetic, and hereditary factors. But these are factors that you cannot control. The other 4 factors listed above are factors that you can choose to control. The latest medical evidence proves that you can unclog your arteries before it's too late by modifying your habits.

5 Ways To Unclog Arteries, Avoid Heart Disease Or A Heart Attack

(1) Give up the use of tobacco products. According to the American Heart Association, smokers are two to six times more likely to have a heart attack than non-smokers.

(2) Mild to moderate exercise (walking is one of the best methods) for at least 3 hours per week.

(3) Manage your stress by using breathing methods, meditation, relaxation, and stretching exercises for 1 hour per day.

(4) Change your diet to include more vegetables and fiber, but less fat and cholesterol. Have yoor blood pressure checked regularly, and be aware of your total cholesterol reading.

(5) Watch your weight. People more than 30 percent overweight are more likely to develop a heart disease even without any other risk factors. The AMA recommends that you keep your weight within moderate limits.

There are a few simple tests that can reveal your risk of heart attacks. These "heart predictors" can show your current status and give you guidance to make changes. These tests are very easy for a doctor to perform.

Breakthrough In Preventing Heart Attacks: Simple Ratio Reveals Your Risk

The recent Physician's Heart Study revealed a simple ratio that can predict your risk of heart attack. This Lipid ratio test measures the ratio of total cholesterol to HDL cholesterol (the good kind of cholesterol).

The higher this ratio is — means that your blood has more of the "bad cholesterol". In the Physician's Heart Study the people with the highest ratio had 4 times greater heart attack risk than those with the lower ratios. So it could pay to have your doctor check this ratio. You could then make lifestyle changes that could lower this ratio.

What You Should Know About Your Triglyceride, Level That Your Doctor May Be Overlooking

Several medical studies have shown that high levels of triglycerides in the blood also leads to a greater risk of heart attacks. Triglycerides are a major type of fat in the bloodstream. A person who has fairly low cholesterol levels but high triglyceride levels could still have an increased risk. Therefore, a number of reputable doctors state that your blood should be tested for both cholesterol and triglycerides. This can help you to locate and correct any potential problems that are caused by the diet that you eat. By making the correct changes in your diet you can make big changes in the level of cholestrol in your blood stream.

Obesity is a common condition that is associated with high triglyceride levels. You can dramatically lower your blood's triglyceride levels by exercise and diet changes. A diet that is higher in vegetables, nuts, fruit, and grains, and low in animal fat will produce quick results. Increased exercises burn more fat and decreases triglycerides in the blood.

3 Vitamins That Help the Heart

Several recent studies reveal that certain vitamins can help to reduce the blood levels of "bad" LDL cholesterol. This could cause a significant reduction in your risk of heart attack. These vitamins include beta carotene (15 to 20 milligrams per day), vitamin C, and Vitamin E. The best source of beta carotene is yellow vegetables, especially carrots.

Read This If You Have A Heart Murmur

A report by Dr. T. Welch states that people who have heart murmurs are in danger of infections of the heart valve. Therefore, they should take antibiotics before, during, and after dental or surgical procedures.

Second Hand Smoke: New Data You Need To Know

A report in the Journal of the American Medical Association states that breathing second hand smoke results in increased heart attack risk. The study shows that non-smokers who are married to smokers have more heart attacks than nonsmokers who are also married to nonsmokers. This could result in as much as 35,000 heart attack deaths each year.

Baldness and Heart Problems

A study by Dr. Carlos Henera of the University of Texas Medical School shows the following. Men who lose their hair quickly also are twice as likely to have coronary heart problems. This is probably due to some genetic factors. It means that these men should pay particular attention to the other high heart attack risk factors. Lowering these other factors could help to normalize or lower bald men's heart risks.

"Wonder Drug " May Help Prevent A Stroke

People at high risk of stroke because of irregular heartbeat may benefit from taking low doses of warfarin, a blood-thinning drug.

According to the results of a recent study published in the New England Journal of Medicine, warfarin can reduce the risk of stroke by almost 80 percent in people at high risk. The drug is already widely used to treat people who suffer from a heart irregularity also known as atrial fibrillation.

Following almost two years of tracking over 500 men with atrial fibrillation, researchers discovered that 23 men had suffered strokes— 19 were in a placebo group and 4 were using warfarin.

Toll Free Heart Information

A toll free number 1-800-345-4278 has been established to answer callers' heart questions. The hours are 10 A.M. to 7 P.M.

8 Things To Prevent Or Heal Osteoporosis

Osteoporosis is known as the brittle bone disease. It can affect both men and women. Osteoporosis develops slowly over many years. Recent studies show that men over 30 years old begin to lose some bone mass each year. This loss could be as much as 2% a year. This could result in brittle bones.

Here are a few tips that you should take during your younger years. They could help produce stronger bones in your later years.

(1) Get adequate calcium in your daily diet. This can be done by including foods like dairy products, dark-green leafy vegetables, salmon, and tofu.

(2) Get enough vitamin D and the trace mineral manganese.

(3) Exercise regularly. This helps to promote bone growth. It also strengthens the muscle which supports the bones.

(4) Avoid smoking, alcohol, caffeine, and high-protein foods.

(5) Aluminum

Avoid antacids that contain aluminum. Aluminum can reduce the amount of phosphorous in your bones and this could weaken them. You may also want to avoid cooking certain high acid foods in aluminum pots. This can could cause some of the aluminum to dissolve into your food.

(6) Caffeine

A number of studies have shown that caffeine can cause calcium loss. Caffeine leaches calcium from the bones and causes it to be excreted in urine. It can also prevent the digestive system from absorbing enough calcium. Thus, you should limit your intake of caffeine containing beverages. This includes, coffee, tea, and many of the popular soft drinks. You do not need to cut these items out entirely but instead limit yourself to 1 or 2 servings per day.

(7) Salt

Too much salt in your diet can have the same effect that caffeine does. It can cause the body to lose calcium in the urine.

(8) Vitamins

Recent studies have showed that Vitamin D is especially important in helping your body to prevent calcium lose.

The New England Journal of Medicine recommends calcium fortified orange juice as a great way to add calcium to your diet. The calcium citrate appears to be helpful in preventing calcium loss from the spine.

Foods That Reduce Risk Of Stroke And Lower Cholesterol

A report in Medical World News states that you can cut your risk of fatal strokes. This method is to increase your intake of potassium by eating more fruits and vegetables. Four studies have indicated that adequate potassium in the diet can lower your risk of fatal strokes.

Vitamin-B complex can reduce your risk of strokes. It works by correcting a defect that can lead to weakened blood vessels. Some vegetables, fruits, and grains have high amounts of vitamin B complex.

Other studies indicate that Vitamin C and Vitamin E can also reduce your risk of strokes. These vitamins can help prevent hardening of the arteries, and lower your cholesterol.

New Treatment For People Who Suffer From Lupus

Recent studies reveal that there are more than 500,000 Americans who suffer from systemic lupus erythematosus (SLE), more commonly known as lupus, a chronic disease which involves a malfunction in the body's immune system. While there is still no known cure, medical research has made significant progress in diagnosis and potential treatment. And even though the exact cause(s) of lupus are as yet unknown, the advances made by researchers have led to the development of more effective treatments which can help reduce the effects that lupus has on some sufferers.

Experts say that there seem to be many things which can "trigger" a flare-up of lupus symptoms, wherein the disease affects the body in a more intense manner. Stress appears to play a major role in triggering a flare-up of lupus symptoms, with stress-related fatigue and the adverse effects of sunburn to the body being frequent factors. However, since each individual is unique, the triggers of a lupus flare-up cannot be overly generalized.

The latest research reveals that sufferers of lupus can help avoid, or at least minimize the number and severity of lupus flare-ups by learning more about their individual triggers. Once you have discovered your own unique triggers, you can take steps to "head them off". You can protect yourself from excessive exposure to the sun, and try to avoid stressful situations. Try not to exert yourself, either physically or mentally, to the point that you become overtired. You do have a certain amount of control simply by being aware of what triggers your lupus flare-ups and doing everything you can to avoid them.

In some cases, drugs may trigger a lupus flare-up. If that occurs, altering the dosage, or stopping the medication altogether usually alleviates the flare. The key in this type of self-treatment is to recognize your triggers and in being alert to any warning signs that might indicate that a flare-up is imminent. Some common warning signs include a low-grade fever with no known cause, weakness and/or excessive fatigue, and, in some cases, frequent chills.

Currently, the most effective general treatment of lupus involves adjusting one's general lifestyle to accommodate specific changes in both behavior and activity to avoid possible flare ups; learning how to control emotions which could lead to added stress; medication to help suppress specific symptoms: and the maintenance of a healthful diet which provides essential nutritional needs. It is important to remember however, that each individual has his or her own unique symptoms and specific reactions to lupus. When your doctor sets up a treatment program for you, it is based on your individual needs.

In order to cope with lupus, the best advice may be to learn all you can about the disease by talking to medical professionals and doing as much research as you can. There are several books dedicated to the discussion of lupus, and one of the best source books on the subject is Coping With Lupus by Robert H. Phillips, Ph.D (Avery Publishing Group, New York, 1991). Another good source is Understanding Lupus by H. Aladjem (Charles Scribner's Sons, New York, 1985).

You can also get more information about lupus and the latest research and treatment by contacting the Lupus Foundation of America, 1717 Massachusetts Avenue, NW, Suite 203, Washington, DC 20036; (800) 558-0121: and the American Lupus Society, 23751 Madison Street, Torrance, CA 90505, (213) 373-1335.

3 Infectious Diseases
That Are Returning To The U.S.

Many authorities thought that some major infectious diseases had been eliminated. But recent statistics show an increasing number of cases of infectious diseases. This may be brought about by: 1. better transportation, 2. expanded population 3. germs becoming resistant to drugs. Here is a list of 3 infectious diseases that are making a comeback.

1. Lyme Disease— This is a disease that is carried by ticks. More than 9000 cases have been reported in the U.S.

2. Streptococcal Bacteria— Some kinds of strep bacteria have mutated into a more damaging and stronger form. Some are so bad that they can cause death within a few days. So you should always treat a strep infection very seriously.

3. Tuberculosis— TB has spread among those who have AIDS because their immune systems become weak. Also there are more drug

resistant TB strains around.

There are many infectious and non-infectious diseases that seriously affect millions of people in the U.S. However you can greatly lessen your chances of getting these diseases by taking certain precautions. In addition, if you maintain good overall health you can reduce your risk of contacting these diseases.

How To Poison-Proof Your Home

Being prepared for potential poisoning can mean the difference between life and death. Here are several ways you can reduce the risk of household poisoning:

1) Post your local poison control center number near your telephone. If you can not find the number in the front of your telephone directory, get the information from your doctor.

If someone in your home has swallowed poison call the poison control center immediately for first aid instructions. Be prepared to give the victim's age (and weight if the victim is a child), the name of the poison, how much poison was swallowed and how long ago, whether or not the victim has vomited, and how long it will take you to get to the nearest hospital emergency department. Have the poison container in front of you when you call the poison control center and take it with you to the hospital emergency room. The poison center will give you precise instructions and you should follow them exactly.

2) Lock up all poisonous substances. Be aware of all the hazardous items in your household and make sure they are out of the reach of children and identified clearly for adults. Make sure that all cupboards containing poisons are secure. Try to keep handbags and briefcases that may contain medicines out of the reach of your children.

3) Always have a supply of syrup of ipecac and activated charcoal powder on hand. These are the two most reliable and effective substances to have in case of a poisoning. Either induces vomiting and both are available without a prescription at a drugstore. However, you should not use either until you have checked with the poison control center.

How To Treat Skin Poisoning

There are some household chemicals that can be absorbed through the skin—they include solvents, strong cleaning agents, insecticides, and weed killers. If any of these come into contact with your skin, you should immediately hold the affected area under luke-warm, running water for approximately 10 minutes. (If a poison has spilled onto your clothing, remove the clothing before you use water on the affected area.) Wash the affected area with soap and water and rinse thoroughly. Once this is done, call your poison control center and follow their directions exactly.

Do not attempt to neutralize acids with alkalis, or alkalis with acids, or you risk dangerous chemical reactions and severe burns.

5 Tips
To Preventing Inhaled Poisoning

Whenever you use insect poisons, weed killers, solvents and strong cleaning agents, take these precautions:

1) Use liquids and sprays only in well-ventilated areas.

2) Some aerosol sprays contain fluorocarbons which, if inhaled, can be extremely dangerous. The symptoms of poisoning by this substance may include hallucinations, panic, lethargy, and coma. Avoid such sprays if at all possible.

3) Wear a mask over your mouth and nose whenever you are spraying paints or pesticides.

4) Cover your skin and wear goggles.

5) Get rid of unwanted pesticides safely. Call the National Pesticide Telecommunications Network—800-858-7378—for disposal suggestions and additional pesticide information.

The Popular Dishwashing Detergent That Could Harm Your Family

When choosing a dishwashing detergent, take care to read the label of contents before taking it home. Try to buy a brand that has the least amount of potentially harmful chemicals. Look for liquid products that contain little or no dye which is sometimes added to make the liquid yellow, pink, blue, or green. Also try to avoid those products that contain "perfume" to give the liquid the scent of strawberry, lemon or lime. The appealing color of the dye and the "flowery" or fresh fragrance can make these products especially appealing to an inquisitive child.

Swallowing these detergents usually results in immediate vomiting which reduces the chances of any serious,or lasting harm. The most common problems with products that contain dye and perfume may be allergies and irritations. The colors of the dyes are primary allergens and can, to a large extent, be avoided by choosing a product without added coloring. It's much harder to find a dishwashing detergent without some sort of perfume. The perfumes are also primary allergens, and most dishwashing detergents contain a certain amount of perfume.

While there may be no completely safe dishwashing detergent, those with little or no dye and the lowest amounts of perfume are probably the safest. It's also advisable to wear gloves to avoid irritating your skin, especially if your skin is very sensitive. You should also rinse all your dishes in warm water to make sure no dishwashing detergent remains.

The Popular Household Spray You Should Never Use In Your Home

Some common antistatic sprays you may use on your clothes so they won't cling to you often contain ammonium chloride, plus a fragrance, and potentially harmful propellants. Such sprays can irritate your skin and eyes. If you inhale the fine mist from the spray, it may also cause irritation to your respiratory tract. If overheated or punctured, the spray can may explode, and the propellant gases in the spray may be flammable.

You may be able to avoid such products by using a fabric softener in your wash. Not only is fabric softener safer, it may also be a good bit cheaper per application. If you continue to use a spray, read the label carefully, and take every precaution to ensure safe use.

Household insecticide sprays all contain specific insect poisons. It makes sense that something which is fatal to an insect also has the potential of having harmful effects on humans. The seriousness of the effect depends on the particular poison being used. Some insecticides contain arsenates which are compounds containing arsenic. If swallowed, these mixtures can be fatal. Aliphatic thiocynates (such as Lethane 384) are chemicals which release cyanide when swallowed or inhaled.

There are a whole host of other toxic chemicals in various insecticides which all pose a potential danger to humans if improperly handled. Some studies have even linked some of the chemicals used to cancer if excessive exposure is involved.

One alternative to the potentially dangerous insecticides is silica gel which is virtually nontoxic to humans. If you use insect sprays, be sure you wear a mask to cover your mouth and nose. Also cover your skin and protect your eyes by wearing goggles. Spray only in well-ventilated areas. Perhaps the safest way to get rid of insects is to hire a professional pest control.

Pesticide Safety
- Wash Your Clothes 3 Times!

If you use pesticides to dust your flower garden, you'll need to take extra care to ensure that potentially toxic substances don't linger on your clothing. You can do that by putting the clothes through three full laundry cycles. That's how long it takes—using warm to hot water and detergent—to reduce even a light, indirect spray of harmful chemicals to safe levels.

Infrequent overexposure to such chemicals can cause a rash, nausea and headache. Regular, repeated exposure has been linked to cancer.

9 Pest Control Tips That Keep "Them" Away

Many common household pests, such as houseflys, spiders, wasps, and mosquitoes, represent a potential health risk if not controlled. The key to keeping such household pests away is to deny them food, water and shelter.

Here are several proven methods of keeping common household pests at bay:

1) Keep food stored in tightly sealed glass or plastic containers.

2) Clean up all crumbs and spills immediately.

3) Keep sink areas clean and dry.

4) Clean garbage cans regularly, and secure their lids.

5) Fill all cracks and crevices, and repair all torn screens.

6) Cover chimney and flue openings with spark-arresting screening.

7) Electric bug zappers, while virtually ineffective against most stinging and biting insects, such as wasps and mosquitoes, do lure other flying insects away from the patio, pool and picnic areas at night.

8) Sprinkle a few broken up bay leaves on windowsills to combat invading ants. If the ants head straight for your flour and sugar bins, place a couple of bay leaves inside. Replace the leaves every month.

9) Don't use "all-purpose" pesticides. They often lack the one ingredient needed to kill a specific pest. For information and advice on how to select the safest and most effective pesticide, contact your local Cooperative Extension Service.

Dangerous Cleaning Solvents You Should Avoid

Any solvent labeled petroleum distillates or petroleum hydrocarbons is flammable. Nonflammable solvents include triethanolamine, perchloroethylene, trichloroethylene, and trichloroethane. Always read the labels carefully before choosing a cleaning solvent for use in your home. And be sure to store all such solvents out of the reach of children. Never transfer it to a container normally used for food, such as a soda bottle or cup.

Simple Way To Test If Your Water Is Safe To Drink, And What To Do If It Isn't

New mail-away home pollutant tests allow you to check your home for pollutants in your drinking water and for radon. To check for pollutants in tap water— lead, minerals, radon, bacteria, and pesticides— you can use a special water test kit and then send a water sample to a lab. Water testing kits are available from the National Testing Laboratories, 800-458-3330; or Suburban Water Testing Laboratories, 800-433-6569; or Water Test, 800-426-8378. If the tests say your water is not safe, these companies will tell you how to correct the problem.

How To Tell If Your Home Is Safe From Harmful Radon Gas

Radon, a colorless, odorless radioactive gas that accumulates inside homes, is suspected of causing between 5,000 and 20,000 lung cancer deaths a year in the United States. The gas is a product of the decay of uranium and it may penetrate through cracks in the walls and foundations of a home. It can also contaminate the household water supply, or it can be emitted through some building materials.

Here are four ways you can reduce the risk of radon exposure:

1) Make sure there is good ventilation throughout your house.

2) Test your home for radon. Levels below 4 picocuries/liter are considered safe.

3) Get in touch with a professional. You can get information and advice from your public health department. Most solutions to reducing radon levels, such as sealing cracks in the basement floor, are relatively inexpensive.

The test for radon requires a specially made charcoal canister which is available at industrial supply houses. The canister is attached to a wall in the basement for a day or a month, depending on the test. You can then call the American Industrial Hygiene Association at 216-873-2442 for names of labs in your area which can test for radon. You can also contact the Radon Information Hotline By Calling (800) 767-7236.

Home Test For Lead Poisoning

Even though restrictions on the levels of lead allowed in paint, cookware and other products are stricter than ever, thousands of Americans still suffer from lead poisoning. Lead poisoning has been linked to decreased coordination and mental abilities, as well as damage to the nervous system, kidneys and red blood cells.

Here are several things you can do to help "lead-proof" your home and reduce your exposure:

1) Don't remove any paint that you suspect may contain lead. Get an expert to test and remove the paint. (Current estimates indicate that nearly 75 percent of American homes built before 1980 have some lead-based paint.)

2) If you have any questions about lead testing or removal, contact your local health department or call the Toxic Substances Hotline, 1-202-554-1404.

3) Test your drinking water for lead. To get testing information, contact the Safe Drinking Water Hot Line at 800-426-4791.

A new, fast and effective home test can help you detect the presence of lead in your dishes and cookware. The home test uses swabs, which change color if lead is present. Although the swabs won't indicate how much lead is present, all dishes or cookware that test positive should not be used for either food or drinks. The Frandon Lead Alert Kit is available from Frandon Enterprises, 511 North 48th St., Seattle, WA 98103 (800-359-9000); Leadcheck Swabs for home use are available from HybriVet Systems, P.O. Box 1210, Framingham, MA 01701 (800-262-LEAD).

4 Ways To Reduce The Risk Of Carbon Monoxide Poisoning In Your Home

Homes with unvented kerosene or gas heaters, leaking chimneys and furnaces, and gas stoves are all at risk of carbon monoxide exposure. Low concentration of carbon monoxide can cause fatigue in healthy people and chest pain in those with heart disease. Higher exposures can cause impaired vision and coordination, dizziness, nausea, and death.

Here are several ways you can reduce the risk of carbon monoxide exposure in your home:

1) If possible, install a vented gas furnace and space heaters.

2) Have a trained professional inspect and clean your central heating system once a year.

3) If you have a gas stove, install an exhaust fan vented to the outdoors.

4) Don't use charcoal indoors because it produces deadly amounts of CO (carbon monoxide).

A new device recently approved by Underwriters Laboratories is designed to prevent death from carbon monoxide poisoning. The new device resembles a smoke detector and is supposed to sound an alarm if the carbon monoxide in the air nears a dangerous level.

Records indicate that most of the 230 cases of fatal carbon monoxide poisoning reported each year are due to faulty appliances or damaged chimneys and vents. Others result from automobile exhaust in houses that have attached garages.

The new carbon monoxide detectors can operate on batteries or they can be plugged into a household electric outlet. Their sensors, unlike those in smoke detectors, must be replaced every 3 to 5 years, and cost from $15 to $20. The detectors themselves sell for $50 to $70.

Currently, there are three carbon monoxide models which meet the standards developed by the Consumer Product Safety Commission and UL: the CMD-1 and CMD-2, marketed by BRK Electronics under the brand name of First Alert; the COS- 200 made by a small Canadian company, Asahi Electronics; and the COS-TAR Model 9B-1, which is made by Quantum Group in San Diego, California. The BRK and Asahi models are available in retail stores, and the Quantum is sold through stores and catalogs which feature camping and marine products.

Home Test For Sulfite

For the many Americans who are especially sensitive to sulfites—additives often used in food, wine and beer to prevent spoilage—a new home test can help reduce the risk of discomforting side effects. The CHEMetrics test indicates the presence and quantity of sulfites in foods and wine. This home test for certain foods and drinks before you consume them can prevent the allergic reactions, headaches, nausea, and asthma attacks that afflict most people who are sensitive to sulfite.

The CHEMetrics home test for sulfites is available from CHEMetrics at 800-356- 3072.

Free Guide To Eliminating Cancer - Causing Abestos

This heat-resistant and insulating material is a carcinogen which is found in fibers used for many years to insulate and fireproof furnace ducts, oven linings, floor and ceiling tiles, siding, and shingles. The cancer-causing potential results from inhalation of asbestos fibers.

Since the mid 1970s, asbestos has been replaced as much as possible by other materials, such as glass fiber. However, older homes can still present a potential danger from asbestos pollution.

A guide for identifying and handling asbestos has been published by the Environmental Protection Agency (EPA) and the National Consumer Product Safety Commission (CPSC). To get a copy of the booklet, titled "Asbestos in the Home", write to the Superintendent of Documents, U.S. Government Printing Office, Washington, D.C. 20402; or call 800-835-6700 for more information.

9 Ways To Avoid Getting Food Poisoning

Food poisoning from eating contaminated food can cause nausea, vomiting and diarrhea. The condition will usually run its course within 24 hours without need for medical treatment. During that time, it is important that you avoid dehydration by drinking lots of fluids, beginning with water and/or weak tea for the first 12 hours, and then gradually add juices, broth and bland solid foods over the next day or so.

You should seek medical treatment if food poisoning occurs in a child younger than 3, if the food poisoning lasts longer than 2 days, if watery diarrhea occurs every 10 or 15 minutes, if it contains blood or mucus, or if stomach pain or fever does not subside.

The most common sources of food poisoning include seafood; poultry; meat that is undercooked, inadequately defrosted, or reheated; and raw or undercooked eggs. However, most food poisoning can be avoided by exercising the following precautions:

1) Wash your hands before handling food and after handling raw meat and eggs.

2) Wash fresh fruit and vegetables in cold, running water.

3) Thaw meat and poultry completely before cooking.

4) Cook meat until the pink completely disappears, poultry until there are no red joints, and fish until it becomes flaky.

5) Keep fresh fish in the freezer, and wash it thoroughly before cooking.

6) Reheat meat quickly and thoroughly.

7) Eat meat as soon as it has been cooked.

8) Store egg dishes in the refrigerator.

9) Throw away food that has become moldy or smelly— also discard damaged cans.

Secret To Prevent Mold In Food

Nothing ruins the appetite quite like pulling mold-covered food, such as cottage cheese and yogurt, out of the refrigerator at mealtime. And mold can be rather pervasive. Tiny mold spores get onto the surfaces of food when you open and close containers. With oxygen and enough time to grow, the little spores can then grow into visible mold. The way to keep mold from growing is to turn the food containers upside down—the mold will then suffocate. Just be sure you get the lids on tight enough to prevent leakage. Even though most molds are harmless, no one enjoys the sight of moldy food.

New Plastic Bread-Bag Danger Revealed

Researchers at the Environmental and Occupational Health Sciences Institute in Piscataway, New Jersey have reported a potential health hazard with plastic bread bags. In a study which involved 18 breads, including white bread, whole wheat, pita bread, and bagels, researchers discovered that paint from the outside of the bread bags can leach lead into food. Based on those findings, researchers recommend that if you reuse such plastic bread bags to hold food, make sure they are right or painted side out.

The federal Food and Drug Administration has previously conducted research which shows that lead-based paint presents no danger whatsoever on the outside of the packages. That's because the paint doesn't come into contact with food.

Eight Common "Poisonous Plants" That May Be In Your Home Right Now

More than 700 U.S. plants can cause poisoning. Some plants, such as wisteria, may cause mild to severe digestive upset. Others like castor beans (the seeds) can be deadly. For proper poison prevention, you should be aware of all the potentially poisonous house plants in your home. Here are the most common house plants with poisonous parts:

1) Hyacinth 2) Narcissus 3) Daffodil (bulbs) 4) Dieffenbachia

5) Elephant ear (all parts) 6) Rosary pea 7) Castor bean (seeds) 8) Philodendron (stems, leaves)

Five Tips For Having A Safe Medicine Cabinet

Whenever you take medicine, do you check the container's expiration date? If you don't, you could be putting your health at risk. While aspirin will usually keep for a year or more, other drugs can become dangerous as they age or deteriorate. For example, when liquid evaporates from codeine cough syrup, it becomes more potent and can cause dizziness. In some people, an aged tetracycline can cause kidney damage. You can avoid such potential problems by exercising the following precautions:

1) Buy only the amount of medication that you expect to use soon, and always cap the bottle securely after using.

2) Keep all drugs in a cool, dry place. Heat and humidity can hasten deterioration.

3) Always check the expiration dates and inspect medication before using.

4) Throw away any drugs that have changed color; prescription drugs you are no longer taking; any tablets or capsules that are discolored, disintegrating, softened, stuck together, or that smell different from the original; any tablets or capsules that are past their expiration dates; and any tubes or creams that have changed their odors or have become hard or discolored.

5) Consult with your doctor or a pharmacist before you use any drugs prescribed for a previous illness— even if they have not passed their expiration dates.

The Line Between Watching TV And High Cholesterol

New research suggests that you should turn off the "Wheel of Fortune" and do something more constructive in order to protect your health. Scientists at Brigham Young University in Provo, Utah say that adults who spend three or more hours a day watching TV are twice as prone to have high cholesterol as those people who watch an hour or less. The evidence also indicates that even those people who watch a moderate one to two hours of TV each day tend to have high cholesterol levels— a risk factor for heart disease.

Watching TV several hours each day indicates a sedentary lifestyle and usually leads to the consumption of an excessive amount of high-fat cholesterol- increasing snack foods. The lack of physical activity and eating lots of high- fat foods are part of the prescription for poor health.

Electric Razors May Increase Risk Of Leukemia

According to a recent scientific study, shaving with an electric razor may double a man's chance of contracting leukemia. The study, conducted at Battelle Memorial Institute's Pacific Northwest Laboratory in Richland, Washington found that men who used electric razors for 2 1/2 minutes a day were more than twice as likely to contract leukemia than men who did not use electric razors at all. The researchers were quick to point out that while the study suggested a possible link between electric shavers and leukemia, it does not prove that such razors cause cancer.

Much of the speculation centers around electromagnetic fields. Such a field is created when electricity passes through a wire. The field becomes more powerful with an increase in current. Some scientists think that electromagnetic fields can trigger cellular changes that lead to cancer. However, there is currently no scientific proof that an electric field can cause cancer.

Researchers at Battelle based their study on the supposition that the closer to his face a man used an electric motor to his face, the greater the risk of cancer.

Small appliances such as television sets, hair dryers and electric blankets are currently being studied because the magnetic fields they generate are relatively potent within several inches. Most such small appliances are used in close proximity with humans. The researchers involved in the Battelle study said that electric razors put out a stronger magnetic field than appliances such as hair dryers and personal massagers.

Another study—this one at the Oak Ridge Associated Universities—indicates that there is "no convincing evidence" to support any link between cancer and the use of small appliances. According to the findings from this study, exposure to the extremely low frequency electric and magnetic fields emitted by sources including household appliances, video display terminals (VDTs) and local power lines, has not been proven to constitute an increased health hazard.

A third study—conducted in Sweden—indicates that children who are exposed to relatively weak electromagnetic fields from local power lines may develop leukemia at almost four times the "normal" rate.

The Swedish study took place at Karolinska Institute in Stockholm and looked at 500,000 children and adults in Sweden who lived near power lines. Researchers discovered that children who were exposed to electromagnetic fields from neighborhood power transmission lines were developed leukemia at the rate of 3.8- in -20,000 instead of the typical rate of 1- in- 20,000.

6 Health Hazards Of Working Working With A Computer, And How To Protect Yourself

1) Eyestrain

More and more people are spending more and more time working on personal computers in their homes, and that could mean an increased risk of eyestrain or fatigue. In fact, if you spend several hours a day staring at a video display terminal (VDT), the risk of eyestrain is relatively high, unless you take some basic precautions.

One way to avoid "VDT eyestrain" is to take regular breaks and get away from the monitor screen. This is especially important if you spend a full work day (6 to 8 hours) working on a computer. Experts recommend that you take a 10 to 15 minute break every 2 to 3 hours and refocus your eyes (some doctors recommend that you take periodic breaks every 20 to 30 minutes and focus on distant objects). You may also consider working from a printout of your screen, rather than the screen itself, whenever possible.

Another way to avoid eyestrain is to work from a darker screen.

Many times computer users operate their VDTs at such a bright level, eyestrain is a frequent result. Try turning the brightness down to a relatively dim level and then adjust the contrast knob in order to make up the difference. If background lighting is not adequate, an adjustable desk lamp may be of help.

You can also cut down on the amount of monitor-screen glare, which can lead to eyestrain, by making a hood to put over your VDT. You can make such a hood, using heavy black cardboard placed on top of your monitor. Both sides of the cardboard should be folded down over the VDT. Filters are also available to help reduce the glare on the screen.

2) Headache

Besides eyestrain, long hours in front of a VDT can also lead to headaches. Rest breaks are important as a means of prevention, and some experts recommend that you wear some type of tinted glasses to reduce the risk of headache from staring at a bright VDT screen.

3) Neck Pain

Many people who work with a VDT all day end up with neck spasms and muscle fatigue. That's usually because the terminal is positioned in such a way that these people have to look up or down all day. Experts recommend that you position your VDT at eye level to avoid the discomfort of neck pain. The height of your desk should also enable you to sit at your keyboard so that your lower arms form a 70 to 90 degree angle to your upper body. The monitor itself should be within a 30 degree viewing angle of your direct line of vision.

4) Backache

Poor posture while working long hours at a computer can contribute to backache. To avoid this problem, you should adjust your chair to suit your height at the desk and to provide adequate support for your lower back. The height of your chair should allow you to sit in a relaxed position with your feet firmly on the floor and your back straight.

5) Repetitive Motion Injury

Sometimes aches can develop in your hands and/or arms after

an extended period of time working on a computer. This discomfort is caused by repetitive motion and can be alleviated only by resting the affected part of the body. If you experience persistent pain you should consult your doctor.

For some people, repetitive motion injury from working long hours at a computer can become serious. An estimated 50 percent of people who suffer from a condition known as carpal tunnel syndrome (CTS) do so because of repetitive hand and wrist movements, such as those necessitated by working at a computer keyboard.

CTS is a compression of the median nerve, which runs along the forearm and down the palm. Its symptoms include loss of sensation and weakness. It has become an occupational hazard affecting thousands of people each year.

The problem can be alleviated by surgery which formerly involved making a large incision down the palm as a means of releasing pressure on the median nerve. The healing time for such surgery can take up to two months with some people continuing to experience pain at the incision location. A new procedure, called endoscopic carpal tunnel release surgery, allows doctors to make 2 small incisions and then insert a tiny probe under the skin. The new procedure relieves the pressure on the median nerve without necessitating a large cut down the patient's palm. Most patients have reported healing time from the new surgery to be within one month. There also appears to be less pain and scarring associated with the new procedure.

6) Radiation Exposure

While no conclusive evidence has yet been found, many experts say there are potential health dangers, including an increased risk of cancer, from exposure to non-ionizing radiation emitted by some VDTs (as well as microwave communication equipment, microwave ovens, television and radio transmitters, electric wiring, electric blankets, and other devices). These experts recommend that people who spend several hours a day in front of a VDT take the following precautions:

A) Test your computer (and other household devices) for non-ionizing radiation emmissions. You can get an effective home test kit from Radiation Safety Corporation, 140 University Avenue, Palo Alto, CA 94301.

B) Have annual eye exams.

C) Pregnant women should work no more than 20 hours a week in front of a VDT.

D) Take 15 minute breaks and reduce VDT screen glare as recommended earlier in this section.

Product Safety Hotline

If you have any questions about the safety of any household product, you can call the Product Safety Hotline— Consumer Product Safety Commission at 800- 638-2772.

43 Ways You Can Save The Environment And Be Healthier At The Same Time

1) Discontinue using products which contain large amounts of phosphates. Phosphates are chemical compounds containing phosphorous, and are found in most detergents. Use a low-phosphate or a phosphate-free detergent.

2) Put a stop to unwanted junk mail. Some statistics suggest that if only 100,000 American families stopped their "junk mail", the nation could save up to 150,000 trees every year. You can have your name taken off mailing lists, and you can recycle the junk mail you already have.

3) Save water by aerating your household faucets. An aerator is a simple device that can be attached to the water faucets in your home and result in a significant saving of water.

4) Use reusable containers to keep food in your refrigerator instead of using aluminum foil or plastic wrap.

5) Avoid using oil-based paint. Such paint is toxic, and the by-products of its manufacture are environmental pollutants. Use latex paint instead of oil- based.

6) Don't leave the water running while you are brushing your

teeth, shaving, or washing the dishes. You can save thousands of gallons of water a year by learning to avoid waste.

7) Since the ozone layer is being depleted by manmade gasses that are common in homes and offices, it is critical that we stop using such products which contain those gasses. Avoid aerosols containing CFCs (chlorofluorocarbons) or halons (found in some fire extinguishers).

8) Keep your car properly tuned up to conserve fuel and help reduce toxic emission.

9) Use rechargeable batteries instead of alkaline batteries to lessen the hazardous waste problem.

10) Don't use polystyrene foam. If you eat at fast food food restaurants, ask for paper cups and plates.

11) You can help conserve energy by making sure your home is adequately insulated.

12) If enough people would plant trees we could reduce CO_2 emissions and energy consumption. So...plant a tree.

13) Whenever possible, use natural pest controls instead of herbicides and pesticides.

14) Try organic gardening and/or buy organically grown produce and grains.

15) Dispose of all household hazardous wastes properly. Do not dump toxics down the drain or into the sewer system. You can dispose of such materials in a number of "safe" ways, including recycling and municipal incineration. You can also call the EPA hotline— (800) 424-9346, to find out who to contact in your state about getting household hazardous waste picked up.

16) You can conserve energy by making sure your home is adequately insulated.

17) Join a car pool.

18) Start your own compost pile. To begin with, you can pile all your leaves, grass clippings, and weeds in a small cornor of your garden.

19) Recycle your motor oil.

20) Recycle all your old newspapers.

21) Use cloth, instead of disposable diapers.

22) Conserve energy in your home by having your furnace "tuned-up" regularly. Gas furnaces should be tuned up every other year and oil furnaces should be tuned up once a year.

23) Recycle glass, such as bottles and jars. Glass which is produced from recycling instead of raw material reduces related air pollution by as much as 20 percent and related water pollution by 50 percent.

24) Contribute and support organizations that are involved in rain forest conservation. Contact the Rain Forest Action Network, 301 Broadway, Suite A, San Francisco, CA 94133. (415) 398-4404.

25) Drive your car as little as possible. If your destination is within walking (or bicycle riding) distance, leave your car at home.

26) Don't throw six-pack holders into the garbage without clipping each circle with a knife or a pair of scissors. Six-pack holders have become an ocean hazard to birds and other marine life. Whenever you go to the beach, pick up all the six-pack ring holders you can find and dispose of them properly.

27) Use rags in the kitchen to wipe up spills instead of using paper towels all of the time.

28) Make sure your water heater is adjusted down to 130 dgrees, which is hot enough to kill bacteria and still save energy. Many modern water heaters have an "energy conservation" setting. If yours does, keep it on that setting.

29) Keeping your automobile tires properly inflated can cut down on your car's gas consumption. Experts say that we could save up to 2 billion gallons of gasoline a year by keeping our tires properly inflated.

30) Instead of using paper or plastic bags, take a cloth bag with you when you shop.

31) Whenever possible, use natural alternatives to toxic products. This is a good way to reduce the risk to your family and the environment.

32) Don't adjust your air conditioner to a colder setting before you turn it on. If you do, you'll be wasting energy and the room won't cool down any quicker.

33) Take care not to litter. Keep a trash bag in your car and get into the habit of using it.

34) Contribute to and support groups and/or organizations dedicated to wildlife conservation. Two such groups are the Earth Island Institute Dolphin Project, 300 Broadway #28, San Francisco, CA 94133, (415) 788-33666; and the World Wildlife Fund, 1250 24th St. NW, Washington, D.C., 20037.

35) You can avoid wasting water every time you flush your toilet by installing a "displacement device" in your toilet tank. This will cut down on the amount of water used by over 15 percent.

36) Get a "low-flow" shower head and reduce the water used when showering by up to 50 percent.

37) You can help conserve energy by turning off all lights when they are not in use.

38) Use compact fluorescent light bulbs. These energy saving light bulbs come on instantly and do not flicker or produce a hum.

39) Get involved in recycling outside your own home by organizing community- wide recycling projects.

40) Buy as many of your foods, such as potatoes, carrots, celery, onions, apples, and so on, loose rather than in plastic containers.

41) Make it a point to recycle paper items at work as well as at home. Studies show that office workers throw away almost 180 pounds of high-grade recyclable paper every year.

42) You can help conserve energy in your home by checking for energy leaks and "plugging" all those you find. Windows should be checked very carefully.

43) Instill in your children the proper respect and reverence for the earth and all its valuable resources.

New Warning About Breast Enlargements

The American Society of Plastic and Reconstructive Surgeons (ASPRS) has issued a warning to American women not to undergo fat injections for breast enlargement. According to the ASPRS, such injections of fat can impede detection of early breast cancer or can produce test results that completely miss cancerous cells.

The fat injection process involves removing fat cells from the abdomen, buttocks or thighs and injecting it elsewhere in the body. The procedure is still experimental and has not been well tested. The ASPRS says that the results of fat injection usually fade after about six months. The number of women seeking fat injections has been on the increase ever since silicone breast implants were removed from the market.

Implants And Mammography And Cancer

Specialists say that implants can make mammography difficult and delay the detection of cancer. This poses a particular risk for those women with a family history of breast cancer. Experts advise women who have had implants to tell the mammogram technician that there is an implant.

How To Increase Your Breast Size
Without Expensive, Dangerous Implants Or Surgery

A natural, safe way to increase your breast size without resorting to implants or surgery is not an impossibility. Many women have discovered that specific exercises, when performed correctly and regularly, can result in a higher, firmer chest and, in effect, a larger breast size. Here are some exercises designed to develop higher, firmer breasts:

1) Assume a sitting position, with your legs crossed and your back straight. Place your hands on the back of your head, with your fingertips touching. Extend your elbows as wide as possible, and to the side.

Bring your elbows together in front of your face (don't raise your shoulders). Swing your elbows back to the starting position.

Inhale as your elbows come together and exhale as you swing them out to each side.

For best results, do 10 repetitions of this exercise.

2) Another good exercise designed to create a higher, firmer chest requires that you sit on a couch and bring your arms in back of you, resting them on top of the couch. Hold this position for 30 to 60 seconds. Focus on the stretch in your chest muscles. This exercise can be done while you're watching TV, during the commercials.

4 Little-Known Ways To Ease Problems Of PMS

1) Research conducted at the U.S. Department of Agriculture's Human Nutrition Research Center in Grand Forks, North Dakota, indicates that calcium added to the diet may help cut down on water retention, menstrual cramps and moodiness.

Researchers kept track of menstrual and premenstrual symptoms in 10 healthy women who had a daily intake of 600 milligrams of calcium during the first half of the study period and 1,300 milligrams during the second half. While on the high calcium regimen, 90 percent of the women reported fewer mood swings throughout their monthly cycles than when they were on a lower intake of calcium. Eighty percent had less water retention, and 7 of the 10 women experienced less pain.

While the researchers can't say for certain that calcium works— more research is needed—they do recommend that every woman should increase her calcium intake up to the Recommended Dietary Allowance of 800 to 1,200 milligrams. The average U.S. woman's intake of calcium is 600 milligrams.

There may also be other nutritional solutions to help relieve PMS symptoms. Some doctors recommend the following:

2) Vitamin C— this vitamin is an antitoxidant which is believed to help reduce stress and may help relieve stress felt during PMS. Vitamin C may also help alleviate allergies that worsen before a period because it is a natural antihistamine.

3) Vitamin E— also an antitoxidant, vitamin E may help relieve painful breasts, anxiety and depression.

4) Vitamins A and D— working together, these two vitamins help to keep your skin healthy. Because of that, they may help to suppress premenstrual acne and oily skin.

Relief For Tender Breasts

Avoiding caffeine may be the best remedy for the almost 70 percent of women who suffer fibrocystic breast change— tender, swollen, and often lumpy breasts, most commonly occurring before menstruation.

While there are no definitive studies to support the advice to avoid caffeine, some medical experts say that as many as 50 to 60 percent of women who stop their intake of caffeine—including coffee, tea, cola, and chocolate—report a significant reduction in fibrocystic breast-change symptoms.

New Study Shows Women Can Build Bone Mass Up To Age Thirty

New findings by researchers show that women keep building bone long after they stop gaining height. In fact, the researchers say that women in their late teens and 20's can add bone mass and most likely reduce their chances of developing osteoporosis later in life by exercising and getting enough calcium. Furthermore, taking birth control pills may also help.

This is the first time that researchers have been able to establish that women add bone mass until near age 30 and that even modest lifestyle changes can increase their gains.

Researchers measured periodically the bone mineral content and density of 156 women. Activity levels were also monitored by instruments which were strapped to the women's waists. The women kept written records of everything they ate. The researchers also updated the subjects' height, weight, family history, and contraceptive use, every six months.

The results of the study show that the women who participated experienced a 12 percent gain in bone mass in their 20's. Regular calcium consumption had the most significant effect on bone growth. Women who consumed 900 milligrams more per day than the RDA of 1,200 milligrams gained an average of 16.4 percent in bone density. Women whose total calcium intake averaged only 700 milligrams per day gained just 3.4 percent in bone density.

Researchers say that exercise was almost as important as calcium intake. Those women in the study who engaged in moderate exercise—walking, jogging or playing tennis—tended to add more bone mass than those who were basically inactive. Oral contraceptives, which contain estrogen, also appeared to help some of these women build bone mass, according to the study.

Douching And Cervical Cancer
- What You Must Know

According to a study conducted at the Uniformed Services University of the Health Sciences in Bethesda, MD, frequent douching may increase a woman's risk of cervical cancer. Until now, scientists had not been able to separate the effect of douching from that of sex—especially from a young age and with multiple partners—which has long been linked to an increased risk of cervical cancer.

To isolate the effects of douching, researchers focused on Mormon women whose religion strictly forbids extramarital sex. The researchers compared the douching habits of over 250 cervical cancer patients and 480 healthy women. The results showed that women who douched more than once a week were almost five times as likely to develop cervical cancer as were women who douched less often. The type of douche made no difference.

The researchers speculate that vaginal secretions and normal vaginal bacteria may protect the pelvic area and that frequently disrupting those secretions by douching may lead to the appearance of microbes which can trigger cancer.

Earlier research had shown that a douche carrys with it the risk of introducing infection into the vagina as well as spread an existing infection into the uterus or Fallopian tubes. Moreover, according to experts, douche is completely ineffective as a contraceptive.

Gynecologists rarely, if ever, recommend douches for any reason anymore, however, for women who feel they need to douche—even though the vagina is normally slightly acidic and cleans itself—a mild solution of vinegar or baking soda may be best.

8 Medicines That Reduce Effectiveness Of The Pill

According to medical experts, the Pill, if used properly, has a success rate of about 99 percent. However, more than 8 percent of women in their first year on the Pill become pregnant. Doctors say that many failures are simply due to missed doses, but that drug interactions can also lower the Pill's success rate. These experts recommend that if you are taking the Pill—especially if it is a low dose formulation— you consult your gynecologist before taking certain drugs including the following:

1) Adrenocorticoids— this is a cortisone-like medicine which is commonly used to treat an assortment of ailments.

2) Antibiotic and antibacterial drugs— these include ampicillin, bacampicillin, chloramphenicol, neomycin, penicillin, tetracycline, rifampin, and sulfa drugs.

3) Anticonvulsants— including carmazepine, phenobarbital, phenytoin, primidone, and valproic acid.

4) Antihistamines and Decongestants— this includes those found in many over- the-counter cold remedies.

5) Cholesterol-lowering drugs.

6) Headache remedies— including prescription drugs.

7) Mineral oil

8) Sedatives and tranquilizers— including barbiturates, chlordiazepoxide (Librium) and diazepam (Valium).

Exciting New Condom For Women

The U.S. Food and Drug Administration has conditionally approved a female condom. The new method of contraception also provides women with protection against sexually transmitted diseases (STDs), such as AIDS.

The new female condom, or vaginal pouch, with the trade name Reality, is manufactured by Wisconsin Pharmacal, of Jackson, Wisconsin, and may be on the market in the near future. It will, for the first time, allow a woman to choose a contraception method she can insert herself. And, similar to the male condom, the female condom will not allow the transfer of fluids during intercourse.

The new female condom is prelubricated and about the same length as a male condom, but wider. It has two rings— an inner ring which is inserted into the vagina in much the same way as a diaphragm fits over the cervix and behind the pubic bone, and an outer ring which stays outside the vagina. The outer ring covers the labia and prevents sperm from entering the uterus.

Studies conducted by the American College of Obstetricians and Gynecologists suggest several advantages to the female condom including the fact that it is thinner than male condoms, permitting more sensitivity; it is more difficult for viruses or bacteria to penetrate because it is stronger than male latex condoms; it can be removed immediately following intercourse; and it does not require either sizing or a prescription.

In the early fall of 1991 an FDA advisory panel gave their conditional approval to Reality and Wisconsin Pharmacal is conducting more studies for the panel. The panel will also make recommendations about the entry of the female condom into the public market. However, the FDA advisory panel can do nothing more than make recommendations— executives of the FDA will be making the final decision on whether or not the new female condom, Reality, is approved for use by the general public.

Women: Barrier Methods Of Contraception Can Lower Your Sexual Disease Risk

A University of North Carolina study indicates that barrier methods of contraception, controlled by women, may work better than the male condom to prevent some sexually transmitted diseases. The findings revealed that those women who used diaphragms and contraceptive sponges were less likely to get gonorrhea trichomoniasis (a vaginal infection) and chlamydia, which is the most common sexually transmitted disease, than women who used no contraception, who were sterilized, or whose partners used condoms.

Incredible New "Hormone Shot Contraceptive" Protects Against Pregnancy For 3 Months

A hormone shot that protects against pregnancy for up to three months has been recently approved by the Federal Drug Administration for use as a contraceptive. The hormonal drug Depo-Provera has already been available in the United States for two decades as a treatment for kidney and endometrial cancer.

Medical experts say that Depo-Provera has been used by women for contraception for many years, particularly women who for one reason or another could not use the Pill. Until now, the drug has not been an approved substance for contraception, but with the FDA approval, it can now be marketed actively as a contraceptive.

Depo-Provera, like other oral contraceptives, has certain side effects. Studies indicate that 55 percent of Depo-Provera users have no menstrual periods for three months or longer the first year they use the drug. There's also the likelihood of a slight weight gain, moodiness, depression, and headaches.

The drug is a synthetic version of the natural hormone progesterone. It works by delivering progestin to the bloodstream to stop ovulation. The shots are given four times a year and are effective 96 to 99 percent of the time, according to medical experts. The shots cost about $25
each.

Little-Known Things Women Must Know About Iron

While as many as 65 percent of young American women have an
iron deficiency, 20 percent of them are actually clinically anemic. An iron
deficiency can be caused by a diet which is low in iron, pregnancy and
lactation, and excessive use of antiinflammatory drugs such as aspirin
and ibuprofen. To get more iron, women are advised to eat iron-rich foods
together with food containing lots of vitamin C, and to use iron-rich grain
products. Cooking in cast-iron pots also helps, as some iron leaches into
the food.

Foods That Can Help Improve Your Memory

Up to 15 percent of all U.S. women of childbearing age are deficient in iron— needed for healthy blood—and zinc which is necessary for
immunity. According to medical experts, correcting those deficiencies can
also lead to memory improvement.

A two month study at the University of Texas Medical Branch in
Galveston, tested the effect of supplements on the memories of 34 iron-
and zinc- deficient women whose ages ranged from 18 to 40. Eleven
other women who had normal levels of both iron and zinc served as a
control group. Each subject had a normal memory range and took a vitamin supplement. Some of the subjects who were deficient in iron and zinc
took 30 extra milligrams of iron and/or zinc. At the end of eight weeks, the
iron and zinc deficient women who had taken one of the supplements had
improved their memory test scores by as much as 20 percent. Women
who had taken both iron and zinc showed only a slight improvement in
memory, while those who took just a common multivitamin experienced
no improvement at all. The researchers explain the disparity by pointing
out that iron and zinc can interfere with each other's absorption when they
are taken as supplements. There is no such interference when the two
are part of a balanced diet.

The best source of both nutrients is red meat, and not eating enough red meat is a typical cause of iron and zinc deficiencies. Iron and zinc can also be found in chicken, fish and beans, but in lesser amounts than in red meat.

New "Heart Attack Signal" Test Available

Research at the Albert Einstein College of Medicine and New York Hospital- Cornell Medical Center has uncovered a potentially more reliable indicator of heart attack than the usual signals such as high cholesterol, elevated blood pressure and smoking habits. Scientists monitored 1717 hypertensive women and men over an eight year period and found that those with high blood levels of the kidney hormone, renin, were 5 times more likely to suffer heart attacks than people whose renin level was too low. Researchers say that renin triggers the release of a second hormone, angiotensin, which constricts blood vessels, cutting off oxygen and precipitating a heart attack. The good news is that doctors can reduce renin levels with certain medications.

Skinless Chicken May Reduce Risk Of Colon Cancer

A continuing study which has already revealed that red-meat consumption may increase the risk of colon cancer, has also suggested that women who eat skinless chicken regularly may reduce their risk of colon cancer. The study, conducted at the Harvard Medical School, analyzed nearly 89,000 women and found that those who ate skinless chicken at least twice a week were 50 percent less likely to develop colon cancer than were those women who ate it once a month or less. The researchers speculate that the reason chicken may reduce the risk of colon cancer is that it contains less saturated fat than red meat, and saturated fat may be instrumental in the formation of cancer-causing compounds in the colon. Researchers say there may also be an as yet undetected substance in chicken which protects against colon cancer.

Further studies are needed, but in light of the most recent evidence, some experts are recommending that women eat lots of fruit, vegetables and fish (which also appears to have some effect on reducing the risk of colon cancer), and using skinless chicken as a frequent substitute for red meat.

New Test May Aid In Diagnosing Bladder Cancer

There's more good news in the continuing battle against cancer. Researchers at the Baylor College of Medicine, Center for Biotechnology, in The Woodlands, Texas, have developed a test that may change existing treatment and possibly extend the survival rate for many of the over 50,000 women and men who are diagnosed with bladder cancer each year.

The researchers discovered that after analyzing tumorous cells, they could determine the status of a "tumor-suppressed" gene. If the gene, called retinoblastoma (RB), is not functioning properly the cancer will grow much faster and will require more aggressive treatment. And in a related study at the Memorial Sloan-Kettering Cancer Center in New York City, researchers found that bladder-cancer patients with malfunctioning RB genes tended to survive for only one year. Those patients with normal RB genes lived an average of eight years.

Experts say that improperly functioning RB genes may also contribute to cancers of the prostate, breast, eye, lung, and blood. The new test, which should be available in the near future, may allow doctors to detect malfunctioning RB genes and replace them with normal genes, thus saving the lives of many cancer patients.

Anti-depressant Drug
May Be Effective Treatment For Bulimia

A common treatment for the eating disorder bulimia involves both psychotherapy and antidepressants. The medications can, however, have harmful side effects, including weight gain and a significant loss of energy. The results of a recent study, conducted at 13 medical centers, suggests that the drug Prozac, which is often used to treat depression, may be the best choice for some women battling such an eating disorder.

The study, which continued for two months, revealed that of the 387 women who were involved, the women who took 60 milligrams of Prozac per day binged and purged 50 percent less than those women who were given a placebo. Prozac also seemed to reduce depression and the cravings for carbohydrates, resulting in a small weight loss. For most of the subjects, the side effects from the medication, such as nausea and insomnia, were relatively mild.

According to the researchers, antidepressants such as Prozac may help control bulimia and depression in some people because both disorders may be due to a deficiency of serotonin— a chemical in the brain.

While some bulimics are helped with antidepressants, experts say there is currently no specific drug treatment prescribed for general usage. However, researchers at the National Institute of Mental Health (NIMH) linked bulimia to excessive levels of a brain hormone called vasopressin. The new information may lead eventually to a specific effective medication for the disease.

Scientists say that vasopressin regulates the body's balances of fluids and salt. It also affects some physical and mental functions including thirst, blood pressure, learning and memory. When under stress, some people produce an excessive amount of the hormone making themselves more vulnerable to illnesses such as bulimia.

According to researchers, continued study of vasopressin may also be of benefit to anorexics who literally starve themselves, and obsessive-compulsive patients who cannot control repetitive thoughts and activities.

Little-Known Things Only Men Should Do For Their Health

Routine maintenance for the human body can help prevent many of life's unpleasantries, and just as women have health concerns that should be addressed in regular doctor visits, so do men. For men, those concerns include blood pressure, cholesterol levels, the health of their hearts, their activity levels, and as they reach middle-age and late-life years, specific tests to detect prostate cancer, colon/rectal cancer and heart disease.

In addition to an electrocardiogram or heart stress test, blood pressure monitoring, cholesterol blood test, immunization, and counseling and discussion, which all follow the same guidelines as women's checkups described earlier in this chapter, men should also perform a monthly testicle self-examination for soreness, lumps and swelling. Starting at age 40, men should also have a digital rectal exam—a physical exam of the rectum and prostate to detect signs of cancer or prostate disease—every year.

Doctors recommend that men between the ages of 20 and 40 should perform a self-examination of their testicles about once a month to look for lumps or swellings that may indicate cancer. Self-examination (in addition to your doctor's periodic examinations) is important because testicular cancer, which is the most common cancer in young men, is one of the most easily curable of all cancers if detected early. The best time to perform the examination is during or after a bath or shower when the scrotal skin is relaxed. Here's what to look for:

1) A lump in either testicle.

2) Pain, swelling or tenderness of either testicle.

3) Ulceration of the scrotal skin.

Here are the steps involved in the self-examination procedure:

1) Standing in front of a mirror, look for obvious lumps or swelling of the scrotal sac.

2) Examine each testicle thoroughly and gently with the fingers of both hands by rolling the testicle between the thumbs and the fingers. Feel for any lump or abnormality in texture or contour. A normal testicle is oval and firm, but not hard, and has a regular surface.

3) Locate and identify the epididymis at the top and back of the testicles (the ropelike structure which collects the sperm). The structure may feel firm but should not be confused for an abnormal lump. Consult your doctor if it is tender or swollen.

Other danger signals to report immediately include a heavy feeling in the testicles, a dragging sensation in the groin, or a sudden accumulation of blood or fluid in the scrotal sac.

New Breakthrough Can Reverse A Vasectomy And Restore A Man's Verility

Doctors at the University of Iowa College of Medicine have achieved a high rate of success in reversing vasectomies—a procedure that until now wasn't often successful. The doctors have achieved an 85 percent success rate in rejoining the duct that carries sperm from each testicle to the urethra (vas deferens). The new method for reversal uses a laser to seal the rejoined ends of the duct. It also reduces the length and risk of the operation, and over half of the patients undergoing the new reversal surgery have gone on to father children.

New Technique For Easier Vasectomies

A new, no-scalpel operation developed in China may prove to be faster and less painful than a standard vasectomy. Experts say the new technique is just as effective as the old procedure and is much faster, taking only 5 to 10 minutes compared with a conventional vasectomy which takes 15 to 20 minutes. The new technique also usually does not require the use of stitches because it employs a tiny puncture instead of an incision.

Reports from doctors who have used the new technique indicate that their patients experience less bleeding and pain, both during and after the operation, compared with men who undergo standard vasectomies.

New MethodsTo Fight Male Infertility

Two new methods of identifying and combating male infertility provide encouraging news to men who have been unable to father children.

At the University of Oklahoma Health Sciences Center in Oklahoma City, a new sperm antibody diagnostic kit is being developed. The kit will enable doctors to identify antibody-related infertility. According to medical experts, abnormal antibodies produced in the male that attack his own sperm can cause sterility. Antibodies in the female which attack all sperm can also cause sterility.

Doctors at the Iowa College of Medicine are currently using

"laparascopic" surgery to remove a varicose enlargement of the veins of the spermatic cord. A varicocele is the most common cause of male infertility. With the new surgical technique, patients have recovered in three days instead of ten to fourteen days.

Zinc Deficiency And Male Infertility - What Sexual Men Need To Know

A diet which is deficient in zinc may lead to infertility in some men, according to recent findings from a study conducted by the U.S. Department of Agriculture (USDA). The study involved 11 men who maintained a diet containing only 10 percent of their RDA for zinc. As a result, researchers say that the subjects' semen volume decreased more than 30 percent compared with semen levels later in the study when the men were consuming adequate amounts of zinc. The findings suggest that while the men's total sperm count did not suffer a significant change, the lowered volume could cause a decrease in fertility by reducing the migration of sperm in the woman's reproductive tract.

According to researchers, when stores of the mineral zinc— which is necessary for proper cell growth and repair—are low, the body may "sacrifice" its capacity for reproduction in order to maintain other more critical zinc- essential operations such as wound repairing wounds.

Since zinc deficiency is difficult to detect, researchers recommend that all men who have fertility problems check with a doctor to make sure they are getting the Recommended Daily Allowance of the essential mineral. In most cases, men should be able to get an adequate intake of zinc through their diets— red meat and dark turkey meat are excellent sources. However, vegetarians may need to take a zinc supplement. In any event, men should consult their doctors before increasing their zinc intake because too much zinc can irritate the stomach and cause vomiting.

Lack Of Nitric Oxide May Cause Impotence

Until recently, many experts thought that impotence was usually due to psychological problems. New research now indicates that, in most cases, the cause of impotence originates in the body instead of the mind.

For the first time, researchers at Clark Urology Center at the University of California in Los Angeles have apparently identified a chemical which has a key role in producing erections. The substance is nitric oxide, which is produced throughout the body and also takes part in the immune response. Researchers speculate that a lack of nitric oxide may be responsible for the type of impotence which affects many American men.

The new information about nitric oxide may lead to its use in more effective treatments for impotence. According to the researchers, the new knowledge may help them develop a convenient pill or skin patch as treatment for impotence, instead of relying on an injection.

New Patch Treatment For Impotence

According to findings from recent studies, nitroglycerin patches may provide effective treatment of impotence for some men. The same type of patches used for years as treatment for angina, appear to allow nitroglycerin to penetrate the skin and widen the blood vessels, resulting in increased blood flow to the penis.

Whether or not the patches will become the treatment of choice for certain forms of impotence remains to be seen. Researchers say that while the patches appear to be effective they can also cause side effects such as headaches.

6 Tips For Preventing Impotence

For some individuals, impotence results from unavoidable accidents or injuries. Scientists have also identified certain genetic factors as being instrumental in many of the physical conditions associated with impotence. For all of those men, prevention is beyond their control. Most men, however, do have several options when it comes to preventing dysfunctions such as impotence.

The six tips which follow, while generally recommended as effective means for maintaining good general health, can also help prevent specific problems, including impotence, from ever occurring.

1) Maintain a balanced diet— poor nutrition can result in impotence in several ways. First of all, a diet which is high in salt and fats can promote high blood pressure, and many of the medications used to control hypertension have been linked to impotence. A diet which is high in fats—especially saturated fats and cholesterol—can result in vascular problems which is a major factor in impotence. A diet which includes an excessive carbohydrate intake is a risk factor in diabetes, which is a major cause of impotence.

Experts recommend a diet which emphasizes fish, chicken, fruits, vegetables, and whole grains as a means of getting essential nutrients. Such a diet, along with control of the consumption of salt-and sodium-containing foods, can help prevent many of the factors underlying impotence.

2) Maintain your proper weight— excess weight has been shown to be a directly contributing factor in both diabetes and high blood pressure. Thus, proper nutrition requires that you maintain not only a well-balanced diet but control of your total caloric intake as well. When caloric intake is excessive, a buildup of fatty substances can occur within the vascular system, and that can also contribute to impotence.

3) Get regular exercise— just about everyone is well aware that even moderate exercise provides certain health benefits. Many people however are not aware that exercise helps prevent impotence, or that it does so in several ways. A proper exercise program can improve and maintain general cardiovascular fitness, help to lower blood cholesterol levels and promote weight control.

4) Don't abuse alcohol and/or other harmful drugs— studies suggest a definite link between excessive alcohol consumption and impotence. While an occasional drink by a nonalcoholic individual does not increase the risk of impotence, consumption that regularly exceeds two drinks per day should be a matter of concern.

In the case of controlled substances, the risk of impotence has been shown to be higher in users than that of non-users. Some legal drugs prescribed by physicians have also been linked to impotence. You should ask your doctor about all possible side effects before you take a prescribed medication.

5) Don't smoke— given the possible cardiovascular consequences of smoking, any man concerned about or interested in preventing impotence would be well- advised not to smoke. While not always possible or practical, it is also a good idea to avoid secondary tobacco smoke and other airborne pollutants whenever possible.

6) Avoid stress— like avoiding exposure to secondary tobacco smoke, avoiding stress isn't always possible, but none-the-less it is an important part of prevention. If you cope with stress by drinking excessively, chain smoking or by overeating, you increase your risk for such diseases as arteriosclerosis, which could lead to impotence.

Incredible New Way To Prevent Impotence

The Revive Systen Corporation of Lake Geneva, Wisconsin has announced a new, patented, effective system to prevent impotence. The Revive System works to prevent impotence before it becomes a problem or to control existing impotence without surgery, drugs, injections, or vacuum pumps. The new system is designed to enhance normal performance and endurance.

To get a report detailing the Revive System, send a #10 SASE to : Revive System Corp., 156 Broad St., Dept., PR, P.O. Box 790, Lake Geneva, Wisconsin 53147.

How A Man's Health And Lifestyle
Affects A Women's Pregnancy

Women who are thinking about getting pregnant are constantly advised to give up habits—drinking, smoking, drugs—or alter lifestyles which could put a baby's health at risk. Recently, researchers have been trying to find out whether the same advice holds true for men as well. Since men contribute half of the genetic material to a baby, researchers have been trying to determine what, if any, effect a man's health or lifestyle has on pregnancy. As yet, no definite conclusions have been reached. However, new studies are underway and experts may soon have some answers to this very important question.

Recent sperm studies have furnished medical experts with the following information:

1) Babies fathered by men who drink alcohol tend to weigh less and have higher chances of birth defects than do babies of non-drinking fathers.

2) Men who smoke tobacco tend to father babies with higher-than-normal rates of birth defects.

3) In some cases, men with lower than average levels of vitamin C produce genetically damaged sperm which could cause birth defects if they fertilize a woman's egg.

4) Men who are exposed to radiation—usually in the workplace—tend to father children with higher-than-normal incidences of leukemia.

Researchers acknowledge that no conclusive evidence exists to date which would lead to recommending that potential or expectant fathers change their habits or lifestyles. However, the circumstantial evidence and additional studies on the long-term genetic consequences of lifestyles and other factors on sperm may very well lead to such a recommendation in the near future.

New Patch For Smokers
Means Quitting Twice As Easy

There's some possible good news on the horizon for smokers who want to quit. Newly developed "one-a-day" patches which administer a timed dose of nicotine may prove to be an extremely effective aid to "kicking" the smoking habit.

In a six-week clinical trial of the new patch, conducted at the West Virginia University School of Medicine, smokers were given either 21-, 14-, or 7- milligram doses each day. A placebo group was given patches with no active medication. During the final four weeks of the trial, subjects with the highest dose were twice as likely to have stopped smoking as those who were given the placebo.

The researchers say that one important advantage of the patch over nicotine gum is that it thwarts withdrawal symptoms. With gum, the individual waits at least 15 minutes before it takes effect. The patch, which is placed on the upper body, provides a fuller, more constant nicotine replacements according to researchers.

The new one-a-day patch is available by prescription only, and should be used as part of a comprehensive stop-smoking program.

WARNING: The Food and Drug Administration is investigating reports that some people have suffered heart attacks as a result of smoking while wearing a nicotine patch. While the patches have been shown to be safe, the packaging does warn against smoking and wearing the patch at the same time. The best advice is to heed that warning, and to consult your doctor to be absolutely certain.

Quit Smoking Easier With This Grocery Store Food

Recent studies suggest that an extract of common oats may help reduce the craving for nicotine. In one study, heavy smokers were given either a placebo or an oat extract. After one month, researchers noted a significant decrease in the number of cigarettes smoked by people who took the oat extract compared with those taking the placebo. According to researchers, the oat extract seems to help diminish the craving for nicotine. While this is encouraging news for people who want to quit smoking, more research is needed before any definite conclusions can be reached.

Is A Drink Or Two A Day Good Or Bad For You? New Study Revealed.

According to a new study, if you don't want to give up alcohol altogether, it's best that you limit yourself to no more than two drinks per day. If you consume more than two drinks a day there's a good chance your blood pressure will increase, and that you'll soon suffer a calcium deficiency. The study, conducted by the American Heart Association, suggests that once a person starts having more than two drinks a day, health problems are usually not far behind.

The study also revealed that once the calcium-draining effects of alcohol have taken their toll, simply taking calcium supplements will not correct the problem. The best advice is to eliminate your consumption of alcohol or drink in moderation— no more than two drinks a day.

Use This Food To Stop Drinking And Wanting Alcohol

While scientific research has yet to verify the potential of Vitamin B3 (niacin) in reducing a person's craving for alcohol, anecdotal evidence suggests that it may really work. Some experts theorize that niacin may work by "freeing" toxic substances which are stored in fatty tissues. The toxins are then propelled in perspiration, generated by strenuous exercise and/or extended saunas. Other anecdotal evidence indicates that niacin supplements, in the form of nicotinic acid, can significantly reduce the craving for alcohol (and drugs) among many people who are addicted to those substances.

While anecdotal evidence is by no means conclusive, scientific research into the possible benefits of Vitamin B3 in reducing cravings for alcohol continue, and could reveal some encouraging results in the near future.

Good dietary sources of niacin include fish, lean meats, and poultry.

"Double Danger" For Men Who Smoke And Drink Alcohol

Smoking and drinking have long been linked with an assortment of health risks for both men and women. Now another possible health problem can be added to the list.

According to a study at Indiana University, men who smoke regularly and who drink may lose bone mass up to twice as fast as men who abstain. This evidence also suggests that smokers and drinkers may be more vulnerable to fractures as they get older.

Want To Get Pregnant?
Here's The Best Sexual Position To Use

If you and your mate want to have a child, experts recommend that you have intercourse as close to the time of ovulation as possible. Another way to increase the chances of pregnancy involves what many experts believe is the best sexual intercourse position, the rear entry position. These experts say that entering the vagina from the rear allows the sperm to be deposited closer to the cervix.

The rear entry position requires that both partners be positioned on their knees, with the man behind the woman.

New Intercourse Position:
It's Simple And Gives Women Orgasms,
Including Multiple Orgasms

Sex therapists report that the most common complaint from women is an inability to achieve orgasm during sexual intercourse. Some studies suggest that no more than 30 percent of women achieve orgasm regularly during intercourse. The good news is that a recently developed technique can help women have an orgasm, even multiple orgasms, during sexual intercourse.

The new technique, known as the Coital Alignment Technique (CAT) was developed by Edward W. Eichel, MA; Joanne De Simone Eichel, MA; and Sheldon Kule, DO; and reported on in the Journal of Sex And Marital Therapy. CAT involves a variation in a standard intercourse position as a means of heightening the sexual response in both men and women. Its developers say that it could also help increase the chance of both partners experiencing orgasm simultaneously.

The new position is similar to the standard missionary position in which the woman lies on her back with the man on top, and facing her. CAT varies from the missionary position in that the man's pelvis should "override" the woman's in a "riding high" alignment. The woman should wrap her legs around the man's thigh's, bending her legs at an angle which does not exceed 45 degrees. She should allow her ankles to rest on the man's calves.

For this position to be successful, the man should let his entire weight be on the woman (he should not use his hands or his elbows to support his weight). Although the woman may find the man's weight uncomfortable at first, it is necessary to ensure that his pelvis does not slide away from hers. The new CAT does not concentrate on a great deal of awkward (and tiring movement) as in conventional intercourse, but rather on the partners' pelvic movement. The position is designed to allow rhythmic movement that is virtually the same for both the man and the woman. The penis and the clitoris are brought together tightly by the pressure and counterpressure created by the couples rhythmic movement. The result is one of maximum stimulation and almost certain orgasm for both the woman and the man.

New For Men:
The One Hour Erection Technique

Sex therapists say that in order to extend sexual response, both partners should learn more about their physical and mental control systems. Mental control involves learning to concentrate by narrowing the individual focus of attention. The goal of mental control as a means of extending sexual response, such as erection, is to filter out and eliminate distractions.

Without our realizing it, our thoughts can be like background noise, causing us to be distracted at the most inopportune moments. One technique for focusing your concentration and taking control of your thoughts is a countdown exercise. Sex therapists recommend this technique because, with practice, it will enable you to eliminate distractions and focus on sexual enjoyment and response.

In the countdown technique, you simple close your eyes and count backwards, slowly, from 20, all the way to zero. If you are distracted by an unwanted thought, proceed with your countdown, taking up with the last number you remember. This technique of counting backwards from 20 as a means of helping you focus your attention, will probably require a good bit of practice before you are able to eliminate all distracting thoughts. The key to maintaining an erection for up to one hour, lies in your ability to concentrate.

Another technique often recommended by many sex therapists is the "Sensate focus technique". The aim of this technique is to make each partner more aware of his or her bodily sensations during intercourse. Men who have practiced this focus technique with their partners have reported great success in extending their sexual response.

The Sensate focus technique involves three basic steps:

1) Each partner gives the other as much pleasure as possible by caressing and fondling any part of the body except the breasts or genitals.

2) This stage of the technique progresses to stimulation of the genitals and breasts, but should stop short of orgasm.

3) The final stage of the Sensate focus technique is sexual intercourse. Both partners should concentrate on pleasure and enjoyment rather than on orgasm. The main goal of this technique is not orgasm, but rather extending the sexual response.

Premature Ejaculation: How To End It

According to many leading sex therapists, premature ejaculation is the most common sexual difficulty in men. It is not, however, an insurmountable problem. There are several proven techniques that are helpful in correcting and preventing the problem of premature ejaculation.

Perhaps the most common technique taught by sex therapists is the "squeeze technique". This technique involves squeezing the tip or base of the penis for a few seconds just prior to ejaculation. The squeeze technique can be applied by you or your partner whenever you want to delay ejaculation.

A second technique often recommended by sex therapists, requires that both partners stop thrusting just before ejaculation. Once the man regains control of the ejaculatory reflex, sexual activity resumes.

A third technique recommended by sex therapists is deep breathing. This technique is based on the theory that deliberate deep breathing helps to delay ejaculation by "diffusing" feelings of arousal throughout the entire body.

The Safest, Most Tear-Proof Condom
- And The Worst Type

If you've been inhibited from using a condom because of stories about tearing, experts agree that your concerns are virtually unwarranted. Research has revealed that condoms are almost always uncommonly sturdy, and will endure rather severe treatment before tearing. In fact, the chances of a popular brand of condom tearing are very remote.

To ease your concerns, experts say that American brands, especially the thicker brands of condoms, are perhaps the safest when it comes to the likelihood of tearing. Some foreign brands, such as Japanese brands, are sometimes thinner than American brands, and as a result may be less sturdy.

If your concerns won't go away, you might actually try to tear a condom. Buy a popular brand and tear several of them. Stretch them as much as you can, clamp one around a water faucet and fill it with water until it bursts. The idea is to see exactly what it takes to tear a condom. After "sacrificing" three or four condoms, you should know whether or not your concerns are warranted.

Health Secrets For People Over 40

Aging is a natural process which doesn't have to result in chronic aches and pains, digestive disorders, diseases, and loss of sex drive. Medical experts agree that people who eat right, stay active and avoid health-damaging habits are likely to enter old age in excellent health. Many of the changes wrought by the aging process seem to begin around the age of forty or so.

Here's what begins to happen in the 40's and beyond, and some suggestions and recommendations to help you "beat the clock":

1) Vision— as a general rule, vision doesn't change much through the 30s, but about the time a person reaches 40, the lens begins to have trouble changing from a flattened to a spherical shape in order to focus on nearby objects. The eye then gradually becomes focused permanently at a relatively constant distance. This condition is called presbyopia and is a form of farsightedness which commonly requires people, beginning in their 40s, to hold a book or newspaper at arm's length in order to read the print.

This natural change in vision doesn't have to be just another sign of the aging process. The problem can be corrected and/or controlled by wearing corrective glasses to do close work. In many cases, bifocal glasses with separate corrections for both close and distant viewing will correct the problem.

While some changes in vision—especially difficulty seeing up close—are a natural and normal part of aging, other problems of a more serious nature, such as sight-threatening diseases like cataracts and glaucoma, begin to take their toll. Cataracts, which are clouds in the lenses that often cause dim vision in the 60s, can be a natural result of lifelong oxidation damage, which is a byproduct of normal body chemistry.

In a study at the Human Nutrition Research Center on Aging at Tufts University, in Medford, Massachusetts, researchers discovered that men and women without cataracts have higher levels of anti-oxidant nutrients such as vitamins E and C and beta-carotene in their blood, getting them more from natural sources— fruits and vegetables—than from supplements.

Glaucoma—abnormally high pressure of the fluid of the eye—seldom occurs before age 40 and generally causes no symptoms until the advanced stages, which is sometimes too late to prevent vision loss. Glaucoma and Cataracts are two reasons that ophthalmologists recommend routine eye exams about every two years after age 40 and every year after age 60.

An ophthalmologist will check both your distance vision and your ability to focus on near objects (accommodation power). Also during the examination, the ophthalmologist will examine the inside of your eyes to look for any changes which may be caused by disease. He or she will also measure the pressure of the fluid inside your eyes to check for glaucoma. Your field of vision should also be checked during these examinations. Regular periodic, professional examinations such as these are the best and perhaps the only way to ensure that the effects of age are detected early and treated in order to protect your vision.

Another, less serious eye problem known as "dry eye", with symptoms such as stinging, scratchiness and unusual sensitivity to smoke, most commonly afflicts women after menopause. This condition can usually be treated successfully with artificial tears.

1) Hearing— according to experts, even by age 20 many people begin to lose their ability to hear high-frequency tones. With increasing age, that loss of sensitivity to high-frequency sounds, may become significantly impaired. However, most people are not seriously affected until they reach their 60s, when they may begin to find speech difficult to follow. This condition is more common in men than it is in women, and studies have revealed that, in general, women are less likely than men to go deaf.

Studies have also shown that a high-fat diet can clog the blood vessels which provide nourishment to delicate hearing organs, and years of exposure to high levels of noise can cause cumulative damage to our hearing. With that in mind, it's a good idea for people in their 40s or older to have a hearing test to find out how their hearing may have been affected over the years. You can receive such a test, free, simply by dialing 1-800-222-EARS (3277). The toll- free number puts you in contact with a national project, which has already provided screening for more than 5.6 million Americans. (The service is also now provided for Canada at 215-5443-7000).

You will need to furnish a project operator with some basic general information such as where you live. The operator will then give you a local phone number to call for your hearing test. There's usually no toll charge involved with the number because you will generally be calling a location within a 50-mile radius of where you live. Once you call the local number, you'll be given recorded instructions during the test which takes two minutes. The actual test includes 8 signals or tones— 4 for each ear. If you have trouble hearing all 8 tones, you should then consider having your hearing tested by a specialist. The operators can also provide you with referrals if you wish.

2) Renal system— from birth to about age 30 the kidneys actually increase in weight, then a reversal of that process begins to take place. A cumulative decline of 20 to 30 percent is not unusual by age 80. In simpler terms, the kidneys filter waste more slowly as we age. Some women in their 40s who have had children may begin to experience a leakage of a few drops of urine whenever they cough or sneeze. That problem can be corrected with some basic exercises which strengthen the stretched pelvic muscles.

3) Coronary heart disease— after the age of 45, the leading cause of death is heart disease. According to research scientists, one American man in five develops symptoms of heart disease by the age of 60. Statistics show that from the age of 40 to the age of 60, heart disease claims more lives than does stroke, bronchitis, and cancers of the lung, stomach, and breast, combined.

Up until menopause women are far less vulnerable to coronary heart disease than men. Estrogen may work as a protector by affecting the "good" cholesterol (HDLs) which keeps the "bad" cholesterol under control. By age 65, women begin dying of heart disease as often as men do.

Studies have shown that a lifelong low-fat diet and exercise program can help prevent coronary heart disease. And it is never too late to change. Regular exercise and good eating habits can give both men and women protection from heart disease, even in the most vulnerable years.

4) Functional capacity— as we get older, our ability to generate energy for work and play decreases. By age 40, many men and women find that hills seem a little steeper and that they run out of energy quick-

er. While the aging process plays a part in this "slowing down", sedentary lifestyles are also often at least partly to blame. Many people in their 40s are under more pressure and stress than they were at 20, and they devote less time to exercise. Research has shown that stress can lead to lethargy and that regular exercise can help people cope better with stress.

As part of a decade-long study, sedentary women from 35 to 65 were enrolled in a program of aerobic exercise. At the end of 10 years, their functional capacities were a full 6 percent higher than when they began.

In another study, a group of men and women with an average age of 90 worked with weights and increased their muscle sizes by 10 percent and nearly tripled their strength. The results seem to indicate that proper training can build muscle and increase or maintain functional capacity at any age.

5) Muscles and joints— a little loss of muscle strength occurs between 35 and 40, but after that, strength tends to decline gradually for both men and women. By the age of 60, a man may lose up to 20 percent of his maximum strength and a woman may lose even more. Medical experts say that the decrease occurs because more protein is being broken down and less is being synthesized. The result is atrophy and loss of muscle fiber. The protein that has been lost is, in large part, replaced by fatty tissue.

Stiff joints also seem to be a fact of life for many people, beginning at about age 40. The health of joints depends on the strength of the muscles supporting them. Regular exercise—walking or running, weightlifting—is essential if you are to hold your own in the battle with aging muscles and joints.

Lower-back pain is also more common among people in their 40s and 50s. Researchers say that a slow, natural degeneration of the disks that cushion the vertebrae and stress can both contribute to back problems in middle-age people. But most people can overcome the pain and prevent further problems by strengthening the lower body and abdominal muscles through exercise.

6) Bone deterioration— strong bones are essential in order to

prevent osteoporosis, a health problem which often afflicts older women. Osteoporosis causes bones to become thin and porous enough to fracture or break easily. The condition accelerates at menopause and affects about 25 percent of women older than 65.

Studies have shown that the stronger a women's bones are before menopause, the better her chances of avoiding osteoporosis. Adequate calcium intake and regular weight-bearing exercise—walking or running—are recommended to all women to ensure dense bones.

7) Sex— for most women, the hormonal shifts of menopause have little or no effect on desire or responsiveness. Many women at menopause, however, find sexual intercourse painful because of a drying and thinning of vaginal tissues. Many experts agree that the best treatment is to remain sexually active. Studies reveal that postmenopausal women who keep sexually active— with sexual intercourse at least once or twice a week—have considerably less vaginal atrophy than sexually inactive women.

As for men, evidence indicates that older men who keep in good physical condition can apparently maintain their output of sex hormones at the levels of young men. In fact, studies show that both men and women can enjoy sex into their eighties and beyond.

Men And Women Over 40 Should Do These Things For Better Health

1) Eye examination— beginning at age 40, you should have an eye examination every two years if you have good vision. If you are at risk—diagnosed as having diabetes or high blood pressure, or if you have a family history of glaucoma—you should have an eye examination about once a year.

2) Cervical (Pap) Smear— this should be done every one to three years for women 40 and older, and every year if you have already been diagnosed and treated for precancerous changes or for herpes or genital warts.

3) Blood pressure— every three to five years, or as your doctor recommends between the ages of 40 and 50. Men and women over 50

should have a blood pressure measurement every year, or as his or her doctor recommends.

4) Blood cholesterol— for anyone over 40, if the result of your last test was normal, repeat in three to five years. If the results were abnormal, follow your doctor's recommendation.

5) Breast X-ray (Mammography)— every one to two years for women between 40 and 50, and every year after 50.

6) Examination of the rectum and colon— there are three separate tests to detect cancer of the rectum and colon:

A) Digital rectal examination— a physical exam of the rectum and prostate to detect signs of cancer or prostate disease. This test should be performed every year in men beginning at age 40.

B) Hemoccult stool test— a microscopic examination of the feces for signs of colon cancer which should be done every year for both men and women. This is the most common screening for colon cancer as it actually detects blood in feces. You can purchase home test kits to screen your stool for occult—hidden blood—which can indicate colorectal (colon or rectal) cancer long before symptoms are present. Anyone using the kit should understand that it detects only the presence of blood and not cancer itself. Some foods, aspirin and other drugs, and hemorrhoids can also cause positive results.

The test should also be repeated on three consecutive bowel movements. If you get a positive result, you should consult your doctor right away. Also, to make sure that the test is reliable, it is a good idea to get written instructions from your doctor and follow all dietary restrictions.

C) Sigmoidoscopy— this is an internal examination of the rectum and colon with a flexible, lighted tube called a sigmoidoscope. The test should begin at age 50 and be repeated every three to five years.

7) Complete Physical Examination— every one to two years (or as your doctor recommends) between the ages of 40 and 65. After 65, you should have a complete physical every year.

Women Need Calcium And Vitamin A
For Strong Bones After Menopause

Recent research shows that women who are at least five years past menopause receive great benefit from maintaining their intake of calcium. Researchers point out that just getting the RDA of calcium—800 to 1,200 milligrams— significantly reduces the the risk of bone loss.

After menopause, a woman's protection against most bone loss—her natural hormones—ends and bone loss accelerates. If the woman's diet is low in calcium the likelihood of bone loss increases even further. According to a study at the Human Nutrition Research Center of Aging at Tufts University in Boston, older women who get less than 400 milligrams of calcium a day get the greatest benefit by increasing calcium intake. The postmenopausal women who were consuming 400 to 650 milligrams of calcium a day did not benefit from the increase.

The study also showed that calcium carbonate did not seem to help women with low calcium intakes, but calcium citrate malate—available only in calcium fortified juices—did.

A recent study by the U.S. Department of Agriculture Human Nutrition Research Center on Aging, in Boston suggests that the process of maintaining healthy bones requires plenty of vitamin D as well as calcium. Researchers say it is especially important for postmenopausal women who live in colder climates. Apparently, women in cold climates tend to suffer bone loss in the winter because they don't get enough sunlight, which helps the body to produce vitamin D.

Women who were involved in the study, and who were getting the RDA for calcium and took 400 IUs of vitamin D each day (twice the RDA for women) suffered less bone loss in winter than a group of women taking only calcium and serving as the control group for the study.

The results of the study led the researchers to recommend that postmenopausal women eat adequate amounts of vitamin D-fortified foods including skim milk and other low-fat dairy products. Some women may even want to consider taking a multivitamin tablet containing the RDA for vitamin D, but should do so only under a doctor's supervision.

Drug May Help Reduce Bone Loss In Women

New evidence suggests that the drug tamoxifen may help reduce the spinal bone loss which is common in post-menopausal women. In a recent study at the University of Wisconsin Comprehensive Cancer Center in Madison, researchers found that the spine density of several post-menopausal women taking tamoxifen increased by more than half of one percent a year. Another group of post-menopausal women who took a placebo experienced a decrease in spine density of one percent a year.

Earlier research had already shown that the drug lowers cholesterol levels and that it may also prevent breast-cancer recurrence.

The National Cancer Institute is conducting a clinical trial in an effort to find out if long-term use of tamoxifen can protect women who are at high risk for breast cancer from developing the disease, and to study other effects of the drug.

Hormone Replacement Therapy And Stronger Bones

According to a recent study, the most effective way for many older women to ward off osteoporosis may be with hormone replacement therapy.

Scientists at Sir Charles Gairdner Hospital in Nedlands, Australia, investigated the effectiveness of three different approaches to retarding bone loss in 120 postmenopausal women whose average age was 56. The methods investigated were exercise, exercise combined with a calcium supplement and exercise plus an estrogen-progesterone replacement.

The results of the study revealed that exercise alone had little effect in reducing bone loss, while exercise plus calcium did reduce the loss of bone. But, exercise and hormone replacement therapy produced the best results—an actual increase in bone density.

While hormone replacement therapy is still somewhat controversial—it can cause side effects, such as tender breasts and vaginal bleeding, and may increase, slightly, a woman's risk of developing breast cancer—the new research suggests that the therapy may be the most effective treatment for postmenopausal women with low bone mass and no history of breast cancer.

What Women Need To Know About Estrogen And Hormone Replacement Therapy

In the continuing debate over the risks versus the benefits of estrogen replacement therapy (ERT), a new study adds more weight to the positive side of the scales. Researchers at the University of Southern California monitored over 8,500 postmenopausal women and discovered that those who at some time had undergone ERT lived an average of 1 1/2 years longer than those who never did. The researchers also found that women who underwent long-term ERT—at least 15 years—lived up to 3 years longer than women who never had such therapy. The results of this study appear to support the many medical experts who are now maintaining that the benefits of ERT outweigh the risks.

Recent studies suggest that low dose estrogen replacement therapy may not be associated with an increased risk of breast cancer. In the study at U.S.C., women who underwent ERT and had any type of cancer were no more likely to die of the disease than those who did not undergo ERT. However, many experts believe that taking estrogen alone causes a slight increase in the risk of cancer of the uterus. But when progestin, a synthetic form of progesterone, is given in addition to estrogen, the risk is reduced. However, such combination therapy can cause continuation of periodic spotting.

Although much of the recent news about ERT is reassuring, the decision to undergo the therapy is still a highly personal one for most women. Experts also warn that ERt is not appropriate for everyone.

Who Should You Have Hormone Replacement Therapy?

Many doctors recommend that women should take hormones only if their menopausal symptoms—especially vaginal soreness, hot flashes, and night sweats—are severe enough to cause extreme discomfort. Other doctors believe that most women should take hormones to protect themselves against the effects of osteoporosis, and other benefits (see chapter 10). The therapy is generally not recommended for women who have a history of breast and/or uterine cancer, stroke, pulmonary embolism, liver disease, or deep-vein thrombosis.

If you are taking hormones, you should follow your doctor's instructions exactly—have regular medical checkups, including pelvic examinations; Pap smears; blood pressure checkups; and mammograms. In order to eliminate symptoms such as hot flashes, most women need to continue treatment for at least one year. If a woman stops her treatment abruptly, the symptoms can reappear in just a few months. Hormone replacement as a treatment to prevent osteoporosis may need to continue for five to ten years or longer.

Benefits And Risks Of Hormone Replacement Therapy

Before you make a decision regarding hormone replacement therapy, you should consider carefully all the known risks and benefits. Get as many competent opinions and as much professional advice as is possible. Discuss the options with your doctor and seek a second or third opinion. In the end, the decision is an individual choice, so you should get as much information as possible and make sure you understand the entire process and its effects.

Known Benefits

1) Very effective for treatment and prevention in the short-term of menopausal symptoms such as hot flashes, sweating and vaginal dryness.

2) May reduce episodes of depression and enhance sleep patterns. The therapy may also provide an overall sense of well-being.

3) Studies suggest that if taken for several years, this therapy slows down the rate of bone reduction. Other research indicates that if taken for at least five years, the incidence of hip fractures is reduced.

4) Some studies show that if the therapy continues long-term, it can help to maintain quality of skin and breast tissue.

5) If the therapy involves estrogen alone, it may help to protect against heart disease or reduce heart disease by 50 percent. However, the

addition of progesterone appears to neutralize some of those benefits.

Known Risks

1) The therapy may cause minor side effects, such as headaches, nausea, bloating, weight gain, breast tenderness, and jaundice. Your doctor can lower your dose to alleviate the side effects.

2) Taking estrogen alone may increase the risk of endometrial cancer. However, that risk is apparently eliminated with the addition of progesterone.

3) While not conclusive, some studies suggest that estrogen may increase the risk of cancer. Also not conclusive, is evidence suggesting that the addition of progesterone gives protection.

4) Although rare with the dosage levels currently in use, the therapy may increase blood pressure.

5) Newer regimens attempt to eliminate monthly periods, but many women report regular spotting with this treatment.

New Study Links Estrogen To Cancer Risk In Some Women

Researchers at the Ohio State University report that recent findings indicate that estrogen replacement therapy (ERT) used as a treatment for menopausal symptoms and in the prevention of osteoporosis, may double the risk of breast cancer in lean women.

In the study, lean women were described as those in the lowest one-third of body mass— a ratio of weight to height. Researchers studied over 600 women who had been diagnosed recently with breast cancer and 520 women who had similar characteristics but no history of breast cancer. While there did not appear to be a link between estrogen replacement therapy and breast cancer in general, researchers say that among lean women the overall difference was significant.

47 percent of the lean patients with breast cancer used estrogen, compared with 31 percent of women who did not use estrogen.

Researchers say that this obvious difference is worth investigating and that doctors should be more cautious about prescribing estrogen replacement therapy, especially for lean women who have a family history of breast cancer.

The researchers point out that the results of their new study should not be considered as an indictment of ERT as being a cause of breast cancer development. They suggest, however, continued studies into the potential effects of ERT among post-menopausal women, and in particular, "among lean women".

Many experts feel that the overall proven benefits of estrogen far outweigh the potential risks. These proponents of ERT cite the fact that it is beneficial in preventing heart disease and osteoporosis, while the risk of breast cancer has never been strongly confirmed. None-the-less, there is general agreement among experts that women taking estrogen should be monitored regularly and carefully with mammograms and other tests.

Hormone Therapy And Arthritis Relief

Women with rheumatoid arthritis who are currently undergoing estrogen replacement therapy appear to experience an improvement in their conditions compared with women who have taken estrogen and stopped or those who have never used estrogen replacements.

Researchers at the University of California studied over 150 post-menopausal women who had rheumatoid arthritis and found that continued use of ERT was associated with significantly milder arthritis symptoms and an overall improvement in the performance of daily activities when compared to ex- or non-users of ERT.

10 Symptoms Of Menopause

Not every woman is affected in the same way or to the same degree by menopausal symptoms. There are many symptoms of menopause—some obvious, some subtle— and you may or may not experience any of them. However, the more symptoms you recognize from your own personal experience, the more you may benefit from medical treatment. For many women, the symptoms of menopause, listed below, are mild or non-existant, while for others they are very real, and very discomforting.

1) A change in monthly periods— studies show that four of every five women notice changes in the frequency, duration, or regularity of their periods. These changes usually occur gradually in the two to three years prior to menopause. The changes are usually the first indication that menopause is approaching.

2) Hot flashes— about 70 percent of menopausal women experience hot flashes— sensations of intense heat, sometimes accompanied by sweating—which usually begin in the chest and spread up to the neck and face.

3) Night sweats— a typical symptom in menopausal women, sometimes to such a degree that a woman will need to change her nightclothes or sheets.

4) Difficulty sleeping— some menopausal women have difficulty sleeping because of troubling emotions, night sweats, and hot flashes.

5) Vaginal dryness or irritation— lower levels of estrogen can cause the walls of a woman's vagina to become thinner. The vagina itself can become more prone to infection.

6) Lost interest in sex— because of vaginal changes, some menopausal women find intercourse to be painful. Hormonal changes and fatigue can also reduce the sex drive.

7) Urinary problems— reduced levels of estrogen may have an effect on your bladder and urethra, causing pain on urination, increased frequency of urination, and urinary incontinence.

8) Sudden changes of mood— some menopausal women experience depression or sudden changes in mood for no apparent reason. This may be due to estrogen deficiency and to a woman's specific response to the changes she is experiencing.

9) Anxiety and irritability— such symptoms, along with a lack of concentration and loss of confidence, may be brought about by fluctuations in hormone levels, stress and fatigue.

10) Dizziness and palpitation— headaches and dizziness sometimes occur in menopausal women as a result of changes in circulation and heart rate.

New Study Reveals How Much Sex Is Average For Your Age

Don't let anyone tell you that growing older means you'll have to stop enjoying sex. It simply isn't true. According to a new study involving two surveys of over 5,500 people, more than one third of married men and women over 60 make love at least once a week. Moreover, the study reveals that 10 percent of those people over 70 make love at least once a week.

Many people find that the later years can provide the opportunity for partners to perfect their sexual skills as well as to be more sensitive to each other's needs. The new study of the sexuality of people over 60 found that not only were older people making love at least once a week, they were far from being routine about it. Many of the people surveyed reported making love outdoors, swimming in the nude, undressing each other, and buying sexy lingerie.

Experts say that once a woman has reached the menopause and pregnancy is no longer possible, both partners often discover renewed interest and pleasure in their sexual relationship. For couples under age 60, the average amount of sex is about 1 1/2 times a week.

The Link Between Coffee And Sex

Here's an unusual bit of information: according to researchers at William Beaumont Hospital in Royal Oak, Michigan and the University of Michigan at Ann Arbor, older people who drink coffee have more active sex lives than those who don't.

The researchers surveyed almost 800 men and women age 60 and older and learned that women who drank at least one cup of coffee per day were more likely to be sexually active than those women who drank less or no coffee at all. Men who drank at least one cup of coffee daily were less likely to be impotent, according to the survey.

Researchers say that caffeine, which is a central nervous system stimulant, may be responsible for boosting sexual drive. They also say that older people who are healthy enough to drink coffee may simply be better able to perform sex than those seniors who are in poor health.

Older Women And Heart Disease
- What You Should Know

The good news is that heart disease in women can be reversed. The bad news is that a surprisingly high number of women, aged 50 or over, don't know that heart disease is the leading cause of death in their age group. Moreover, even though 80 percent of those women surveyed said they had taken a cholesterol test, only 50 percent knew that 200 was a desirable cholesterol level. This lack of awareness of basic health knowledge could prove to be very dangerous in light of the recent studies that show that, given the proper attention, it may be possible to control heart disease in older women.

In one study, lovastatin, a new and promising cholesterol-lowering drug, seems to work well in women. The drug has already been proved effective in men. According to researchers, the main benefit of lovastatin is that it reduces "bad" cholesterol (LDL) which has been linked to heart disease.

Another study, involving both women and men with existing heart disease, discovered that when LDL levels were lowered, blockages of the arteries that serve the heart also decreased. It is known that if one or more of these vessels is blocked it could result in angina, heart attacks, and other serious problems.

In still another study, conducted at Harvard University, researchers have learned that the lower doses of estrogen may be just as effective as heavier ones in reducing heart-attack risk in postmenopausal women. The study showed that a dose of .625 milligrams provides just as much protection against heart attack as twice that dosage does. Researchers say that the smaller dose reduced LDL levels by 15 percent within three months. The smaller dose also raised HDL or "good" cholesterol levels. For every one percent drop in LDL, there is a two percent drop in heart-attack risk, according to the researchers.

People Over 65 Can Get Free Eye Care. Call This 800 Number

With the importance of comprehensive eye examinations to help cambat the aging process, member doctors of the American Academy of Ophthalmology have agreed to provide a complete medical eye examination and care for any diagnosed condition to U.S. citizens or residents 65 and older who don't have the means or the access to see a doctor he or she has seen in the past. The examination and treatment (if warranted) are being provided free of charge (eyeglasses, prescription drug, and hospital care are not covered). To find out if you are eligible to take advantage of this cost-free eye care, call 800-222-3937.

Vitamin D And Calcium Deficiency May Lead To Strokes In Older Women

The results of a study involving over 40,000 women at the University of Iowa College of Medicine in Iowa City suggests that older women who are deficient in both vitamin D and calcium have a higher risk of strokes than those who consume adequate amounts. The two-year study found that out of 101 women who suffered strokes, 35 percent were free of cardiovascular disease, a contributing factor. However, when the researchers compared this group of women to another group who did not have strokes they found that the stroke victims consumed less calcium and vitamin D.

Nutritionists say that both deficiencies are easy to avoid—low-fat dairy products, such as skim milk and yogurt, and salmon and sardines with the bones, provide good dietary sources of vitamin D and calcium. In some cases supplements may be helpful, but you should consult your doctor first.

6 Secrets To Reduce Prostate Pain

Prostatitis, the most common prostate trouble, is an inflammation of the prostate often caused by bacteria or by congestion. Men who suffer from this condition frequently experience pain on urination or sexual intercourse, frequent urination, and aching in the groin, testicles, and lower back. This is not an unconquerable problem because there are several ways to relieve the discomfort of prostatitis.

1) Avoid foods and drinks such as coffee, both caffeinated and decaffeinated; tea; cola; cocoa; alcohol; chocolate; spicy foods; and nuts, especially cashews.

2) Don't sit for long periods of time or take bouncy rides in trucks, on motorcycles, and so on.

3) Take sitz baths twice a day for 10 to 20 minutes at a time, sitting in 6 to 10 inches of very hot water.

4) If your prostatitis is not caused by bacteria, consult with your doctor about engaging in sexual intercourse. Ejaculation may help relieve the inflammation.

5) If you suffer from acute prostatitis which is caused by bacteria, you should try to avoid sexual arousal until the condition is under control. You should also take your medication exactly as your doctor has prescribed, even if you begin to feel better before the recommended treatment is complete.

What Every Man Over 45 Sould Know About Prostate Enlargement

After a man reaches the age of 45 or so, his prostate gland tends to increase in size. As the gland grows, it may begin to press against and compress the urethra, creating a frequent, urgent need to empty the bladder and/or make urination more difficult. In some cases, the retention of urine can lead to an inflammation of the bladder and possible kidney damage.

Often called benign prostatic hypertrophy (BPH), this is a noncancerous condition, whose exact cause is still a mystery. Symptoms usually develop gradually as the prostate continues to compress and distort the urethra. And according to some studies, as many as 80 percent of men 55 and older may experience at least one of its symptoms—most typically a frequent need to urinate or having a difficult time with the passage of urine.

The first thing you should do if you experience symptoms of BPH is to see your doctor and have the condition checked out, because some of the same symptoms may signal cancer of the prostate. It is also sometimes necessary to have surgery in order to remove the enlarged section of the prostate.

Mild symptoms of BPH do not usually require extensive treatment. Men who do require surgery may have the option of one of several procedures, depending on the nature of their condition. And while surgery has been an effective long- term solution for many men, it can also have certain "side effects", such as retrograde ejaculation wherein men who have had the operation no longer ejaculate out of the penis but rather up into the bladder. The condition presents no health or sexual performance problems, but it does result in infertility. In some cases, surgery may also lead to impotence.

The most common surgical procedure for BPH is transurethral resection of the prostate (TURP). The procedure requires a 3 to 5 day stay in the hospital, followed by a two week recovery period. With the patient under either general or spinal anesthesia, the surgeon passes a resectoscope up the urethra so the prostate can be seen. A tiny cutting instrument is then inserted through the resectoscope and used to cut away enough of the prostatic tissue to allow urine to flow normally. The tissue that is removed is then examined to detect the presence of any cancerous cells. According to many medical experts, TURP is far more likely to provide long-term relief from BPH than drugs or any other alternative treatment.

Get Prostate Relief From Amazing New Techniques

A rather recent alternative to surgery for BPH is a treatment, approved by the Federal Food and Drug Administration, which involves having a tiny balloon inflated inside the urethra. Instead of having any tissue cut away, the inflation of the balloon compresses the overgrown prostate tissue, allowing the urethra to open. While the balloon treatment takes much less time and doesn't seem to cause the bleeding and retrograde ejaculation that surgery does, follow-up studies indicate it may only provide short-term relief. And since the procedure doesn't remove any tissue, doctors can not perform a cancer biopsy.

Studies are also underway investigating other potential treatments for BPH. One potential treatment—microwave hyperthermia—involves heating the prostate to about 110 degrees in order to shrink the overgrown tissue. According to researchers, the heating treatment utilizes a catheter with a small microwave heating element. Initial results suggest that this method would allow patients to be treated on an out-patient basis. While the research on this potential treatment continues, researchers speculate that it may one day be the best alternative for men in poor health or who otherwise may shun surgery.

Another potential treatment is laser surgery. This too is in the investigative stages, and involves passing a small telescope-like devise through the penis, then inserting a laser fiber through the telescope. The laser is then fired for about one minute at each of four sites. The tissue which has been irradiated by the laser is cast off in the urine over a period of four to six weeks. Early indications are that this new laser surgery technique could prove to be an effective treatment for BPH.

Some treatments using drugs have also proven to be useful in treating mild to moderate enlargements of the prostate. Recently, the FDA approved Proscar for such treatment. The drug works by blocking an enzyme which is a contributing factor in the enlargement of the prostate gland. Studies have shown that Proscar can be effective in improving the flow of urine and in reducing the size of the enlarged prostate for some men. But the drug takes time to work— at least three to six months before symptoms begin to improve. Experts tend to agree that, while Proscar may be a viable treatment for some men with mild to moderate BPH which doesn't require surgery, it can also have some disadvantages, and you should consult with a competent urologist before you decide if the treatment is right for you

In some cases, urologists are recommending the use of Proscar along with the hypertension drug Hytrin. The drug, while lowering blood pressure, also relaxes the muscle tissue in and around the prostate, allowing urine to continue flowing. The FDA has only approved Hytrin as a means of treating high blood pressure, but some studies suggest it can also be effective in treating mild to moderate symptoms of BPH. One possible drawback to Hytrin is that is does not shrink the prostate and therefore would have to be taken on a daily basis or the symptoms will most likely return.

If there's any good news in all of this, it's that treatment alternatives for BPH are continuing to evolve. Whereas surgery once seemed to be the most effective long-term solution, researchers are developing alternatives which may give men a choice of treatments. For now, the best answer is to consult with your doctor or urologist for his or her advice.

Early Prostate Cancer Detection

The American Cancer Society recommended recently that mean age 50 or older should get an annual blood test in order to detect prostate cancers as early as possible.

The recommended blood test measures a substance known as prostate specific antigen (PSA). When the prostate is enlarged, PSA levels—secreted by the gland—are elevated. Medical experts say that's a sign which may mean cancer.

The new American Cancer Society recommendation says that PSA testing should be done along with a digital rectal examination every year on men over 50. However, screening should begin at a younger age in blacks or those men who have a strong family history of prostate cancer.

According to the Cancer Society, almost 80 percent of all prostate cancers are diagnosed in men 65 or older. And the Society is recommending the PSA testing even though mass screening for prostate cancer has not been shown to reduce the number of deaths from the disease.

Nasal Spray Warning
For Men With Enlarged Prostates

Some men with enlarged prostates may experience complications when using decongestant nasal sprays. Researchers say that some of the most commonly used nasal sprays can cause urinary retention in men who suffer from moderate prostate enlargement.

The researchers recommend that such men consult their doctors before using decongestant nasal sprays to combat a cold.

Seniors: Vitamins
Can Reduce Your Illnesses Up To 50%

New evidence suggests that people over 65 who take modest daily amounts of a variety of vitamins, minerals, and other supplements have stronger immune systems and a better chance of fighting off infections than those who don't receive them.

The evidence comes from a new Canadian study involving 96 healthy men and women who were living on their own. Researchers examined the effect of 18 vitamins, minerals and other supplements thought to influence the immune system. All of the subjects were evaluated before the study began, and most of them had normal blood levels of the essential nutrients. The researchers aren't sure which nutrients resulted in improved health.

Half of those participating in the study took supplements, while the other half didn't. Among those who took the supplements, infection-related illness occurred an average of 23 days per year— the average was 48 days among those who did not take supplements. Also, the group which received the supplements needed fewer prescriptions for antibiotics than those people in the control group.

While scientists are encouraged by the new information, they agree that before any firm conclusion can be reached about the findings, more extensive and longer studies need to conducted. That's because the positive effects initially ascribed to vitamins, minerals and other supplements may in fact have been influenced by other, as yet unknown, factors.

Aging Problems? Senility, Memory Loss And Muscle
Coordination Can Be Helped By This Incredible Vitamin

Studies suggest that a deficiency of vitamin B12 may be at least partly responsible for declining mental ability and muscle coordination in some older people. And experts say that about 25 percent of people over age 60 no longer have the ability to make enough stomach acid to absorb sufficient amounts of vitamin B12 from food.

Until recently, injections have been the most common treatment for B12 deficiency. Now, oral B12 supplements may provide help for some people. As part of a recent study, oral B12 supplements were given to eight people who had low stomach-acid production and eight "normal" elderly people. Neither group had any difficulty absorbing similar amounts of the vitamins. The results suggest that when B12 supplements are taken separately from meals, the recipient may overcome his or her absorption problems, at least in the early stages. Reversing B12 deficiency could also lead to reversing any related mental and/or physical problem.

Early Diagnosis For Alzheimer's Disease

Until now, the most common method of diagnosing Alzheimer's disease was by eliminating all other possibilities. Some studies indicate that doctors may misdiagnose between 10 to 20 percent of those patients. Most doctors agree that what is needed is a test which will accurately diagnose the disease in its early stages.

According to researchers at SIBIA Inc., of San Diego, they may have developed just such a test. If the new test proves to be both effective and accurate, it would allow patients to plan for long-term care. It would also allow for earlier treatment of Alzheimer's disease which has been diagnosed in over 4 million Americans.

Researchers are also working on the development of a new test to determine those people who are most vulnerable to Alzheimer's disease. According to initial findings, a little known substance called beta amyloid protein may form the brain plaques which are responsible for the disease.

Scientists speculate that beta amyloid protein buildup over an individual's lifetime could make him or her more susceptible to Alzheimer's disease. If researchers are successful in developing a "susceptibility test" they may also then be closer to uncovering ways to reduce the risk of having Alzheimer's disease.

The Alzheimer's Disease Society can provide more information about Alzheimer's disease and the latest scientific developments. Write to the Society at 2 West 45th Street, Room 1703, New York, New York,

---

10036, or call (212) 719-4744. You can also call the Alzheimer's Disease and Related Disorders Association at 800-621-0379.

The Importance of Flu Shots

Influenza, the viral infection more commonly called the flu, can be especially hard on an older person. An annual flu shot is recommended in the fall for men and women over 65, especially those who have a chronic illness, such as heart disease, bronchitis, emphysema, or diabetes. A flu shot provides six to eight months protection for up to 60 to 90 percent of those who receive it. The vaccine itself is changed every year to contain any viruses that are most likely to spread.

To protect yourself against pneumonia, experts now advise that you get a once-in-a-lifetime vaccination. This shot contains strains of the pneumococcal bacteria that are largely responsible for causing pneumonia. Everyone over 65 is advised to get this shot. The vaccination is especially important for men and women who have chronic respiratory disease.

If the number of influenza and pneumonia cases are combined, they rank as the sixth leading cause of death for all Americans and the fifth leading cause of death in people over 65.

13 Things You Can Do To Live Up To Ten Years Longer

1) Watch your diet— a recent study at the University of Texas in San Antonio may provide some valuable insight into the effects of diet on the aging process. The study was conducted on a colony of laboratory rats who were placed on diet restrictions. Researchers found that by cutting the caloric intake of the rats by 60 percent of normal, and preventing malnutrition from occurring, they were able to lengthen the rats' life spans by as much as 50 percent. The researchers are now studying this information, in hopes of finding ways of applying it to humans. to stay young and healthy. The experts recommend that you choose foods that are rich in vitamins and minerals, and stay away from those foods with empty calories from sugar and fat. The key is cutting your total caloric intake, while getting enough essential nutrients. One way to do that is to increase your intake of vitamins A and C.

2) Maintain a desirable weight— a study at Harvard School of Public Health links obesity—being 20 percent or more above desirable weight—with premature death. It is also known that obesity can contribute to adult onset diabetes, heart disease, arthritis, respiratory problems, gall bladder disease, menstrual abnormalities, and high blood pressure. If you need to lose weight, you should follow a moderate diet designed to take off 1 or 2 pounds a week (see chapter 4).

3) Exercise regularly— exercise leads to fitness which in turn provides defense against disease. It is also important that you maintain as much flexibility as possible to avoid stiffness and back trouble. Even if you can't get a full work out, you should do some lower-body stretches for 5 minutes each morning and upper-body stretches for 5 minutes during the day. The more sedentary and out-of-shape you are, the older you'll feel, and the faster the aging process will be working on your body.

4) Don't smoke— you'll have practically no chance of slowing down the aging process and staying young longer if you smoke. There is enough hard evidence to prove that cigarette smoking will shorten your life by causing heart disease, emphysema, cancer, and a multitude of other health problems. Smoking is an excellent way to grow old before your time.

5) Take time for rest and relaxation— there is a world of difference between being a couch potato and relaxing. A daily battle with anxiety, tension, and stress can make you feel as if the "weight of the world" is on your shoulders. It can also sap your strength and wreak havoc with your immune system, leaving you vulnerable to all sorts of health disorders. In short, stress is another factor that can rob you of your youth and speed up the aging process. The best way to deal with stress is by learning to relax (see chapter 7). You should learn and practice daily a relaxation technique.

6) Avoid overexposure to the sun and cold— as we get older, we also become more vulnerable to the excesses of heat and hypothermia, because the aging body doesn't handle temperature fluctuations as efficiently as it once did. Whenever you are exposed to the sun, you should use a sunscreen with a protection factor of 15, especially during the late morning and early afternoon when the sun is at its strongest.

7) Mentally challenge yourself— just as allowing your body to "go to seed" can speed up the aging process, allowing your mind to go

unused can also be debilitating. A continuing research project into the intellectual abilities of over 200 men and women who have gone from middle to old age, suggests that those people who retain their mental abilities over an extended period of time, tend to lead more stimulating and involved lifestyles than those people who experienced reduced mental capacities. It is important that you stay involved and pursue environmental stimulation, and that you continue to think and to mentally explore the world around you.

8) Maintain a positive outlook— this is one of the most powerful secrets of staying young. If you have a positive outlook on life and expect to live a long time you'll actually have a much better chance of doing so. Your attitude in both sickness and health, plays a significant role in determining both the quality and duration of your life (see chapter 7). Think positive. Think young.

9) Don't abuse alcohol or other drugs— alcohol can damage the heart, liver, nervous system, and brain, as well as other organ systems. It also increases the risk of developing cancer of the larynx, the esophagus, and the pancreas. Alcohol and drug consumption are also significant factors in accidents on the road, at work and in the home. Alcohol abuse is essentially an assault on your body which can result not only in premature aging, it can also lead to premature death.

10) Find what makes you happy and do it— your satisfaction and pleasure in life is essential to the maintenance of good health, youthful vitality, and in achieving long life.

11) Maintain warm social relationships— studies in both Michigan and Ohio have shown that stable relationships can boost an individual's immune function as well as lower his or her risk of dying from any cause at any age.

12) Maintain a high level of independence— according to research at Harvard- Yale, maintaining a consistent level of autonomy may help lead to a longer, healthier life.

13) Don't give up on sex— the happiest people in America, according to a recent study conducted in Chicago, are married couples who have frequent sex after age 60. People who are happy, generally tend to have longer lives than those who aren't.

7 Tips To Have Or Maintain Younger-Looking Skin

The ravages of time are nowhere more apparent than in the condition of the skin. As you get older, the colagen tissues in your face begin to break down, causing your skin to wrinkle and sag. While nothing can prevent this process from occurring, there are several basic ways you can slow it down.

How young or old you look depends largely on how young or old your skin appears. By taking good care of your skin and by giving it the protection it needs, it will retain its youthful appearance, and so will you. On the other hand, if you neglect your skin, or otherwise care for it improperly, you will not be able to slow down the obvious signs of aging. By following some basic guidelines, you can have smooth, firm, youthful skin.

1) Cleanse— every day your skin is attacked by germs, grease, grime, perspiration, oils, cosmetics, and pollutants, so it is important that you do all you can to keep it clean. When you wash your face you should avoid extreme temperatures—use water that is warm, lukewarm or cool, but not hot. Excessive heat can cause a great deal of damage to the skin.

The soap you use should be mild. Since soaps are alkaline, they can cause drying even though they contain fats such as coconut and palm oil for lathering. If you have sensitive skin, you should try a soap containing additional fats. New, synthetic-detergent soaps may work well for you, as they seem to cause less irritation than conventional soaps, and they leave less residue.

To cleanse your face properly, you should make a soapy lather in your hands— don't use a wash cloth or sponge—then smooth the lather lightly over your skin and rinse thoroughly with luke-warm water. Gently pat dry with a clean towel.

2) Moisturize— a common affliction of aging skin is dryness, and while dryness does not cause wrinkles, it does make them appear to be more pronounced. The key to combating such dryness is moisturizing. The purpose of a moisturizer is not to provide moisture on its own, but to remain on the surface of the skin and seal in whatever moisture is already there. That means you will want to apply a moisturizer when your skin is already moist. The best way to do that is to allow the bathroom to get

steamy before you take a bath or shower. Then soak or shower for 15 minutes or longer to let the water seep deeply into your skin. Don't towel your skin completely dry because you will want to apply a moisturizer to your still damp skin. Smooth the moisturizer over all areas which are likely to be exposed during the day.

Most commercial moisturizers are relatively inexpensive and work quite well. Many dermatologists recommend using a moisturizer containing such effective moisturizing substances as petrolatum, which has plenty of ability to lock water into the skin, and glycerin, which draws water up from the lower skin layers. It may be necessary for you to experiment with different kinds of moisturizers in order to find the formulation that works best for you.

3) Protect yourself from the sun— this is the most important step you can take in order to have healthier, younger-looking skin. Experts say that 80 percent of all skin damage, including wrinkling, roughening, discoloration, broken blood vessels, sagging, and skin cancers, is caused by chronic exposure to the sun. The only way to protect your skin from such damage (other than remaining indoors) is to use an effective sunscreen. No matter how light or dark your natural skin is, you should use a sunscreen on all sun-exposed areas of your body whenever you plan to be out in the sun for more than a few minutes.

FDA regulations require sunscreens to be labeled with sun-protection-factor (SPF) numbers. Whenever you are going to be outdoors in bright sunlight for any length of time, you should use a product with a SPF of 15 or higher. In general, the higher the SPF number, the higher the protection. The sunscreen you choose should also be waterfast. Apply the sunscreen liberally to dry skin before you use a moisturizer, and 15 to 20 minutes before you plan on going outside. You should reapply the sunscreen after heavy sweating or after swimming.

Even when you acquire a tan very gradually using a high-potency sunscreen— either outdoors or in a tanning booth—your skin is being damaged. That's why many dermatologists recommend that instead of exposing yourself to the skin- aging and-damaging power of the sun, you apply your own tan with a bronzer. It's the safest and surest way to protect your skin from the sun and to keep it looking smooth, young, and healthy.

4) Don't take chances— there are numerous medical skin treatments used by Americans every day. Some of the treatments are relatively effective, but none is without a certain amount of risk. Even so, some reports indicate that about 100,000 people in North America had collagen injected into their skin to eliminate acne scars and wrinkles on the cheeks and around the eyes. No one can say for certain how long the results of these injections will last— some say six months to a year, and others say not nearly that long. And just recently, many people have begun reporting side effects, ranging from temporary allergic reaction to disease and permanent disfigurement. As of now, the debate continues whether or not collagen injections present a serious risk, but it is a treatment you should investigate as thoroughly as possible before trying.

Liquid silicone injections are also causing quite a stir. Even though the FDA has not yet given its approval of liquid silicone for dermatological use, some doctors are still injecting it into patients' skin to smooth out wrinkles and scars. Experts say that since silicone lasts forever, complications such as autoimmune disorders are difficult to correct. Silicone can also swell and harden tissues inside the body, causing permanent disfigurement and damage to internal structures.

5) Stop smoking— besides all the other health problems attributed to smoking, a study at the University of Utah Health Sciences Center in Salt Lake City suggests that cigarette smoking causes premature facial wrinkles.

Researchers studied 132 men and women with an average age of 47 and found that those people who had smoked an average of two packs a day for 25 years were 5 times more likely to get facial wrinkles than were non-smokers.

6) Drink plenty of water— some medical experts recommend that you pay attention to how much water you drink because it can make a difference in the overall appearance of your skin. You should try to drink at least 6 to 8 glasses of water or other noncaffeinated fluids every day to help flush out toxins and to help keep your skin moist and young looking.

7) Exercise— studies show that physical exercise, if sufficiently vigorous, can have a beneficial effect on your skin. Through exercise, your skin receives a better flow of blood, making you look healthier, younger and more attractive. According to researchers, their findings from

a study of several age-matched pairs of sedentary and active people show that there is a pronounced difference in skin tone and texture between the two. The skin of those who exercised looked smoother, more supple, and had fewer wrinkles and better color than the skin of those people who did not get regular exercise.

Eat These Foods For Younger -Looking, More Attractive Skin

A diet which is severely deficient in essential vitamins can lead to skin disorders which can dramatically affect a person's appearance. On the other hand, nutritionists insist that a well-balanced diet with plenty of nutrients can produce a smoother, healthier, younger-looking skin.

Both vitamin A and zinc play important roles in assuring normal, healthy skin. While vitamin A helps to replenish skin cells, keeping the skin supple and preventing dryness, zinc helps the skin repair itself. To get more zinc in your diet, you can utilize these food sources: beef, seafood, eggs, milk, whole-grain cereals and breads, and legumes.

Dark green leafy vegetables have plenty of beta-carotene, which the body converts into vitamin A. Other good food sources of vitamin A include carrots, cantaloupes, winter squash, sweet potatoes, sweet red peppers, apricots, and mangoes.

Another nutrient, vitamin C, aids in improving the blood supply to the skin. It also helps in forming collagen, the protein which gives the skin a smooth appearance. Good food sources of vitamin C include citrus fruits and juices, cauliflower, Brussels sprouts, snow peas, broccoli, watermelons, honeydew melons, and tomatoes.

The nutrients obtained from the vitamin B complex help to prevent scaling and cracking of the skin. There are a number of food sources for B-complex vitamins including organ meats, peas, potatoes, fish, green leafy vegetables (the darker the leaves the more nutritional value), fruits, nuts, whole-grain products, cheese, tuna, dairy products, beef, poultry, oysters, mushrooms, and yeast.

As an antioxidant, vitamin E may help to protect skin cells against the damage of abnormal oxidation. It also helps in the process of healing the skin. Good food sources of vitamin E include dried beans, margarine, vegetable oils, and green leafy vegetables.

The Make-Up You Should Use To Have Skin Like A Model's

It's really not too difficult to keep your skin gorgeous and young-looking. You'll need to be willing to take precautions against sun damage 12 months a year, and make an effort to keep your skin from becoming too dry. One way to avoid dry skin is to eliminate caffeine and nicotine from your system. You should also make sure you drink lots of fluids.

Another important factor in protecting your skin is the type of make-up you wear. Many of the best-selling brands of make-up are designed with only one thing in mind— making you look better. That means that safety is sometimes not a high priority, and that some best-selling make-up products have additives that could actually be bad for you. You can protect yourself and your skin by using these little-known make-up secrets, recommended by many of today's top models:

1) Cornstarch can be used as a face powder. It has the advantages of being free of additives, and just a dab can cover up a shiny nose.

2) An egg white, either straight from the shell or whipped, makes a great, inexpensive and safe face masque. An egg white contains proteins that should bring dirt and other foreign matter to the surface of your skin. Once you've washed off the "egg white masque", your skin should look smoother and younger.

3) Mineral oil can be used instead of commercial lip gloss. The oil is actually the active ingredient in all commercial lip glosses, and it doesn't have any potentially harmful additives.

4) One way to get rid of undereye circles and puffiness is to apply moistened tea bags, or cold cucumber or potato slices for about ten minutes while you close your eyes and relax.

5) Cornmeal or oatmeal, mixed into a paste, is a safe and effective way to remove dead skin cells. Some models recommed a mixture of two teaspoons of cornmeal or oat meal with enough honey to form a

paste. Apply the paste to your face gently in a circular motion and rinse with luke-warm water.

6) The common avocado works great for smoothing and drying skin. It contains its own natural oils that are safe and effective in making your skin look smooth and fresh.

New Way To Get A Beautiful Tan Without Harmful Sun Or Tanning Beds

Someday soon, you may be able to get a beautiful tan without exposing yourself to the damaging power of the sun or frequenting a tanning booth. Researchers are currently working on a way to allow people to get a safe tan by taking a shot or an injection.

Initial findings indicate that a synthetic hormone may make tanning possible without exposure to the sun. It may also provide protection against continued sun damage.

In a recent study, some of the men participating, received 10 injections of a synthetic version of melanocytestimulating hormone (MSH) while others were given an inactive saline solution over 12 days. Several of the men in the study were known to tan easily and others sunburned easily.

The results of the study showed that the skin of the men who received the hormone actually darkened. Some of these men even stayed tan up through a seven-week observation period which followed the injections.

Researchers say that the drug works by stimulating an enzyme which in turn triggers the production of melanin— the substance which is responsible for skin color. Studies into the feasibility of "tanning injections" continue.

Little-Known Effects Of Cold Weather On Your Skin

It's not only during the hottest days of summer that your skin can be seriously damaged by exposure to the sun. Dermatologists say you are just as vulnerable to sunburn and sun damage to your skin throughout the coldest days of winter as you are during summer. The reason the skin is in year-round danger from chronic exposure to the sun is not because of the heat from the sun, but rather the real danger stems from the sun's ultraviolet light which streams down in every season of the year. For example, snow can reflect the potent untraviolet rays and increase their danger just as easily as warm summer sand can.

To protect your skin from burning during cold weather, continue to use a potent sunscreen, just as you did during the summer months. Obviously you won't be spending as much time outdoors when it's cold, but when you do go outside, you should make sure your skin is protected.

Since your skin must be kept moist in order to maintain its healthy, youthful glow, it is necessary to take some extra precautions during cold weather. The dry outside air during periods of cold weather can draw the protective moisture from the skin, causing it to become chapped, rough, scaly, and sometimes badly cracked. Even soap and water can cause damage to the skin in cold weather, because it removes fats and oils. You can control the damage, keeping it at a minimum by taking fewer baths, using lukewarm or tepid water instead of hot water. You can also help protect your skin from cold-weather dryness by using creams and lotions containing oil. These products work by providing a film of oil which prevents natural moisture from evaporating from the skin. As an anti-aging strategy, protecting your skin in cold weather is just as important as protection during the heat of summer.

3 Common Products
That Worsen Dry Skin Problems

People commonly use such products as after-shave lotions, astringents and toner because they provide a feeling of freshness. But some dermatologists say that, except on very oily skin, such products have little value and may in fact cause a dry skin problem to worsen. The experts say that if you use such compounds, go with those that have the lowest percentage of alcohol, and avoid putting astringents on irritated skin.

These Delicious Foods Will Help You Have Longer, Thicker Hair

Having a healthy, shining head of hair is almost as important as having vibrant skin when it comes to giving a person a youthful appearance. Many of the problems we have with our hair can be traced to an unbalanced diet. Medical experts say that when a diet doesn't contain an adequate amount of amino acids—the basic structural units of all protein—there is a dramatic increase in hair loss, because the body must break down its own protein.

To get more amino acids into your diet you can consume meats, eggs, milk, grains, and legumes. Since the body can not store protein, foods high in protein must be consumed every day.

There are also many simple and safe ways of "keeping the gray away" and maintaining youthful hair color at its peak. Some people find graying hair to be a distinguishing characteristic and don't mind relinquishing their "youthful" hair color. But for many others, both men and women, gray hair simply means they are losing their youthful appearance. For those people, there is a wide range of effective and inexpensive hair-color products available at most drugstores and supermarkets. If you don't choose to do the coloring yourself, let a professional hairdresser do it for you.

The Best Ways To Eliminate Unsightly Facial Hair

There are several methods for getting rid of facial hair. Here are some of the most effective treatments recommended by experts:

1) Tweezing— this method can be painful and is not recommended for large areas or extremely sensitive spots such as nipples or the stomach. Tweezing can be effective for getting rid of isolated facial hairs, and regrowth is slow.

2) Depilatories— this treatment is good for eliminating hair on the upper lip. It requires some waiting time and may dry and irritate the skin. The treatment should be done in a well-ventilated area.

3) Electronic tweezing— this is an excellent treatment for small facial hairs. Its results usually last from two to three weeks. Regular tweezing is usually just as effective and less time-consuming and costly.

4) Electrolysis— this is the only proven method of permanent hair removal, and is best for small to medium-size areas. The treatment requires a skilled operator. It is expensive, time-consuming, and sometimes painful.

Secret To Needing Bikini Waxing Done Only About Half As Often

Insiders say that to cut down on the number of times you need to wax in order to get your bikini line set to bare can be reduced by half with professional electrolysis. As mentioned earlier in this chapter, electrolysis must be performed by a skilled operator and often results in permanent hair removal. Instead of waxing or tweezing between visits to the electrolysist, it is recommended that you shave.

If electrolysis is too expensive, or simply not for you, here are tips for waxing:

1) For best results, powder your skin before you wax.

2) Before using the wax, test its temperature on the inside of your wrist.

3) After waxing, apply a mild astringent to soothe your skin and reduce any swelling. Avoid sunbathing and chlorine for several hours.

How To Protect Your Eyes From Aging Sign

The aging process can be especially noticeable in the area around your eyes. That's because the skin around your eyes is thinner and more delicate than on any other part of your body. To slow the aging process in the area around your eyes you must do everything you can to protect the entire area— including your eyelids.

There are several routine factors that cause wear and tear around your eyes. By avoiding or minimizing these factors you can maintain your smooth, youthful skin, and, in effect, a youthful appearance around your eyes.

1) Friction— done often enough, even a minimal amount of rubbing can cause injury to the skin around the eyes. That's why it is important that you avoid, as much as possible, the common habit of rubbing your eyes, especially when they feel tired or sleepy. Rubbing your eyes in such a manner causes friction and could produce or worsen bags under the eyes because the skin stretches. Often, people who rub their eyes frequently, end up looking weary even when they are not.

2) Applying and removing makeup— the application and removal of certain kinds of eye makeup can also cause stretching, and lead to the appearance of "tired eyes". Whenever eye shadow or eye liner is applied and whenever makeup remover is used to remove waterproof mascara and liner, the skin is bound to be stretched. Some cosmetic consultants recommend that you use only an eye-brow pencil and non-waterproof mascara on the area around the eye, except on special occasions. Neither product involves the application or removal of cosmetics to and from the skin, and both come off easily at the end of the day with just a little soap and warm water.

3) Squinting— even a natural adaptive response such as squinting can eventually help make you look older. Most people squint instinctively as protection against excessive light. You are also likely to squint when you are trying to focus on something you are not able to see very well. While it may seem rather innocuous, such squinting simply "engraves" squint lines, or crow's feet, around your eyes.

The best way to prevent squinting and the resulting damage to the skin around your eyes, is to wear tinted glasses to protect your eyes against bright light while you are outdoors, and glasses or contacts indoors or out to correct any vision problems.

Since wind and extremes of temperature compound the damage caused by chronic sun exposure, wearing glasses can also provide a shield against the elements. Even if you wear contact lenses for general use, it's a good idea to have a pair of tinted or plain glasses on hand to wear whenever you go outside to help prevent the signs of aging around your eyes.

The disadvantages to AHAs are the same as those for Retin-A, although they are not quite as drying. AHA treatment costs the fee of an office visit, plus about $50 for the prescribed cream.

New Treatment For Facial Wrinkles

A quick and inexpensive treatment for facial wrinkles may have been discovered in a most unlikely source— botulinum toxin. Until now, this toxin's main claim to fame was that it often causes serious and sometimes fatal paralysis when it contaminates food. Although it sounds nasty, new research indicates that small doses of the toxin—known as botox— may be an effective treatment for facial wrinkles.

In earlier studies, researchers have found that botox, when injected into muscles around the eyes, eases certain spasmodic conditions. It has also proven to be an effective therapy for abnormal contractions or tics in the face, neck, and arms and legs. While studying the treatment of those disorders with botox, researchers discovered that the toxin also seemed to smooth out the patients' facial wrinkles.

According to the researchers, botox does not "distort" the face as does collagen and silicone. It works by weakening underlying muscles which can cause wrinkles by tugging at the skin. The researchers also say that botox treatments must be performed every four to six months, but that after an accumulation of injections, the benefits may begin to last longer.

New studies are now underway as researchers continue to investigate the potential of botox, how to determine correct dosages, and how to correct any side effects, such as increased local muscle weakness, as experienced by some patients in earlier studies.

Immune Boosters To Combat Aging
And Fight-Off Disease

The immune system is one of the primary factors involved in the aging process. As we get older, the body's ability to recognize and ward off foreign invaders deteriorates, leaving us increasingly vulnerable to many serious health disorders, including cancer. Scientists have been trying for several years to find a way to strengthen the immune system—ideally, to make it somehow impervious to the effects of aging.

With biotechnology, researchers may have recently taken a step in that direction by making it possible to isolate and mass-produce substances that bolster the immune system. Many of these immune-boosting substances, such as interleukin 2, have been tested on cancer and AIDS patients, but some experts believe that small doses of certain "immune boosters" may also slow down the aging process. Whether or not these current immune boosters being tested prove to be effective in combating aging remains to be seen, but initial results are encouraging.

Other studies of the immune system suggest that aging and decline in immune function may result, at least in part, from damage to cells caused by certain toxic compounds known as free radicals. Researchers say that antioxidants, such as vitamins E and C and beta carotene, may be able to counteract or impair the ability of free radicals to attack healthy cells. If true, anti- oxidants will help to avoid some of the cell damage.

Vitamins E, C, and beta carotene have already been credited with being powerful disease-fighters, with the ability to slow down or prevent a number of ailments usually associated with aging. If the new information proves true, and these antioxidants can help slow down the decline of the immune system, their reputations will be even more firmly established.

The Great Truth About Vitamin C

New research suggests that vitamin C may help reduce the risk of heart disease, thereby leading to a longer life. The recent findings indicate that men and women who get high levels of vitamin C every day may live longer, more youthful lives.

A decade-long study involving over 11,000 adults revealed that women who had the highest level of vitamin C intake experienced a 10 percent lower overall death rate and a 25 percent lower heart disease death rate than women taking a lower amount of vitamin C. Men in the high vitamin C group (intake averaged 300 milligrams per day—50 or more milligrams from food, and a regular intake of supplements) experienced a 41 percent lower death rate during that ten year period, compared with men who were taking 50 milligrams naturally. Men in the high vitamin C group were also 45 percent less likely to die of heart disease than were men in the low-intake group.

The researchers say that vitamin C may help prevent heart disease by using its antioxidant properties to block the activity of unstable molecules of oxygen, which damage cells and may trigger heart disease. While vitamin C appears to have an independent effect on preventing heart disease, researchers say it is more likely to be effective when combined with other healthful practices.

How To Feel Better And Look Younger By Losing Cellulite

Cellulite— the excess fat that collects under the skin—is a reminder to many people that they are not as young as they used to be. For those people, getting rid of cellulite is often a way to reclaim a youthful appearance. It can also be a very difficult thing to do. Massages, creams and gels, all claiming to be the answer to cellulite, have proven to be ineffective in the long-term.

Experts say the best way to get rid of fatty deposits is to maintain a low-fat diet along with a regular program of aerobic exercise. Properly followed, such an eating and exercise routine can prevent the storage of fat as well as help bring about fat mobilization. Fat cells which produce cellulite tend to grow or shrink depending on the ratio of the body's storage of fat to its mobilization of fat.

To inhibit fat storage, try a low-fat diet which is high in complex carbohydrates. The best way to bring about fat mobilization and lasting weight loss is to complement your diet with aerobic exercise, ideally, performed four times a week. The areas of the body in which you lose fat more quickly are determined by genetics, but a concerted effort on your part—proper diet and exercise—can eliminate cellulite and help you to maintain a more youthful appearance.

Here is a "hopping" exercise, recommended by some experts as an addition to a 20 minute aerobic workout, that may be of benefit in your battle against cellulite:

1) With your feet placed close together and your arms near your sides, begin hopping on both feet.

2) Pause for a few seconds, then begin hopping on your right foot while you touch the floor with your left heel, in the direction of your left side.

3) Return to step one and hop on both feet, finally reversing the procedure by hopping on your left foot, with your right heel touching the floor toward your right side.

The Benefits And Risks Of Cosmetic Surgery

Each year, millions of American men and women undergo plastic surgery. In many cases, the surgery is performed in order to improve appearance and provide a "youthful look". For many people, such surgery is an anti-aging strategy designed to remove excess skin and fat and any unflattering wrinkles or marks that are a result of the aging process. The surgery is most commonly performed on the eyelids, face, breasts, and stomach. Here are several of the most common "anti-aging" cosmetic surgery techniques:

1) Liposuction— this cosmetic procedure is performed more often in the United States than any other type of plastic surgery. Figures from the American Society of Plastic and Reconstructive Surgeons (ASPRS) indicate that almost 110,000 liposuction procedures were performed in the U.S. in 1990. The procedure removes fat deposits from various areas of the body. Muscles are not affected by the surgery, and fat is removed from below the skin— no skin is removed.

The area of the body to be liposuctioned is anesthetized and a suction instrument (cannula) is inserted through a small skin incision (about 1/2 inch) and moved back and forth under the skin to break up large areas of fat which are then suctioned through the instrument. The entire procedure usually takes about 45 minutes for any specific part of the body. After the fat has been removed from various areas of the body, those areas should look smaller, more defined, and consequently more youthful.

Minor scarring from the procedure may occur, but hardly any

stitches are needed. However, the procedure usually results in pain, numbness or discomfort for several days. There will also most likely be some dimpling of the skin, swelling, and discoloration of the skin for six to eight weeks. It should also be noted that the total amount of fat which can be suctioned at one time is limited, and the procedure can not be used as a substitute for proper weight control.

Having the liposuction procedure performed on your face will cost anywhere from $2,500 to $3,500; stomach, $3,000 to $6,500; hips, $3,000 to $6,000; and other areas, including the buttocks and thighs, from $3,500 to $7,000.

2) Face-lift— this procedure is a cosmetic operation to smooth out wrinkles and lift sagging skin to give the face a more youthful appearance. Depending on a patient's needs, the skin and muscle layers are both tightened, and the layer of fat is removed or shifted or injected into other areas. A face-lift is often performed on an out-patient basis, and unless there are complications, patients can return to their normal activities in a week to ten days.

The procedure may cause some bruising of the face, but there is usually no pain. There may also be some bleeding below the flaps of the skin that were lifted and tightened. The area should be drained or washed out thoroughly in the operating room to cut down on the risk of infection.

3) Eye-lift— this procedure has become a very popular anti-aging technique as it removes deposits of fat and excess skin to give the eye area a more youthful appearance. Two separate operations are required for the upper and lower eyelids.

While the surgery allows a patient to return to normal activities after a couple of days, it may also leave behind some fat. If that occurs, a second operation is required. There is also the risk of the surgeon removing too much skin. Eye-lifts are usually priced from $1,500 to $5,000.

4) Abdominal Wall Reduction (Abdominoplasty or Tummy Tuck)— this is a contouring operation in which excess skin and fat are removed from the abdomen. The most common abdominal wall procedure is performed using a general anesthesia and may require a hospital stay of two to three days. The surgeon makes a horizontal incision along

the bikini line and another around the navel. The skin is then pulled away from the abdominal wall and raised above the rib cage. The loose tissue which covers the abdomen's large vertical muscle is then pulled toward the center of the abdomen, where the surgeon sutures it together, tightening the muscles and providing a firmer abdominal wall and a more youthful looking narrow waistline. The flap of skin is then pulled downand the excess is removed.

Following this procedure, most people experience some soreness and discomfort. Scars caused by the surgery are permanent, however they usually lighten within three to six months. A tummy tuck costs, on the average, from $1,100 to $8,500.

5 Keys To Find A Good Cosmetic Surgeon

The most recent statistics show that well over 3 million Americans undergo plastic surgery each year. Most of the people who have such surgery—to improve their appearances or correct damage caused by accidents or disease— report that they experience no serious side effects and are completely satisfied with the results.

Even so, experts are recommending that anyone who is considering cosmetic surgery should take some common sense precautions in finding a qualified and skilled practitioner. Since this is an almost $4-billion-a-year industry, some unethical and unqualified people have "taken up practice". The result has been tragic for the thousands of people who have been mutilated and swindled out of millions of dollars.

There are only about 4000 physicians who are properly board-certified in plastic surgery, and finding one of those can be quite time-consuming. How can you be sure of getting one of these properly certified, skilled doctors to perform your cosmetic surgery? Here are several expert suggestions to help you make the right choice:

1) Inspect the doctor's credentials. You can find out if the doctor has been certified by calling the American Board of Medical Specialties at 800-776-2378 or the American Society of Plastic and Reconstructive Surgeons at 800-635- 0635. If the doctor objects to such a background check, mark him or her off your list and find someone else.

You can also find out whether or not the doctor is a member of the staff of a major hospital— practically all hospitals require that their doctors carry malpractice insurance. If the doctor is on the staff of a hospital, you can ask if he or she has the hospital privileges to perform the procedure you want, even if the surgery is to be done in the doctor's office. If the doctor has no such privileges, find another doctor.

2) Ask the doctor to give you "references". Request the names of people upon whom the doctor has performed the same procedure that you are considering. Talk with these former patients and find out whether or not they are satisfied with the doctor and their surgery.

3) Be suspicious of any doctor who talks exclusively of miraculous results, and a safe, quick surgery, never mentioning any possible risks and complications.

4) Make sure there will be adequate emergency equipment and an experienced anesthetist on hand if the surgery is to be performed at a doctor's office or at a surgical center.

5) The doctor should take your complete medical history and give you a thorough physical examination. It may also be prudent to bring along to the consultation an objective friend or family member to provide another perspective.

Extend Your Life Through Meditation?

There may not be a fountain of youth, but the ancient practice of meditation might hold a key to slowing the aging process. According to a new study at the Maharishi Ayur-Veda Health Center for Behavioral Medicine and Stress Management in Lancaster, Massachusetts, people who meditate regularly may have levels of an age-related hormone similar to "non-meditators" who are 5 to 10 years younger.

The study, reported in the Journal of Behavioral Medicine, focused on transcendental meditation (TM), which is the most commonly practiced type of meditation in the United States. TM involves sitting quietly with eyes closed while thinking of a "meaningless sound" called a mantra. This type of meditation is usually practiced for at least 20 minutes each day.

Chromium May Help You Live Longer

While it works for rats, researchers can't say for certain that dietary supplements of the metal chromium can extend a human life span. But, according to the researchers from Bemidji State University in Minnesota, the findings are promising.

During the study, researchers gave a special chromium supplement to ten rats and compared them to 20 rats that received chromium in a form less readily absorbed. After almost 3 1/2 years, the researchers reported that 80 percent of the rats that received chromium picolinate were still alive, while all the other rats were dead. The results show that the rats that received the supplements lived an average of one year longer than the others.

Until now, research had uncovered only one factor which could produce substantial increases in life span in animals— a significant reduction in caloric intake. The new information about chromium supplements changes all of that because the supplements can produce an equally large increase in life span without any dietary restrictions.

According to one expert, more than 90 percent of adult Americans have a chromium deficiency, mostly because it is not readily absorbed from many foods. Recently, researchers from the USDA developed and patented a form of chromium, called chromium picolinate that is easily absorbed. That's the form the researchers used in the 3 1/2 year study.

4 Ways To Get More Attention And Better Service From Your Doctor

How many times have you come away from a visit to your doctor more confused or in the dark about your condition than you were before the consultation and prescribed treatment? Actually, that sort of unsettling experience happens to many people who subsequently feel they may not have received the best care possible. The best way to avoid such an experience is to be prepared. Here are several suggestions that may help you get more out of your doctors' visits:

1) Keep a diary of symptoms to show to your doctor. Such a diary or list will be a great help to the doctor in making a proper diagnosis and prescribing the right treatment.

2) If possible, do advance reading and research on your condition and symptoms to help you ask informed questions.

3) Carry a notepad to write down important information.

4) If there's something you don't understand—an explanation that isn't clear- -ask the doctor to go over the information again.

How Doctor's Can Be Dangerous To Your Health

If you want to be sure you're getting the best care from your doctor, you shouldn't be afraid to ask questions and/or provide the doctor with any pertinent information. That's the advice of researchers from Harvard University who recently conducted a study into the patient/physician relationships.

According to the study, doctors can become so intent on writing prescriptions and ordering the latest tests that they completely overlook providing patients with even the most basic information. In order to get the information you need about any medical problem, you must ask questions.

Over 500 physicians were involved in the study which presented a specific case scenario, requiring the doctors to indicate what questions they'd ask the patients and what treatment they would prescribe. In the hypothetical case, the patient was a man with stomach pain, and a test indicated stomach inflammation but not ulcer. Fully one-third of the doctors responded to the case scenario by saying they would not ask questions and would prescribe drugs, even though they were openly encouraged to ask for further information.

Researchers say that if those doctors had asked the patients a few questions, they would have found out that the patient took aspirin on a regular basis, was a heavy drinker and smoker and had recently gone through the death of a child— all factors which could contribute to the problem of stomach pain.

In order to avoid such "distracted" treatment and get the information you need, patients are encouraged to provide information and to ask their doctors questions, and doctors are advised to ask questions and to listen to their patients.

Two Things You Should Never Tell Your Doctor If You Want Correct Diagnosis And Treatment

Full communication with your doctor is essential if you want to receive the best treatment. Since much of a doctor's information comes from what you tell him or her, it is essential that you provide information as accurately as possible. Anything less could result in an improper diagnosis and treatment.

The first thing to remember is that you should never try to diagnose your illness for the doctor. Describe your symptoms, but don't tell your doctor what you think your illness is. While most doctors will investigate thoroughly before making a diagnosis and prescribing treatment, some may simply take your "diagnosis" without investigating. For example, if you tell your doctor you have a kidney infection, you may receive treatment for that condition when there may actually be something else wrong with you. Unless you have a medical degree, you aren't trained to diagnose illnesses— your doctor is. Tell your doctor, as accurately as you can, what's bothering you without offering your own diagnosis— diagnosing is the doctor's job.

You may also get an incorrect diagnosis if you don't reveal potentially important information, or if you don't answer your doctor's questions honestly. For example, if you have been taking any drugs, don't hide that fact from your doctor, or tell him or her "no" if the question is asked. Drugs such as Valium can produce Parkinson-like symptoms if taken in large enough doses over a long period of time. Withholding such information, or lying about it, could lead to an incorrect diagnosis and treatment.

11 Common Illnesses That Doctors Misdiagnose And Treat Wrong The Most Often

There are several factors which can affect a doctor's ability to diagnose a patient's symptoms. Sometimes a doctor's lack of knowledge of a disease can place certain limitations on his or her ability to diagnose a specific problem. At other times the elaborate array of tests doctors now have to help in making their diagnoses aren't always conclusive, and doctors sometimes have trouble interpreting them.

To further complicate the process, the specialist may not have a complete medical history and physical exam to refer to. There are also many diseases that have similar symptoms, making their diagnosis difficult. As a result, diagnosis is not an "exact" science. Here are several of the most commonly misdiagnosed, or hard to diagnose diseases and illnesses:

1) Osteoporosis— in a study conducted at the University of Kansas in Kansas City, researchers evaluated 180 women who had either had or were suspected of having osteoporosis. The researchers learned that in 46 percent of the women involved in the study, there were other health factors that could cause or worsen the disease but that had gone undetected by their doctors. Among those factors: menopause before age 40, thyroid disease, asthma or other lung diseases, and a loss of calcium through the kidneys. The researchers recommend that women should furnish their doctors with a complete and detailed medical history.

2) Food sensitivity— this involves an abnormal reaction to food or a food additive. It may or may not be caused by a food allergy. The illness can cause vomiting and/or diarrhea; hives; headaches and stomachaches; fatigue; respiratory problems; and severe cases can result in a life-threatening allergic reaction.

The symptoms are vague and may be hard to diagnose because they can suggest any number of illnesses. It is also difficult to track down the precise food causing the problem.

The American Academy of Allergy and Immunology, 611 East Wells Street, Milwaukee, WI 53202, can furnish you more information on food sensitivity. Write, or call, 414-272-6701.

3) Rheumatoid arthritis— this is an autoimmune affliction that causes inflammation of the joints. Its symptoms may include pain when moving; swollen, tender and painful wrist, knuckle or finger joints; stiffness; and difficulty forming a fist.

The problem can be hard to diagnose because blood tests may produce false- negative results. The symptoms are also similar to many other autoimmune disorders.

To get more information, you can write to: Arthritis Foundation, P.O. Box 19000, Atlanta, GA 30326, or call, 800-283-7800.

4) Fever— a recent study of persistent, unexplained fevers in children discovered that doctors who used an assortment of imaging tests, such as X- rays or Catscans, failed to make a diagnosis 66 percent of the time. The finding suggests that doctors should pay more attention to the symptoms, rely on basic laboratory findings and observe the child over time, in order to properly diagnose fevers.

5) Parkinson's disease— a degeneration of the nerve cells in the brain, the symptoms of this disease may include tremors, rigidity, and a shuffling gait. It can be hard to diagnose because the symptoms in the early stages can appear similar to those of other afflictions, including stroke.

More information about Parkinson's disease is available by writing to the National Parkinson's Foundation, 1501 Northwest Ninth Avenue, Miami, FL 33136, or by calling 800-327-4545.

6) Clinical depression— this is a disorder which is caused by a biochemical imbalance in the brain. It involves serious mood disturbances which impair the person's ability to function.

There are many possible symptoms of clinical depression including persistent sadness, emptiness or anxiety; loss of interest or pleasure in ordinary activities including sex; fatigue; changes in sleeping patterns; sudden fluctuations in weight; inability to concentrate or make decisions; forgetfulness; apathy; and thoughts of death or suicide.

The problems in diagnosing clinical depression arise from doctors who are not trained to detect a major depressive disorder. Such doctors are apt to misdiagnose the condition about half of the time. In many cases it is diagnosed as a "low" mood brought about by a stressful situation. Other times it is attributed to physical problems. Among elderly people, the symptoms of clinical depression are often misdiagnosed as the early stages of senility.

For general information about depression, you can write to the National Foundation for Depressive Illness, P.O. Box 2257, New York, NY 10116, or call 800-248-4344.

7) Multiple sclerosis— a progressive central nervous system disease which is thought to result from the breakdown of the myelin sheaths which protect and insulate nerve fibers in the brain and spinal cord.

The most common initial symptom of multiple sclerosis is numbness or tingling in the hands or feet. Other symptoms may include visual disturbances, muscle weaknesses, poor bladder control, balance problems or dizziness, or tremors.

The main problems involved with diagnosing this disease are that the early symptoms can easily be mistaken for other disorders, and the symptoms often disappear after a few weeks and then return months or years later.

To get more information write: National Multiple Sclerosis Society, 733 Third Avenue, Sixth Floor, New York, NY 10017, or call 800-624-8236.

8) Hypoglycemia— this is a condition in which the sugar content of the blood is abnormally low. The condition, which is common among diabetics can also be due to an underactive thyroid, improper diet or allergies, or emotional problems.

Two to five hours after each meal, a person with hypoglycemia may experience weakness, trembling, dizziness, sweating. fatigue, hunger, craving for sweets, and anxiety.

Current tests for hypoglycemia are not always conclusive. Some doctors may also be skeptical that such a condition exists at all, causing the illness to go undetected and unchecked.

Write to National Hypoglycemia Association, P.O. Box 120, Ridgewood, NJ 07451, or call 201-670-1189 for information about hypoglycemia.

9) Irritable Bowel Syndrome— a chronic gastrointestinal disorder which is made worse by emotional stress, some foods, and infections or illnesses. The condition is twice as common in women as it is in men. The symptoms may include diarrhea, often alternating with constipation; abdominal pain; bloating; heartburn and nausea; and mucus in stools.

Doctors may miss a correct diagnosis for this problem because its symptoms provide no clear cut possibility. In some cases the same symptoms can also be a normal reaction to a single episode of stress in many people who do not have irritable bowel syndrome. Usually, doctors diagnose irritable bowel syndrome by eliminating all other reasonable possibilities.

10) Subacute Bacterial Endocarditis— this is a bacterial infection of the valves of the heart, often the result of an upper respiratory tract infection or dental work. Its symptoms include weakness; fatigue; inter-mittent, low- grade fever; night sweats; chills; aches; and weight loss.

This condition is more commonly found among AIDS patients and in IV drug users. Doctors who are inexperienced in such cases may have difficulty recognizing the condition.

The American Heart Association at 7320 Greenville Avenue, Dallas, Texas 75231, has more information. Or call 214-373-6300.

11) Early Onset Emphysema— Lung specialists say that about one in three thousand people have alpha- antitrypsin deficiency, also known as early onset emphysema. The deficiency is often misdiagnosed because it is not well-recognized by many physicians. According to experts, if physicians are not lung specialists, they might not even know about the deficiency. In many cases it is confused with and misdiagnosed as asthma or bronchitis.

The deficiency is caused by an inherited lack of the protective protein, alpha-antitrypsin, and can be detected through a simple blood test. Experts say that not everyone who has the deficiency develops emphysema, and while the deficiency has no cure, researchers are hav-ing some success in developing a potential treatment to slow the progress of the disease. The treatment which is currently being tested involves giving patients back the missing protein intravenously through a substance called prolastin. The substance is derived from human plasma and according to researchers, has no significant side effects. Researchers need to conduct more tests with the new treatment before they can say for certain that it will slow the disease.

Early diagnosis is essential, otherwise the deficiency can devel-op into chronic asthma and lead to death. (Researchers say that smok-ers will die 20 years sooner than non-smokers who have the deficiency).

People who have a family history of emphysema or with symptoms including shortness of breath, excessive coughing, difficulty exhaling, wheezing, and a decreased ability to exercise, should be tested by a physician.

Warning:
Heart Catheterization May Not Be Necessary

A new study reveals that as many as 500,000 heart catheterizations performed each year to diagnose heart disease may be unnecessary.

The catheterization procedure involves inserting a catheter and injecting a dye-like substance in order to check for blocked arteries. It is the first step toward balloon angioplasty or bypass surgery. Researchers say that many people who have undergone the unneeded catheterizations have subsequently been subjected to unnecessary heart operations.

The findings—reported in the Journal of the American Medical Association—are based on a study of 160 people who were informed by doctors that they needed the catheterization procedure, but who subsequently sought a second opinion.

7 Ways To Protect Yourself From Medical Fakes

According to a nationwide poll, as many as 1 out of every 4 Americans has tried a "quack" or "miracle" treatment. In 1990, the House Committee on Health and Long-Term Care estimated that fake medicines and cures bilk consumers out of as much as 10 billion dollars each year.

Another report, issued by the American Medical Association's Council on Scientific Affairs in 1990, estimated that 4 to 5 billion dollars a year is spent on unapproved and questionable cancer tests and treatment. The report also estimated that as many as 30 percent of all cancer patients paid for and underwent "worthless" treatments. Experts say that if people seek "traditional" treatment as soon as possible after being diagnosed, they stand a good chance of recovery in many cases. But, if you succumb to a promise of a "miracle cure" before you get conventional treatment, you may be risking your life.

Here are several things you can do to protect yourself from medical charlatans and worthless products.

1) If you need a specialist, get a referral from your family doctor or some other physician you trust. You can also get reliable referrals from hospitals that are affiliated with medical schools.

2) Discuss any treatment you are considering with your family doctor before you make any decisions.

3) Contact your state medical board if you have any questions about a specific doctor. The medical board will be able to tell you if any charges have been made against the doctor in question.

4) You can find out about cancer treatments and clinics by calling the National Cancer Institute's Information Hotline— 800-422-6237.

5) Don't buy any unconventional products before you check them out thoroughly with the nearest FDA office, local consumer agency, or Better Business Bureau.

6) Be suspicious of advertising and phrases such as "miracle cure", "secret formula", and "amazing health care breakthrough".

7) Stay away from any doctor who prescribes expensive vitamins and supplements, or who sells them in his office.

How To Avoid Long Waits In The Doctor's Office

Doctors are usually pretty busy people which often means that patients spend a lot of time waiting for their appointments. In order to avoid waiting to see your doctor, many experts recommend that you try to have your appointment scheduled at a time when there may not be as many other patients with appointments. This may mean going in as soon as the office opens in the morning or, in some cases late in the evening, depending on the doctor's schedule.

Talk with your doctor about the best times to schedule your appointment. You may be able to avoid sitting in the waiting room for 45 minutes or an hour if you are scheduled as the first patient the doctor sees, or possibly the last appointment scheduled for the day. If you have a good relationship with your doctor, don't be afraid to ask about scheduling your appointments at those times when he can see you without delay. You should also phone the doctor's office before leaving for your appointment to see how long the current delay in seeing patients is - you may be able to leave later and wait less!

How To Cut Your Doctor Visits In Half And Enjoy Better Health

While it's nice to know that doctors are there when you need them, it's even better to know that you don't need to visit them very often. You do have a good deal to say in the matter because, to a large extent, you can control the state of your overall health. By following several guidelines, you can cut down on your trips to the doctor and enjoy good health.

1) Adopt a healthy life-style, and increase your awareness of health risk factors.

2) Maintain a healthful diet with plenty of fruits and vegetables.

3) Get regular exercise— at least 3 or 4 times a week.

4) Don't smoke or abuse alcohol or drugs.

5) Get regular health check-ups by medical professionals.

6) Ask the nurse for suggestions over the phone for problems that are not serious.

7 Proven Ways To Cut Your Health Care Costs

While it may be impossible to decipher the language of politicians as to who knows more about health care costs and who can do more to reduce them, the average American has several clear-cut options in order to save money. Here are several things you can do to cut the cost of your health care costs:

1) Get itemized bills. That is the only way to ensure that you (and your insurance company) are actually getting what you pay for. You should know exactly what you pay for, and how much. Before you visit your family doctor, find out what the charges will be for the office visit and other necessary services.

2) Don't go to a specialist unless it is absolutely necessary. Many people make the mistake of paying a specialist for routine treatment which could have been taken care of just as effectively, and at a lower cost, by a family doctor. Check with your family doctor before you see a specialist.

3) Don't pay for insurance coverage you won't collect. Before you buy extra insurance to cover a specific disease, make sure you understand your regular health insurance coverage. Many times, extra or "special" policies duplicate coverage which is already provided by your regular health insurance policy, and your insurance company will not let you collect more than 100 percent of the cost.

4) Get more than one opinion. Whenever you have to decide on surgery or from among different methods of treatment, you should get, at least, a second opinion. You can ask your doctor for referrals, or you if you feel uncomfortable doing that, you can contact your county medical society and get a list of physicians in your area. Many specialty groups, such as the American Academy of Dermatology and the American Academy of Pediatrics, will also provide referrals.

If the second opinion differs from the first, then you get a third opinion.

5) Make sure you and your family get all your vaccinations. Such immunizations can prevent many illnesses and conditions that require expensive medical treatment. Be sure you keep accurate records, and get boosters as they are needed.

6) Practice preventive care. Whenever it comes to your health, you should exercise as much control as possible. By doing all you can to prevent health problems—quit smoking, control your blood pressure, maintain your ideal weight, eat sensibly, and get regular exercise—you improve your health and as a consequence, reduce the amount of money you have to spend on doctors and medicine.

7) You can also join a Health Maintenance Organization (HMO). These organizations encourage preventive care and their services often cost less than conventional ones. Also don't be afraid to go to younger doctors who charge less. They are fresh out of school and know all the latest information.

How To Save Up To 62% On Your Prescriptions — Both Regular And Generic

It is difficult enough to meet everyday living expenses without having to pay sky-high prices for prescribed medication. For those people who must take some type of medication on a regular basis, the additional expense can be an extreme financial burden. Some experts say that, in general, prescription prices are increasing almost twice as fast as other consumer prices. There are, however, several ways that you can cut the cost of medication, in some cases by over 60 percent. Here are some money-saving suggestions which could help you cut the costs on medicine you must use regularly:

1) Start with a small amount of medication. Rather than buying a big supply of medicine you have never used before, ask your doctor to prescribe a small amount. This is especially important if you've had discomforting side effects from any medication in the past. By purchasing a small quantity on a "trial" basis, you can avoid spending money on pills that are either ineffective or produce uncomfortable side effects.

2) Buy medicine in bulk. This is a saving technique only if you will be taking a medication for a long time, such as maintenance medication to control high blood pressure. By getting a 60-day or 90-day supply of such medication through a retail druggist or mail-order pharmacy, you can get substantial discounts.

3) Take advantage of mail-order pharmacies. Many times you can get prescription drugs from a mail-order firm for less than you would pay at a pharmacy. These firms can't provide refills as quickly as a pharmacy, but that's usually not a major problem. You can find out about the availability and prices of mail-order drugs by calling Pharmail at 800-237-9827; Media- Mail, 800-331-1458; Action Mail-Order Drug, 800-452-1976; and the American Association of Retired Persons (AARP), 800-456-2279. The AARP service is available to members who are 50 or older

and who remit an annual fee of $5.

4) Buy generic drugs. Both over-the-counter and prescription generic drugs can cost considerably less than brand-name products. They also have the same active ingredients as their brand-name counterparts, and are almost always as safe and effective.

Generic drugs that are generally considered to be safe include generic painkillers, congestion/allergy medication, constipation and diarrhea formulas, and antibiotics. Generic drugs considered to be somewhat risky include those for heart and thyroid problems, hormones, blood thinners, and seizure medication. Ask your doctor to prescribe generic drugs when they are available.

5) Be sure to take all of your medication. Often times we begin to feel better before we have taken the entire prescription. Many of us then just stop taking our pills. More times than not, whenever a person stops taking medication short of the number of prescribed pills, he or she runs a very high risk of having a relapse. When that happens, you end up spending more money on a refill. The best advice: do exactly as the prescription and your doctor direct.

6) Be aware of drug interaction. There are some drugs that don't interact well together. Some cancel each other's effectiveness and others become dangerous when taken together. Taking incompatible drugs at the same time can not only be a waste of money, it can also be dangerous to your health. You can prevent such a problem, and such an expense, by making sure that your doctor(s) and pharmacist(s) know all the drugs you are taking.

9 Things You Must Know About Any Medication

Before You Take any medication—whether over-the-counter or prescription—you should be able to answer the following questions:

1) What is the name of the medicine?

2) What positive effect is the medicine supposed to have?

3) Are there any side effects?

4) How often should you take the medicine— before or after meals?

5) How long should you take the medicine? Should you continue to take the medicine once you start feeling better but while there's still some left?

6) Are there any other medicines you should not take while you are taking this one?

7) What, if any, foods or beverages should you avoid while you are taking the medication?

8) Is it alright to have an occasional alcoholic drink while you are taking the medicine?

9) Can you get the prescription refilled without another appointment?

If you are uncertain about the answers to any of those questions, ask your doctor or pharmacist before you take the medication.

8 Tips For Taking Medicine

1) Dampness, heat and light can speed the deterioration of most drugs. Therefore, rooms such as the bathroom are not the places to keep your medication. The best place is outside the bathroom in a small closet or cabinet which can be locked or is not within the reach of children. If the label on the medication advises that it be refrigerated, make sure that's where it is kept.

2) Make sure that your medicines haven't expired, by checking the expiration dates on the medicine bottles frequently.

3) To remind yourself to take medication that must be taken at certain times, set your clock or alarm watch for the correct interval of time between dosages, and then listen for the alarm to go off. Or, you can purchase one of the new electronic beepers discussed elsewhere in this chapter.

4) To avoid having drips or spills ooze over the labels of bottled medicines, making the directions hard to read, keep the label side facing up when pouring.

5) You should not tell children that medicine tastes good or that it is or tastes like "candy". That may lead your children into thinking that all medicines are good tasting or candy and they'll try to find them while you aren't looking. Accidental poisoning is always a possibility with medication. Don't try to hoodwink your children about the medicine's taste. You can also give them a little juice and/or a cracker before and after they take the medicine.

6) A good way to give liquid medication to an infant is to put the prescribed amount in a nipple and give it to the baby just before feeding time. Most infants will be so hungry they won't even notice that they've swallowed medicine.

7) Another way to give medicine to your baby is with a plastic dropper placed against the baby's cheek. When you squeeze the dropper slowly, most babies will begin to suck automatically.

8) Another tip for giving liquid medicine to a child is to hold a small paper cup under his or her chin. Any medicine that dribbles into the cup can be mixed with a little water, and your child can then drink the rest.

New Way To Swallow Pills Without Choking

One solution for taking a hard-to-swallow pill is to crush it and mix it with your food. However, there is a catch to this solution. Crushing destroys the coating on a pill, which could be dangerous. Talk to your pharmacist or doctor before you crush any pills in order to find out what, if any, risk is involved. You can also get a list of about 200 pills not to crush by sending a stamped, self-addressed envelope to: Trademark Medical, Department MC, 1053 Headquarters Park, Fenton MO 63026-2033.

Instead of crushing a hard-to-swallow pill, you can also ask your doctor or pharmacist if the medication is available in liquid form, in a capsule, or perhaps in a smaller pill. You can also try a new "swallowing" technique. If you are unsuccessful bending your head back as you attempt to swallow the pill, try tilting forward, or try bending your head back if you've tried tilting forward without success.

Average Shelf-Life Of Common Medicines

1) Nonprescription painkiller tablets— 1 to 4 years.

2) Cold tablets— 1 to 2 years.

3) Prescription antibiotics— 2 to 3 years.

4) Laxatives— 2 to 3 years.

5) Travel sickness tablets— 2 years.

6) Prescription antihypertension tablets— 2 to 4 years.

Health Warning: Studies Confirm
These Ten Over-The-Counter Medications Can Hurt You

Although we don't usually think of over-the-counter drugs as being harmful, they can be if used improperly. Many over-the-counter drugs can, taken incorrectly, cause physical and psychological dependency. Here are the most common ones you should use with care:

1) Laxatives— as surprising as it may be, experts estimate that millions of people become "hooked" on laxatives. Laxatives that are the most habit-forming contain phenolphthalein, and work by irritating the lining of the intestines, which in turn irritates the nerves that cause the muscles to contract. With continued use the nerve cells can degenerate permanently, making the constipation worse than it was before you began taking laxatives.

If you use laxatives too often, you'll soon have to take them in increasingly larger amounts in order for them to be effective. The problem is, the more you take, the worse your constipation becomes.

It usually takes several months to taper off gradually from the overuse of laxatives. In some cases people substitute bulk-type laxative because it works more naturally than the stimulant type. It is also important, both during and after "withdrawal", to maintain a high-fiber, low-fat diet with plenty of fluids, and to get regular exercise. If you do need a laxative, be sure you read the packaging and labels before you make a decision. Be especially careful with those that have the obvious warning that "frequent or continued use may result in dependency".

2) Nasal spray— such sprays work by shrinking blood vessels in the nose. If the spray is used too often, the blood vessels become fatigued and it takes larger and more frequent dosages to make the vessels shrink. Continued use usually ends up causing more congestion.

To end such dependency, you can try switching from long-acting 12-hour brands of nasal spray to short-acting kinds, and then finally to a more diluted children's formula. You can also try a "homemade" solution consisting of baking soda and salt. Dissolve one half teaspoon of salt and one half teaspoon of baking soda in a quart of cool water. Use this solution several times daily, until the inflammation ends. Also, pay attention to the nasal spray packing directions and take seriously any warning such as, "...shouldn't be used for longer than 3 days".

3) Sleeping pills— once again, read the product packaging carefully. You'll find that over-the-counter sleep aids are approved by the FDA "for occasional use only". According to some experts, many people try to "anticipate" insomnia by taking a sleeping pill just in case a sleepless night is in store for them. This kind of usage, according to the experts, can lead to psychological dependency.

Most sleeping pills generally contain antihistamines, usually used to treat allergies. Used in sleeping pills, antihistamines can produce such side effects as nausea; vomiting; dizziness; fatigue; dryness of the mouth, nose and throat; and double vision, and are best used on an infrequent basis.

4) Codeine cough medicine— while codeine is a relatively safe drug, some people who take large quantities can become nauseated and constipated. Other people can develop a tolerance to those unpleasant side effects, and become addicted to codeine. Such an addiction is serious and requires treatment under the supervision of a doctor.

5) Eye drops— if you use eye drops three or four times a day for several weeks, you may suddenly find that you need them every few

hours to alleviate eye redness. That's because, when you try to stop, your eyes tend to get redder than they were before you first started using eye drops.

According to many ophthalmologists, the best way to quit using eye drops is to stop, cold-turkey. The doctors admit that it will take up to a month for your eyes to get back to normal, but continued use would only exacerbate the condition. Occasional use of eye drops is fine, but overuse can lead to problems.

6) Antibiotics— whenever you take antibiotics to treat bacterial infection, you must take the entire course or risk a recurrence of the infection. You may also increase your chances of bacterial resistance to further treatment when you use antibiotics.

Some antibiotics, such as tetracycline, are rendered ineffective when they are taken with antacids containing calcium, magnesium or aluminum. Dairy products, such as milk, can also keep some antibiotics from working.

Women who are treating a sinus infection, strep throat or bronchitis with antibiotics run a high risk of developing a vaginal yeast infection. Symptoms which can include itching, burning, pain during sex, and vaginal discharge, can begin two days to a week after you first begin taking an antibiotic.

7) Antacids— these drugs to relieve indigestion and heartburn generally shouldn't be taken within one or two hours of any other oral medication because they may prevent the other drugs from working. If you suffer from congestive heart failure, you should stay away from antacids which contain calcium and sodium bicarbonate. You should also avoid consuming large amounts of dairy products, otherwise you'll increase your risk of constipation, nausea, and other side effects.

8) Antidepressants— the best advice is to avoid alcohol and to be cautious when driving or doing any kind of hazardous work when you are taking such a drug. The side effects from such drugs—especially when you first start to take them—can include dry mouth, blurred vision, drowsiness, dizziness, insomnia, palpitations, shaky hands, headaches, and nausea. The effects vary from person to person, but used incorrectly, antidepressant drugs can cause some serious problems.

9) Anticoagulants— these drugs, such as warfarin, help maintain normal bladder flow in people who have an increased risk of clot formation— such as people who are bedridden or who have heart failure. Foods rich in vitamin K, including broccoli, lettuce, and spinach, tend to reduce the effectiveness of warfarin, Coumadin and other anti-coagulants. Antacids can also neutralize their effect.

10) Antiseizure medicine— drugs such as Tegretol, Dilantin, and Phenobarbital can all cause dependence. If you want to stop taking them, you should do so under a doctor's care and guidance.

9 Side Effects Of Commonly Used Drugs

A recent study of the possible side effects of many common drugs found that at least 40 percent of all patients experience some kind of negative reaction to the prescription medication they are taking. The study also indicates that the majority of side effects are not serious and most don't last very long. Here are some of the most common side effects and the drugs which may cause them:

1) Diarrhea— this is one of the most commonly experienced side effects of drug treatment. Many drugs, including antibiotics and anti-cancer drugs, which can affect the lining of the intestine, can cause diarrhea.

2) Drowsiness— antidepressant drugs, tranquilizers, sleeping pills, narcotic painkillers such as codeine and morphine, anti-anxiety drugs, anticonvulsant drugs, and any other drug that has a depressant, can cause drowsiness.

3) Rash— this type of a reaction indicates an allergy to the drug being taken. The reaction can be caused by almost any drug. Drugs used to treat infection, such as penicillin, ampicillin, and the sulfonamides, are commonly associated with this side effect.

4) Nausea and vomiting— opiates, anti-inflammatory drugs, antibiotics, anti-cancer drugs, and hormones are just some of the many drugs which can cause these side effects.

5) Dizziness— some drugs such as streptomycin, quinine, and aspirin can affect the part of the inner ear that controls balance and cause this side effect.

6) Headache— this side effect is associated with a wide range of drugs including nitroglycerin, which is used to widen blood vessels in the heart.

7) Wheezing or difficulty breathing— this side effect is caused by drugs which create a narrowing of the small airways (bronchioles). An allergic reaction to aspirin can cause wheezing and some beta blockers can cause wheezing in people who have respiratory disorders.

8) Hives— this side effect is characterized by itchy, raised white patches of skin, surrounded by red inflamed skin. The condition, as a side effect, is most commonly due to an allergic reaction to a specific drug. Many drugs can trigger such an allergic reaction.

9) Itchy skin (Pruritus)— this is a common side effect of narcotic pain killers such as codeine. It may also be associated with rash, caused by an allergic reaction to a drug.

Avoid This Medicine If You Have Diarrhea

Medical experts warn those people afflicted with diarrhea that they shouldn't use an anti-diarrheal medication if they are also taking an antibiotic. Doctors say that such a combination is likely to worsen the condition.

It seems that sometimes antibiotics can not tell the difference between the normal bacteria in your body and the actual cause of the infection. Diarrhea occurs when the antibiotic eradicates the normal bacteria in your intestinal tract. Treating diarrhea with an anti-diarrheal medication will likely prevent the intestinal tract from purging itself of the remaining bacteria and the subsequent toxins.

20 New Drug Breakthroughs

Several new drugs which could have far-reaching beneficial effects on the health of millions of Americans have recently been approved by the FDA. Here are some of the most important drugs to get approval by the FDA for treatment of everything from heart disease to lead poisoning:

1) Videx— used to treat adults and children with advanced HIV infections who are unable to take AZT or who aren't showing any signs of improvement with AZT use.

2) Foscavir— a medication used to treat inflammation of the retina in patients who have AIDS.

3) Zofran— this drug helps to prevent nausea and vomiting associated with chemotherapy treatments.

4) Fludara— helps to relieve discomfort brought about by the symptoms of chronic lymphocytic leukemia, a cancerous blood disease.

5) Nipent— provides treatment for adults who have hairy cell leukemia, another cancerous blood disease.

6) Zocor— a drug used to lower high cholesterol levels that won't come down, even with a healthful diet.

7) ISMO— helps to prevent the chest pains caused by angina.

8) Ticlid— used to reduce the risk of a stroke in patients who have blocked arteries.

9) Relafen— provides pain and inflammation relief from both osteoarthritis and rheumatoid arthritis.

10) Altace, Accupril, Monopril, Lotensin, and Plendil are all newly approved drugs used for the treatment of high blood pressure.

11) Chemet— used to treat high levels of lead in children.

12) Zoloft— provides an alternative drug treatment for depression.

13) Biaxin— used to clear up respiratory tract infections as well as lung diseases such as pneumonia and chronic bronchitis. May also be helpful in treating some skin infections.

14) Penetrex— for adult use only against some sexually transmitted diseases and urinary tract infections.

15) Zithromax— used for treatment of infection of the respiratory tract and skin. Also used for some sexually transmitted diseases in patients over 16.

16) A new drug called acyclovir is now being used to treat chicken pox. Acyclovir, an anti-viral drug which is also used to treat herpes and some severe or complicated cases of shingles, shortens the recovery period and lessens the severity of Chicken Pox in most cases, according to medical experts. In order for acyclovir to be effective it must be taken within twenty-four hours after chicken pox has been diagnosed.

17) A new drug, sotalol hydrochloride, has been approved by the Food and Drug Administration to treat irregular heartbeat. The drug has one side effect— it may sometimes cause the condition it is intended to treat—and will be used only in severe cases.

According to the FDA, sotalol hydrochloride may help about 150,000 people each year who experience potentially fatal ventricular arrhythmias. However, it is not recommended for people who have non-life-threatening arrhythmias because it can cause dangerously irregular heartbeats.

The FDA says that the drug changes the way the heart conducts electrical signals and reduces the effects of nerve impulses on the heart.

18) Recent findings from a study at Boston's Children's Hospital suggest that nitroglycerin, a drug which is commonly used to treat heart disease, may also provide protection for nerve cells.

The Boston study indicates that nitroglycerin protects nerve cells from the brain chemical glutamate. The chemical, in increased levels, is partially responsible for the damage experienced in conditions such as head trauma and stroke.

19) A new drug which doesn't cause serious side effects may soon be available for the treatment of migraines. The new drug, called sumatriptan, is still being tested, but in initial clinical tests, researchers report that almost 70 percent of patients experienced a drastic reduction or elimination of headache pain within one hour of taking the drug. Clinical trials of the new drug are still underway to determine just how effective and safe it is.

20) A report presented to the American Heart Association says that wider use of clot-dissolving drugs for heart attack patients could triple the number of lives saved each year.

A recent study concluded that clot-dissolving drugs, which break up blood clots that cause heart attacks, can prevent heart damage if given quick enough. However, doctors are sometimes hesitant about using these drugs because they can trigger dangerous, uncontrolled bleeding.

The "Wonder Drug" Aspirin: 4 Ways It Can Help You

A potent drug found in most medicine cabinets, aspirin seems to provide more and more health benefits as medical research studies continue. Here are some of the latest promising developments concerning aspirin:

1) Heart attack and strokes— studies have shown that aspirin, taken every other day by men and women who have had heart attacks, chest pain and strokes caused by clogged blood vessels, can reduce the risk of a second heart attack and lower overall death rates. However, it should be noted that the study also suggests that aspirin may promote those strokes caused by bleeding in the brain.

The major study, conducted by researchers in Boston, concludes that aspirin is as good as clot-dissolving drugs and high-tech procedures for controlling angina, the dangerous chest pain which afflicts 750,000 Americans every year. The study involved almost 1,400 patients and is, to date, the largest ever conducted in order to determine the best treatment for unstable angina— the leading cause of admissions to hospital coronary-care units.

2) Pregnancy— researchers at Case Western Reserve University School of Medicine in Cleveland report that daily low doses—1/5 to 1/2 of a tablet—of aspirin can help prevent pregnant women from developing high blood pressure or from giving birth to low-weight babies.

Studies by French researchers suggest that aspirin may help women who have had previous miscarriages deliver a healthy baby. However, since aspirin can cause bleeding in the late stages of pregnancy, it is not likely to be used except in high-risk cases.

Caution: Although these studies suggest that aspirin may provide some benefits to pregnant women, you should not take the drug without first getting your doctor's permission.

3) Cancer— a study conducted by the American Cancer Society suggests that aspirin may reduce the risk of colon cancer. The study tracked over 650,000 people for a period of six years. Those men and women who reported taking aspirin at least 16 times a month had about 1/2 the death rate from colon cancer as those people who took no aspirin at all.

4) Immune system— a link between taking aspirin and a more effective immune system is suggested in findings from a study by researchers at George Washington University Medical Center in Washington, D.C.

The results of the study indicate that aspirin may increase the production of certain elements in the blood which, in turn, increase the potency of disease- fighting cells.

While most of the news about aspirin is encouraging, researchers caution that none of their findings are conclusive. Furthermore, while aspirin is generally safe, taken steadily over a long period of time, it can cause stomach irritation, intestinal pain and bleeding ulcers. Researchers also say that parents should be reminded that children under 18 should not be given aspirin, especially those who have a viral illness such as the flu, because it can lead to the liver disease Reye's syndrome.

5 Important Pain Killer Warnings

Here are some things you should know about over-the-counter pain killers:

1) Don't use over-the-counter pain killers for longer than 48 hours before you seek medical advice.

2) Avoid taking aspirin for a few weeks before you are to have surgery.

3) Do not give aspirin to children or teenagers.

4) If you are allergic to aspirin, you may also be allergic to ibupro-fen, so don't take either.

5) Don't take ibuprofen if you have kidney disease.

New Source For Prescription Drug Information

People wanting to get information on a specific prescription drug can now take advantage of a 900 line phone link with the Physicians Desk Reference (PDR)— a highly respected source of such information. The phone service is available to the general public at 1-900-680-7771. After dialing that number, callers should then punch in the first five letters of generic or brand-name drugs. Once that's done, the caller will hear a tape of two to five minutes duration, which has been approved by the PDR'S panel of doctors and pharmacists. If you seek information about a drug which has the same first five letters as several other drugs, a recording will provide you with a choice of actual drug names.

The recordings include clear instructions on the proper dosages for more than 500 different drugs. The caller will also be provided with information regarding common side effects and potential hazardous inter-actions when patients take more than one drug at a time. The call to the PDR costs $1.50 per minute.

New $4 Electronic Beeper
Serves As Medicine Reminder

When a doctor prescribes medication it is important that you take it exactly as directed. However, according to the United States Food and Drug Administration, over 800 million prescriptions are taken incorrectly each year. Many people simply forget to take their prescribed medicines at the appropriate times. To help solve that problem, a new electronic beeper designed to remind people when it's time for them to take their medication is now on the market.

The beeper, called the Mediaid AdvisRx, is a device that is small enough to be carried wherever you go or it can be taped to a bathroom mirror or pill bottle. There are five versions, programmed to beep one to five times a day, without the need for setting a clock. The beeper costs about $4 and is available at most pharmaceutical chains. It has an expected life of about two months.

Cancer Patients May Suffer Unnecessary Pain

A recent study at the City of Hope National Medical Center in Duarte, California discovered that as many as 80 percent of advanced cancer patients experience pain that could be prevented or controlled.

The researchers discovered that patients are afraid of becoming addicted to pain medication, and that fear may keep them from asking for relief. The researchers pointed out that those fears are generally unfounded because such addiction rarely happens.

Experts say the problem is exacerbated by doctors who are concerned only with dealing with the disease, not pain, and by nurses who spend very little classroom time on pain management.

The news isn't all negative, however. Recent efforts initiated by several states are helping to develop an awareness of the problem across the country. Also, federally sponsored guidelines for medical personnel are being created and numerous advances in pain treatment have been made in the past several years.

In the meantime, experts advise patients who experience persistent pain to request relief, and to be clear and decisive in making their needs known to family members and to hospital staff.

How To Reduce Infection And Pain After Surgery

The study revealed that patients who had received antibiotics up to two hours before surgery were as much as 50 percent less likely to develop infection than those patients who received antibiotics either earlier or after their operations.

The researchers say that the two-hour period prior to surgery is the optimum time to give the patient antibiotics because it can help reduce the risk of post-surgery infection and pain, as a consequence reduce the patient's hospital bill by thousands of dollars by reducing the time of recovery.

New Study:
98.6 May Not Be The Normal Body Temperature

It seems as if sooner or later everything changes, and that may be the case with the century-old idea that 98.6 is the "normal" human body temperature.

New research at the Veteran's Affairs Medical Center and the University of Maryland in Baltimore suggests that normal temperature may actually vary from individual to individual. The researchers took more than 700 temperature readings from about 150 healthy adults over a three day period and found no meaningful link of 98.6 to human body temperature.

According to the findings, normal temperatures for individuals ranged from 96 to 99.9 degrees, and the average was 98.2 degrees. The researchers say that a temperature of 98.9 in the early morning and a temperature of 99.9 overall should now be considered as the upper limit of the normal oral temperature range in healthy young adults.

The 98.6 degree mark is credited to the 19th century scientist Carl Reinhold August Wunderlich, who reportedly used awkward thermometers pressed against the subjects' armpits to get more than 1 million temperature readings. Today's researchers say that their "measuring" instruments are far more reliable than the method used by Wunderlich.

Good News If You Hate Shots And Needles

Patients who suffer from severe allergies or diabetes may not have to face the needle much longer.In a study at Johns Hopkins Asthma and Allergy Center in Baltimore, researchers discovered that a liquid form of ragweed was easily swallowed by test subjects, and that it also produced the same protective antibodies as allergy shots.

New diabetes research may also lead to less painful alternatives to a needle injection. At Hadassah-Hebrew University Medical Center in Israel, scientists are testing a new insulin pill. Early reports indicate that the new pill can withstand harsh stomach acid and that it also effectively boosts insulin levels.

In other research at the Diabetes Research Laboratories in Oxford, England, an insulin solution taken from a pen-size nasal sprayer tested as more effective than pre-meal injections. And, a new battery-powered device which would allow diabetics to shine infrared light through their fingers rather than pricking themselves to measure blood-sugar levels is awaiting approval by the FDA. Key: Always ask if there is an alternative to a shot.

New Sensor For Early Detection Of Birth Defects

Research into fiber-optics, at the University of Michigan, has led to the possible development of a device that could locate birth defects in an embryo shortly after conception.

Researchers say that the new device—actually a sensor—provides accurate measurements of acid levels in animal cells without causing them any damage. It also could be used to monitor a cell's DNA— the genetic code for producing a human plant or animal. The sensor may eventually allow doctors to test for birth defects at a much earlier stage than is now possible.

According to researchers, the new device functions at a level 1,000 times smaller than existing fiber-optic sensors. It is also 100 times more responsive.

10 Ways To Ease Allergy Problems

When your body detects an invading substance it doesn't like, it reacts— usually by sneezing, wheezing, dripping, and itching. The best way to treat an allergy is to avoid whatever you are allergic to. While that is sound advice, it is not always practical or possible. Most allergies fall into three basic categories: food, contact, or inhalation allergies. Four typical causes of inhalation allergies—the most common allergies we experience—are pollen, house dust, pet dander, and mold.

Even though avoidance isn't always possible, there are several things you can do to relieve the symptoms and ease allergic discomfort. Here are 10 things you can do:

1) Try antihistamines— over-the-counter antihistamines, which are available at your local pharmacy, can be very effective in treating a drippy nose and red, itchy eyes. In order to get the greatest benefit out of antihistamines, you have to take them before you are exposed to allergens. Some allergists say that during your allergy season, you should have antihistamines in your system constantly. They also recommend that, if your allergy persists for more than a week, you should see your doctor. Allergy shots may be the answer.

2) Avoid alcohol and smoking— if you are already a little stopped up, alcohol consumption can cause you to become more congested. You can also create a potentially dangerous sedative effect if you mix antihistamines with alcohol. And according to allergy experts, smoking can promote hay fever.

3) Air-condition your house— this strategy will go a long way in alleviating pollen, and it can also reduce the risk from dust mites and mold. Keep your windows closed, and allow the air-conditioning to seal the house from the outside pollen-laden environment.

4) Air-condition your car— it works on the same principle as having your home air-conditioned. If you don't have air-conditioning in your car, you'll have the windows down and the pollen in.

5) Maintain clean air-conditioning units— to keep mold from growing in your air-conditioner, you should clean the filter and water pan on a regular basis.

6) Don't sun-dry your clothes on a line. When you do that, your clothes accumulate pollen.

7) Do something about your pets— of all pets, cat dander is usually the biggest problem. The most obvious solution would be to give your pet away, but most people simply can't do that. For those people, an alternative would be to isolate your pet from your bedroom, which should be effectively "sealed" off from the rest of the house.

8) Keep your lawn mowed short— a close-cropped lawn won't have a chance to pollinate. If you have to mow the lawn yourself, wear a pollen mask or scarf over your nose and mouth.

9) Stay indoors between 5 a.m. and 10 a.m.— that 5 hour period is when pollinating plants are their most active.

10) Dust-proof your bedding— you can do this by sealing it in plastic. This will help bring relief from dust mites.

If You Have Allergies, These Two Foods Can Help Better Than Drugs

Allergy sufferers may be able to get some relief with honey. Some medical experts say that ingesting traces of the pollen found in honey may desensitize a person to allergies the same way allergy shots do. Research conducted into the potential of honey as a remedy for some allergies provides some credible evidence indicating that honey may indeed help some people.

Yogurt is a good milk substitute for people who are allergic to milk. Many people have a problem digesting lactose (milk sugar) and as a result cannot drink milk. Yogurt is a good source of calcium, contains less lactose, and is easier to digest.

Arthritis: 7 Self-help Techniques That Lessen The Pain

According to a recent nationwide survey conducted by the Centers for Disease Control in Atlanta, as many as 6 million Americans, out of an estimated 40 million who have arthritis, are not seeing a doctor for their condition. While it is important that you get a doctor's diagnosis and care, there are also many things you can do at home to complement a doctor's treatment.

1) Maintain your ideal weight— as is the case with many other health problems, being overweight can cause added distress with arthritis. Excess weight places more stress and pressure on your joints, with

the end result being more inflammation, swelling and pain. By losing that excess weight, you will reduce a great deal of the stress and pain you experience.

2) Get regular light exercise— while exercise is important for everyone, it is especially important for people with arthritis. Exercising will help keep your joints flexible, your muscles strong, and help alleviate pain by activating the release of endorphins, the body's own natural painkiller.

Many doctors advocate swimming and walking as two of the best exercises for people with arthritis. If possible, you should engage in a variety of light exercises designed to build strength, stretch the muscles, and increase flexibility in the joints.

3) Relax— according to recent research, stress worsens arthritic pain by causing people to contract their muscles. You may benefit from sessions with a professional stress-management teacher. You can find such a professional by asking your family doctor for a referral and/or by contacting a local hospital or your city or state psychological association. Books and audiotapes teaching relaxation techniques are also available at most bookstores. The key is in learning to relax and removing your focus from the pain.

4) Use heat and cold— many experts recommend using heat— either in the form of a warm bath, an electric blanket, or a hot water bottle wrapped in towels— to relieve arthritic pain.

On days when your joints are especially inflamed and hot to the touch, applying cold may bring some relief. Some people use a homemade "cold pack" made out of a bag of frozen peas wrapped in a towel.

Alternating hot and cold treatments may also be helpful. Dip your hand or foot in warm water, then cold, then warm, and so on.

5) Wear stretch gloves at night— this will help to reduce or eliminate morning arthritic pain, stiffness and joint swelling.

6) Take advantage of vitamin C— this is an especially good treatment for people with rheumatoid arthritis, who are usually deficient in vitamin C. Before you try vitamin C therapy, consult your doctor.

7) Watch what you eat— studies within the past several years have shown that fish oil can be an effective treatment for joint tenderness and fatigue for some people. Studies have shown that avoiding foods which may trigger allergies can also be beneficial in treating arthritis. Before you embark on a "fish oil" treatment or food avoidance diet, visit your doctor and get his or her recommendation and advice.

7 Tips For People With Asthma

More than 10 million Americans have or have had asthma during their lives. It is a condition in which "twitchy" overactive bronchial tubes narrow, swell, and become clogged with mucus. The condition is usually triggered by pollens, house dust, animal fur and other common substances. Stress and anxiety can also play a role in bringing on an asthma attack. Sometimes even exercise can trigger an attack.

Regardless of what triggers an asthma attack, there are several precautionary measures you can take to lessen both the frequency and severity of attacks.

1) Breathe clean air— this is often easier said than done, but just about any assault on the respiratory tract can trigger an asthma attack. Avoid such irritants as paint fumes, pine oil, insect spray, household cleaners, strong cooking odors, and smoke of any kind.

2) Avoid allergens— if you suffer from asthma, the chances are about 3 to 1 that you are allergic to one or more substances. If you can avoid the most common allergens—dust, mold, and pollen—you may be able to protect yourself from asthma attacks (see allergies, elsewhere in this chapter).

3) Stay out of the cold— according to medical experts, cold air can trigger asthma. The best thing to do when it's cold outside is to stay indoors, but if that isn't possible, you should keep your mouth and nose covered with a mask or a scarf.

4) Watch the foods you eat— pay attention to the foods you eat and give up any that seem to be followed by breathing difficulties. Be especially wary of eggs, milk, nuts, some meat products and seafood.

5) Watch what drugs you take— you should take drugs only under your doctor's supervision. Among the drugs most likely to trigger asthma are penicillin and related antibiotics. Avoid aspirin and all aspirin-containing compounds because you are most likely sensitive to the pain reliever.

6) Know how to use an inhaler— whatever type of an inhaler you may have—one bought over-the-counter, or one prescribed by a doctor— you must be able to use it correctly.

The proper position for an inhaler is 1 to 2 inches from your lips with your mouth wide open. Inhale deeply as you squeeze the canister down; hold your breath for 3 to 5 seconds.

7) In an emergency, use caffeine— some studies have shown that the amount of caffeine in two cups of coffee can help ease an asthma attack. Doctors say that caffeine and some popular asthma drugs are so much alike that your body can't tell the difference. While caffeine is not a recommended substitute for medication, nor a recommended treatment , many experts say the caffeine in two cups of coffee or a couple of chocolate bars can be used effectively in an emergency when your medication or inhaler is not available.

How To Prevent And Get Rid Of Athlete's Foot

You don't have to be an athlete to contact this common skin condition in which the skin between the toes becomes itchy and sore. Sometimes the skin will crack and peal away and, on occasion blister. The culprit is a fungal infection which thrives in warm, moist conditions. Sweaty footwear is often the breeding ground for this painful and annoying foot menace.

Here are some suggestions on how to prevent athlete's foot and how to treat it once you've got it:

1) Buy two pairs of shoes— if possible, never wear the same pair of shoes day after day. It normally takes shoes at least 24 hours to dry out completely. You can also try keeping the insides of your shoes dry and clean with frequent use of antifungal powder or spray and by wiping them with a disinfectant, such as Lysol, occasionally. Shoes that allow evaporation of moisture are best.

2) Change your socks— if your feet have a perverse tendency to perspire a lot, it's a good idea to change your socks two or three times a day— cotton socks are best. To prevent the organism from breeding, it's important that you make its living conditions as inhospitable as possible— clean and dry.

3) Dry your feet— after a shower or a bath, make sure your feet are allowed to dry thoroughly before you put them into shoes and socks. Once you're sure your feet are dry, apply powder to help them stay that way.

4) Don't go barefoot in public— you can help reduce the risk of contracting athlete's foot by wearing slippers and/or shower shoes whenever you are in places where other people often walk around barefoot— swimming pools, health clubs, spas, gyms, locker rooms, and so on.

5) Wash your feet— once you have it, careful hygiene is often treatment enough, without having to resort to drugs. At least twice a day, you should wash the space between your toes with soap, water and a cloth. Be sure to dry the infected area thoroughly with a towel— especially the painful area between the toes. And always put on clean, dry socks.

6) Try aluminum chloride— a twice-daily application of a 30 percent aluminum chloride solution is often effective treatment because of its drying and antibacterial properties. Have your pharmacist make up the solution and use a cotton swab to apply it between your toes at least two times a day. Continue the treatment for two weeks after the condition has cleared up.

7) Use over-the-counter medications— once the infection has cleared up, you should take every precaution to keep it from recurring. One way to do that is to apply over-the-counter antifungal cream or lotion.

Gain Relief From Boils

A boil is an inflamed, pus-filled area of skin— usually a blocked oil gland or hair follicle. The inflammation and pus are a result of a pitched battle between the body's immune system and staphylococcus bacteria which have invaded instigating the fight. The next thing you know, you have a boil. These "battle scars" are common on the arms, groin, back, and buttocks, and just about anyplace where the skin gets rubbed.

Boils are both unattractive and painful, and they sometimes leave scars. Here's how you can treat them yourself and get some relief.

1) Apply warm compresses— at the first sign that a boil is developing, begin applying warm compresses over the boil several times a day. Leave the compress on the boil 20 to 30 minutes at a time. This treatment should bring the boil to a head. Continue to apply warm compresses for a few days after the boil opens to help drain the pus.

2) Take a shower instead of a bath— doing this helps to minimize the likelihood that the infection will spread to another area.

3) Keep your hands clean— it is especially important that you wash your hands well before you handle food. That's because the germs which caused the problem can multiply in warm food and produce toxins that can cause food poisoning.

4) If the boil fails to open, or if you are plagued with recurring boils, consult your doctor.

Bronchitis: How To Get Rid Of It

Acute bronchitis is not ordinarily a reason for major concern. It may be discomforting but most of the time it will go away by itself in a week or two. Chronic sufferers can have the problem for months. Although there is not a lot you can do about acute bronchitis except let it have its way, there are some things you can do to make the experience less unpleasant.

1) Don't smoke— if you are a chronic smoker, you should stop. If you do, your chances of getting rid of your bronchitis increase dramatically. What's more, doctors say that 90 to 95 percent of chronic bronchitis cases are directly related to smoking.

2) Avoid fatigue— sleep in a warm bedroom which is free of drafts.

3) Drink plenty of fluids— warm liquids and/or water help make the mucus easier to cough up. Avoid diuretics such as caffeine and alcohol, which will make you urinate more, making you lose more fluids than you gain.

4) Steam treatment— fill the bathroom sink or a pan with steaming water. Then drape a towel over your head and the sink/pan creating a tent. Inhale the steam directly from the hot water for 5 to 10 minutes.

5) See a doctor— it's time to see a doctor if your cough has become worse after about seven days, if you have a fever or are coughing up blood, or you are short of breath and have a very profuse cough.

3 Step Method To Heal Bruises Faster

There's no way to avoid bruises except to wear padding over your entire body. Sure, you can try not to be as clumsy, but there will always be malicious chairs, stools, desks and other inanimate objects lurking in darkened rooms, just waiting for a tender ankle or shin. The best way to deal with bruises is to try to shrink and heal them. Here's how:

1) Apply a cold compress— this is the first thing you should do whenever you sustain an injury which might lead to a bruise. Use an ice pack on the injured area at 15 minute intervals. This will constrict the blood vessels, and may help minimize the swelling and reduce the pain.

2) After cold, try heat— wait about 24 hours before you begin applying heat to dilate the blood vessels and improve circulation in the injured area.

3) Get more vitamin C— some studies show that people who are deficient in vitamin C are more prone to bruising than those people who get an adequate amount of the vitamin. Before you take any vitamin C supplements, consult your doctor.

6 Ways To Ease Bursitis Pain

Bursitis is what happens when a small, fluid filled sac called a bursa becomes inflamed. These sacs of fluid are located throughout the entire body— primarily in the joints. When they are inflamed they become swollen and very painful. Treatment can be a matter of whatever works best. Here are some possible remedies that may help relieve the pain of bursitis:

1) Rest— this is the most typical treatment and often bursitis will subside in a couple of days. It is important for a speedy recovery that you stop whatever activity is causing the pain, and "give it a rest".

2) Ice it down— if the joint is hot to the touch, applying an ice pack may help relieve the pain. Doctors recommend that you alternate 10 minutes of ice, 10 minutes of rest, 10 minutes of ice, and so on.

3) Try heat and cold— a moist pad can be used when the pain isn't too bad and the joint isn't hot to the touch. When that's the condition, alternate cold and heat treatments— 10 minutes each.

4) Take ibuprofen or aspirin— both will help reduce inflammation.

5) Treat the pain with castor oil— once the pain is no longer acute, usually after 4 or 5 days, you can apply a new treatment involving castor oil and heat. Here's how it works: cover the afflicted joint with castor oil, then put cotton over the area. Finally, apply a heating pad to the area.

6) Exercise— following an attack of bursitis it is important that you perform regular stretching exercises to get the afflicted joint moving in a complete and natural way.

Gain Relief From Cold Sores

These small skin blisters anywhere around the mouth are caused by the herpes simplex virus. The strain of the virus which usually causes cold sores is herpes simplex virus 1. Experts say that 9 out of 10 people worldwide have, at sometime in their lives, been infected by HSV1.

You can usually tell when you're about to get a cold sore by a familiar tingling in the lips. The blisters are small at first but soon enlarge for the whole world to see. They sometimes cause itching, irritation, soreness, and a dull social life. If you're lucky, a cold sore will disappear within one week. Here are several expert tips on how to deal with cold sores:

1) Don't pick at it— as long as the cold sore isn't much of a problem, you're better off just leaving it alone. Keep it as clean and dry as possible, but otherwise, don't mess with it.

2) Get another toothbrush— your toothbrush can shelter the herpes virus for several days. This could lead to reinfection after your present cold sore heals. The best way to prevent that from happening is to throw your old toothbrush away and get a new one.

3) Apply a lubricant— to protect your cold sore, you can apply some petroleum jelly over the entire sore area. It is best to use a fresh cotton swab each time you dip into the petroleum jelly.

4) Turn to zinc— some recent studies suggest that a zinc and water solution, applied as soon as you suspect a cold sore is developing, might help to heal the subsequent cold sore faster. Zinc is available at health food stores.

5) Don't eat foods containing lots of arginine— experts say that the herpes virus needs arginine as a vital amino acid for its metabolism. That means you should avoid arginine-rich foods such as chocolate, peas, grain cereals, peas, peanuts, cashews, and beer.

6) Don't discount witch hazel— some people have experienced success with witch hazel. These people say breaking a sore and using witch hazel to dry it up can be quite effective.

11 Secrets To Cutting The Time You Have A Cold In Half

1) Get juiced with vitamin C— studies have shown that vitamin C can help make colds easier to live with by reducing sneezing, coughing and other symptoms. It may also help reduce the life of a cold, in some cases from 7 days to 2 or 3 days. In doses of 500 milligrams four times a day, vitamin C has been shown to diminish many of a cold's symptoms and the length of the cold by half or more. But before you take a vitamin C supplement to combat a cold you should consult your doctor.

The best way to get additional vitamin C into your system during a cold is by drinking it in any number of fruit juices, including orange, grapefruit and cranberry.

2) Watch what you eat— you may not feel much like eating at all, but when you do eat, you should avoid fats, meats, and dairy products,

which can be harder to digest than fresh fruit and vegetables.

3) Try zinc lozenges— sucking on zinc lozenges can also help cut the symptoms and duration of a cold. Studies in the U.S. and Great Britain suggest that zinc lozenges can reduce symptoms such as dry, irritated throat significantly. You should check with your doctor before trying this treatment and get his or her recommendation. Taken in large enough doses, zinc can be toxic.

4) Get some rest— don't try to keep up with your normal routine because you simply won't have the energy or the concentration. Stay home from work and take it easy. The extra rest will give you more strength to stand up to your cold.

5) Don't smoke— if you are a smoker, you should at least stop when you have a cold. Smoke irritates the throat and increases the chances of infection invading your lungs.

6) Gargle a saltwater solution— by gargling three times a day a solution consisting of 1/2 teaspoon of salt in eight ounces of warm water, you can relieve the irritation in your throat.

7) Bundle up— try to stay as comfortably warm as possible to protect yourself from any chills that may accompany your cold.

8) Try petroleum jelly— just a dab inside each nostril can relieve the rawness caused by blowing your nose frequently.

9) Take aspirin or acetaminophen to relieve aches and pains— this is an adult remedy only and shouldn't be given to children because of the risk of Reye's syndrome. This also includes cold medications containing aspirin.

10) The herbal way— some people recommend drinking herbal tea as a way to relieve the symptoms of a cold. For example, licorice root tea can soothe an irritated throat and relieve coughing if used daily.

11) Some chicken soup couldn't hurt— downing a bowl of hot chicken soup can actually help clear mucus particles from your nose and, in effect, help relieve your cold symptoms.

Footaches: Natural Cures
Provide Fast Relief For Sore Feet

According to medical experts, most footaches are caused by an imbalance in the muscles. If your feet hurt, you may be using your foot and leg muscles improperly. Or you may be wearing shoes that go against the natural shape of your foot. Here's what you can do to alleviate most footaches:

1) Elevate and relax— after a long day, treat your feet by elevating them at a 45 degree angle on an ottoman or chair, etc. , and exercise your toes. Twenty minutes a day should do it.

2) Try a salts-water-soak— this is a proven method of easing the discomfort of a footache. Just put your feet in a basin of warm water and two tablespoons of Epsom salts. Afterwards, rinse with clear, cool water; pat your feet dry; then massage on a moisturizing product.

3) Give yourself a foot massage— it's also nice if you have someone to massage them for you, but either way, getting your feet massaged with baby oil can turn your day around completely. Here's how you do it: gently squeeze your toes, then proceed to press in a circular motion over the bottom of your foot. Once you get started, the right technique will come to you.

4) Switch to low-heel shoes— wearing high-heels tends to tighten the calf muscles. The result is usually foot fatigue.

5) Get thick soles— shoes with thick, shock-absorbing soles can protect your feet from just about every surface, no matter how rough.

How To Prevent & Treat Frostbite

Frostbite can affect any part of the body that is exposed to extremely cold temperatures, but it most commonly "gets" the nose, ears, fingers, and toes. If only the skin and underlying tissues are damaged, complete recovery is possible. If, however, blood vessels are affected, the damage is permanent.

Relatively mild forms of frostbite can occur suddenly in very cold weather when you are shoveling snow or taking a walk. It is important that you know not only how to treat frost bite, but how to avoid it altogether. Here are several tips from some medical experts.

1) Know the symptoms— the first symptoms usually include a pins-and-needles sensation followed by complete numbness. The skin will most likely appear white, cold and hard, and then become red and swollen. Following warming of the tissue, peeling and blistering may occur.

2) Stay out of the wind— your exposure to extreme cold is made worse if it is also windy. Wind-chill factors play an important role in contributing to frostbite.

3) Take advantage of your own body heat— you can warm your fingers and hands by placing them under your armpits. This is a measure you can use if you can't get indoors right away.

4) Don't warm the affected area with dry, radiant heat— frostbitten skin is easily burned and you should be properly warmed by immersion in lukewarm water— 104 to 110 degrees F.

5) Avoid alcohol and smoking— in the case of frostbite, instead of making you warm, alcohol actually causes you to lose more heat. Smoking only makes your extremities more vulnerable to the cold by reducing circulation.

6) Don't rub frostbite with snow or ice.

7) Don't touch metal— if you touch freezing metal with your bare hand your skin may freeze to the metal and tear badly when you pull it away.

8) Dress for the cold— wear several layers of light clothing rather than one bulky or heavy garment.

9 Ways To Eat Less Harmful Fat

Here are nine proven ways you can reduce dietary fat in your diet:

1) Eat whole-grain and freshly baked breads and rolls.

2) Instead of butter or margarine, use jam, jelly or marmalade on bread and toast.

3) Stay away from whole milk. The best way to do that is to drink only skim milk.

4) Consume more pasta, potatoes, rice, vegetables, and grains.

5) Eat lean meat, fish and poultry. Chicken should be skinless.

6) Use low-fat or fat-free salad dressings on all your salads.

7) If you must snack, do so with fresh fruit and vegetables, plain popcorn, pretzels or rice cakes, rather than high-fat items such as potato chips and cookies.

8) For dessert, choose from a variety of fruit or angel food or sponge cake.

9) Avoid ice cream. Instead, substitute low-fay yogurt or sherbet.

8 High-Fat Foods To Go Easy On

1) Pork, sausage, brown and serve (3 oz. cooked)— 330 total calories, with 297 fat calories.

2) Veal, loin chop, untrimmed of visible fat (3 oz. cooked)— 360 total calories— 277 fat calories.

3) Butter (1 tbsp.)— 100 calories— 100 fat calories.

4) Cheesecake (1/8 of 8-inch cake)— 417 total calories, with 238 fat calories.

5) Mayonnaise (1 tbsp.)— 99 total calories— 99 fat calories.

6) Macadamia nuts (12 medium)— 218 total calories, with 207 fat calories.

7) Cream, whipping, heavy (1 oz)— 99 total calories— 95 fat calories.

8) Tartar sauce (1 tbsp.)— 70 total calories— 70 fat calories.

How Wives Can Help Husbands Eat Less Fat

A study conducted by the Fred Hutchinson Cancer Research Center in Seattle, Washington suggests that when wives eat less fat, their husbands also cut back. The study included 188 husbands of women who had been taught how to eat lower-fat diets and 180 husbands of women who hadn't. According to the researchers, women who were taught about fat lowered their intake from 40% to 26% after 15 months— their husbands ate an average of 33% fat.

The research nutritionists say that the husbands were cutting down on fat because they were eating what their wives were feeding them. However, when men went out on their own, they usually did not choose lower-fat foods or eat their vegetables.

Cholesterol Tests:
When To Get, How To Read Results

If you are 20 years old or older, The American Heart Association recommends that you have your cholesterol checked. If your test results show a cholesterol level within the borderline range— 200 to 230 milligrams per deciliter— you should have a second test done and average the two results. If the average of the two tests still indicates that you are in the high-risk group. you should begin immediate steps to lower your cholesterol level. A few changes in your diet may be all that's needed to bring your blood cholesterol level down into a safe range.

If your cholesterol level is in the borderline-high range you should be tested once a year. If your is cholesterol level is 240 or higher, prompt medical attention is advised. However, if your cholesterol reading is below 200 mg/dl, you are within the desirable range, and need only be tested every five years or so, along with regular health care as appropriate.

Both The National Heart, Lung, and Blood Institute and the American Heart Association have determined that a relatively safe level of cholesterol is under 200 milligrams per deciliter of blood. The high-risk range is 240 mg/dl or above. More than half of all adult Americans are believed to be over the borderline-high cholesterol level of more than 200 mg/dl.

Lower Your Cholesterol
To Reduce Heart Attack Risk

According to a recent study conducted in China, a relatively small drop in blood cholesterol could mean a significant drop in the risk of having a heart attack— even if your cholesterol level is already within the safe range. Results from the study indicate that a 4 percent drop in cholesterol level may mean as much as a 21 percent drop in the risk of having a fatal heart attack.

The key words in the Chinese study appear to be "relatively small". Research conducted in the United States suggests that those people with extra-low cholesterol levels are more likely to die in later years from a variety of causes, including certain cancers, liver disease and lung disease, than those people with "normal" cholesterol levels.

The latest findings do not question the standard recommendation that people with high cholesterol should go on diets or, in extreme cases, take drugs to reduce their levels. The concern is for people with extremely low cholesterol- -160 units or less. The research appears to indicate that to reduce certain health risks an individual's cholesterol level should be neither too high nor too low.

Reduce Your Cholesterol Up To 50%
Without Dangerous Drugs

If your cholesterol level is abnormally high, your doctor may choose to put you on medication. While it is advisable to follow your doctor's recommendations exactly, there are some people who may be able to lower their cholesterol naturally, without having to go on medication. Here are five ways you may be able to lower your cholesterol naturally:

1) Follow a strict low-cholesterol diet. Most doctors agree that many people may be able to lower their cholesterol levels by making prescribed dietary changes. Some people have experienced as much as a 30 percent improvement after following a strict diet for slightly less than one month, and ultimately experience a cholesterol reduction of up to 50%.

2) Practice weight control. It is important that you maintain your proper weight.

3) Be sure to get regular checkups. This is the only way to keep track of your cholesterol level and other matters related to your health.

4) Maintain a regular program of exercise.

5) If you smoke, quit.

The Truth About Low-Cholesterol Eggs

A reevaluation of the cholesterol content in regular eggs suggests that there is no "significant difference" between those eggs and the relatively new low- cholesterol eggs. According to the Nutrition Composition Laboratory of the United States Department of Agriculture, there's really not much difference between low-cholesterol eggs and regular eggs. The cholesterol content of a regular egg is about 213 miligrams—considerably less than the 274 milligrams previously attributed to regular eggs— while low-cholesterol eggs contain about 180 milligrams of cholesterol. The 30 milligrams of cholesterol difference between low-cholesterol and regular eggs is not large enough to be significant. And, low-cholesterol eggs are more expensive than regular eggs.

The cholesterol count of regular eggs was revised from the previous 274 milligrams because of better testing methods and egg industry breeding practices. The revision motivated the American Heart Association to raise its recommended weekly limit of egg yolks—both regular and low-cholesterol—from three to four. The recommendation does not apply to persons on a cholesterol- restricted diet.

Aggressive People May Lack "Good" Cholesterol

For well over 30 years, scientists have suspected that people with aggressive or "Type A" personalities are more vulnerable to serious heart problems, such as heart attacks, than are people who are more "laid back". But until now, the scientists had little scientific evidence to explain why this might occur. With the release of the results of a new study, medical experts say that low levels of high-density lipoprotein (HDL), the so-called "good" cholesterol, in Type A people may be responsible for the increased risk.

The study, directed by Dr. JoAnn Manson of Brigham and Woman's Hospital in Boston revealed that the HDL levels in Type A's were about 10 points lower than the level in Type B's. Lowering HDL by a mere one point is believed to increase the risk of heart attacks by about 3 percent.

For the purposes of the study, people were considered Type A if they: try to achieve several poorly defined goals; thrive on competition; crave recognition and advancement; are usually in a hurry; have intense concentration and alertness; and/or become angry easily.

While the study does not prove cause and effect, researchers indicate that the stress which is common among Type A's causes their bodies to produce a surplus of hormones that lower the HDL level.

Scientists agree that more research is necessary to know for certain whether low HDL actually causes the heart attacks experienced by aggressive personalities. However, if further research confirms the link between low HDL levels and heart attacks, it will provide more evidence to support the theory that stress reduction is good for the heart.

Warning:
Be Sure You Eat At Least This Much Red Meat

According to British researchers, there is a place for red meat in a healthy diet. The researchers say that as long as the meat is lean and all visible fat is eliminated, it may be added to a diet designed to lower cholesterol.

The study suggests that 6 1/2 ounces of lean red meat (with no visible fat) a day, as part of a low-fat, high-fiber diet can help produce a decrease in cholesterol level.

Vitamin E, Fish, And Heart Disease

According to two major studies presented at the 1992 annual meeting of the American Heart Association (AHA), vitamin E supplements may help reduce the risk of heart disease. However, the scientists involved in the studies stopped short of recommending that everyone take the supplements. The scientists say that while they have found a statistical relationship between the intake of vitamin E supplements and a reduction in the risk of heart disease, no physical proof exists as yet.

Also presented to the AHA meeting were the results of a study into the possible association of the consumption of fish and a reduction in the risk of heart disease. The results of the study were somewhat surprising as they suggested that while fish is an important part of a low-fat diet to prevent heart disease, it doesn't appear to have protective capabilities in and of itself. The researchers say that after following over 20,000 men for 4 years, it appears that consuming fish may not necessarily result in a lowered risk of heart disease.

Is Margarine Really Good For You?

The U.S. Department of Agriculture (USDA) recently concluded a $1 million study which uncovered some potentially troubling news for margarine users. The study, which was partially funded by the shortening industry, found that oils used in margarine, vegetable shortening and many other products, including cookies, cakes, and crackers, may raise blood cholesterol levels which could in turn promote heart disease.

The potential problem appears to center around trans fatty acids which are produced when food manufacturers convert vegetable oils to margarine or shortenings that are solid or semisolid. According to the Agriculture Department's study, the trans fatty acids raised blood cholesterol levels in almost the same way as certain saturated fatty acids. An earlier Dutch study had indicated that trans fatty acids tend to increase the harmful elements in cholesterol and lower its protective elements.

While this new data released by the USDA is rather disturbing, experts say it is still too early to make a definite link between the increase in cholesterol levels and heart disease. Researchers caution that the USDA's findings are preliminary, and should not lead consumers to avoid products such as margarine and vegetable shortening altogether. The best advice is to watch your overall fat intake and eat a balanced diet.

6 Ways To Cut Down On Salt Intake

The most commonly recommended limit for sodium is 2,400 milligrams per day or 1/2 to 1 1/2 teaspoons per day (1/8 to 1/2 for children). Here are six proven ways to help you keep from exceeding that amount:

1) Use herbs and spices, not salt, for cooking and for use at the table.

2) Look for low-sodium, reduced sodium, or unsalted products. Low-sodium foods contain less than 140 milligrams of sodium per serving; reduced sodium indicates that normal sodium levels have been reduced by up to 75 percent. (Milk and yogurt are lower in sodium than most cheeses.)

3) Try to avoid processed, packaged and ready-to-eat foods. Such foods contain large amounts of sodium. When you cook things yourself, you can control the amount of sodium used in the preparation process. Try halving the amount of salt in your favorite recipes. Also, be sure to taste food before you salt it, adding a pinch at a time.

4) Rinse canned vegetables before you use them and wash away some of the sodium.

5) Avoid salty condiments such as soy sauce, pickles and green olives.

6) Use salt substitutes. While substitutes are available they should be used carefully. People who suffer from diabetes, heart or kidney disease, or who are receiving other medical treatment should consult with their doctors before using a salt substitute.

A $20 Automatic Teeth Flosser
For People Who Don't Like To Floss

Flossing every day is now easier because a new automatic flosser has made "hand" flossing virtually obsolete. The automatic flosser is specially designed to floss between all your teeth—even the hard to reach places, making the routine much more effective. The flosser has a unique head which vibrates thousands of times per minute, flossing your teeth automatically and removing plaque. The new automatic flosser is priced at about $20.00 and is perfect for both children and adults. You can order this automatic flosser, or get a free brochure by calling: 1-800-832-2464.

Fluoride And Hip Fractures

While it may sound like a strange connection, a new study suggests that exposure to fluoride at levels commonly found in drinking water may lead to hip fractures in elderly people. According to a University of Utah study, fluoride may cause the formation of weak hip bones.

The researchers say the effect appeared in a water system fluoridated to one part per million. Previous studies had associated hip fractures with higher levels of fluoride sometimes found naturally in water supplies.

4 Ways To Get Rid Of A Tooth Ache Fast

Although toothaches can be torturous, they don't always have to be immediately treated by a dentist in order for the pain to be alleviated. Quite often you can treat your own toothache and get fast relief. Here are several things you can do to get rid of a toothache without going to the dentist first:

1) Use a pain-relieving gel— use a gel with eugenol or benzo-caine. Both gels can numb an aching tooth with their mild anaesthetic action. An effective gel costs about $3.00 a tube at most drug stores.

2) Use zinc oxide putty— this is effective as a temporary filling in a bad tooth when you can't get in to see your dentist for a few days. Zinc oxide putty has the numbing agent eugenol that will give you relief until your dentist can see you. While the product is effective, you should get to a dentist as soon as possible. Zinc oxide putty costs about $3.00 at most drug stores.

3) Use oil of cloves— you can get this temporary remedy over-the-counter at most drug stores. Apply a small amount of the oil directly onto the offending tooth, or put a drop on a small piece of cotton and press lighly against the ache.

4) Use a floss pick— it isn't always convenient to carry dental floss wherever you go. Floss picks, which are actually plastic tooth picks with a taut length of floss attached to one end, make it more practical and easier to dislodge pain-causing particles wedged in a tooth or caught under a denture. Floss picks are priced at about $1.50 at most drug stores.

While the above four suggestions will help ease the immediate pain of a toothache, you should also heed professional warnings about toothaches. Experts advise that you see a dentist if your toothache lasts longer than several minutes. If your tooth is simply sensitive to cold or sweets, the ache should pass momentarily. But, if your toothache is unprovoked and it lingers, it could be a sign that a more serious problem exists. Pain relievers should only be used for immediate and temporary relief until you can see your dentist.

Tooth Whitener Warning

If you've been buying an over-the-counter tooth whitener in hopes of attaining A "gleaming white smile" without seeing a dentist, you may be taking a potentially "damaging" risk. The American Dental Association (ADA) warns that regular use of such products may cause temporary damage to the soft tissue in the mouth. There's also some concern over possible permanent damage to tooth enamel. The ADA has also expressed concern over other possible damage from using the products, including cell damage.

The Food and Drug Administration (FDA) warns that there is no definite proof that any of these over-the-counter tooth whiteners can actually make good on their claims to bleach teeth. There's also no conclusive proof that the products are safe, according to the FDA. Therefore the FDA recently ordered that tooth whitener kits be taken off the market until the products can be proven safe and effective.

Until the matter is resolved, dental experts recommend that you avoid all tooth whiteners which contain any type of peroxide, such as hydrogen peroxide, which is the main ingredient in many of these products. To be safe, visit your dentist and let him or her apply whiteners that will not cause any damage. Such professional treatment requires 4 or 5 trips to the dentist and is a good deal more expensive than a whitening kit, but it's safe.

Five Ways To Find A "No-Pain" Dentist

If you're one of those people who fear dentists, scheduling an appointment for even a regular checkup may be a traumatic experience. The thought of facing the drill can cause some people to stay away from dentists altogether. There are, however, several proven methods of finding a good, "pain-free" dentist. Here are five keys to finding such a dentist:

1) Preventive Dentistry— the type of preventive screenings a dentist performs on your initial visit can tell you a lot about that dentist— good and bad. The four kinds of screening you should expect from a good dentist during your first visit include an oral cancer screening, a screening for jaw disorders, a periodontal screening for gum disease, and a tooth by tooth screening to find out if you have any visible cavities or any

fillings that are about to fall out. A good dentist will also supplement your first visit with a full set of x-rays. You can find out if a dentist is prevention-minded by asking, before your first visit, if the four basic screenings will be performed. Also find out if the dentist takes proper care to prevent the passing of serious contagious diseases from one patient to another. The dentist and the staff should always wear protective gloves and masks during a patient's treatment.

3) Sensitivity— you should be able to tell a dentist, on the first visit, not only about your dental history, but about any unpleasant or painful dental experiences you've had. A good dentist will be sensitive to any fears you have about pain and be exta-careful to be as gentle as possible. A good dentist is one who is understanding and caring— aware of the patient's fears. If a patient is in pain during treatment he should be able to alert the dentist with a mutually agreed upon signal for the dentist to stop.

4) Communication— a good dentist will tell the patient exactly what he/she is going to do, including the risks and benefits involved, how long the treatment will last, and how much the procedure will cost. The dentist should also tell you about treatment alternatives. If, upon your first visit to a dentist, you are unable to get such information, or the dentist doesn't seem interested in helping you make an informed decision about your dental care, find another dentist.

5) Respect— another characteristic of a good dentist is a respectful attitude toward your needs. This respect should be shown by being aware that your time is valuable too. Unless there is an emergency, you shouldn't be made to wait a long time in a dentist's waiting room. The dentist should also be available for any follow-up treatment or emergencies that need immediate attention. And, the dentist should have a clean, friendly office with hours that fit your personal schedule.

The Best Way To Stop Getting Cold and Canker Sores

Some gels used to ease the pain of a toothache may also help in the treatment of cold and canker sores. Gels containing benzocaine or eugenol can numb the sores, bringing some relief to the sufferer. For more information about the causes of and treatments for cold and canker sores you can get a free booklet titled, "Cold Sores, Fever Blisters, and

Canker Sores". The booklet is available free by sending a self-addressed, stamped envelope to: American Academy of Otolaryngology-Head and Neck Surgery, "Fever Blisters", One Prince St., Alexandria, VA 22314.

5 Proven Ways To Get Rid Of Oily Skin

Oily skin is a problem that just about everyone has at one time or another. Most people associate oily skin with adolescence, but factors such as hormones, stress, extreme heat, and hectic schedules can make it a problem for adults as well. Since the skin is a mirror of the inside of a person's body, proper nutrition and exercise are just as important as they are to your general health. If your general health on the inside is not good, your skin will simply be a reflection of that poor health.

In most cases, oily skin is not a problem that needs medical treatment. The sheen you may see on your face if you have especially oily skin is, in part, due to perspiration that mixes with the oil. Exactly what you do to control oil depends on how far you want to go, but there are methods of controlling the problem. Here are five proven ways to get rid of oily skin:

1) Aluminum Chloride— if your skin oiliness is especially severe, making you uncomfortable, there are several topical preparations which contain an active ingredient found in many antiperspirants—aluminum chloride. Such preparations will help shut down some of the activity of the sweat glands and alleviate the unattractive sheen on your skin. Aluminum chloride preparations should only be used to treat extreme cases, and only then under the supervision of a dermatologist.

Glycolic acid can also be used as an effective oil-control measure. This acid works by removing dead cells that might clog pores and prevent oil from being distributed evenly. Available without a prescription, glycolic acid can be a very effective measure against oily skin.

2) Cleansing— controlling mature oily skin requires a method of cleaning without drying out the skin. Oily skin should be cleaned with fingertips rather than stiff washcloths and other types of scrubs. This type of cleansing should only be done two or three times a day with sensitive skin cleansers. It is best to avoid cleansers that are designed for acne. Also avoid astringent or abrasive cleansers. Look for a cleanser labeled, "syn-

thetic", which is designed to not leave deposits on your skin if you use hard water.

Removing soap reside is the final part of the cleansing process. This should be done with a mild astringent in order to avoid overdrying. Most skin-care- product companies now feature a line of astringents that are especially designed for this part of the skin cleaning process.

3) Moisturizers— Modern moisturizers help the skin hold onto its own moisture rather than adding it on from the outside. These moisturizers are available in oil-free formulas that help skin maintain its balance, allows better make-up application, and protects the skin from the sun's ultra violet rays. If you choose to use a moisturizer, be sure to read the label and select only those products that are designated for use on "oily skin".

4) Water-based Make-up— most women with oily skin also experience problems with make-up. The solution is to use only makeup for oily skin that is water- based. Today's water-based foundations allow a woman with oily skin to achieve whatever type finish she desires. If you want lots of coverage to hide imperfections, you can choose completely oil-free make-up designed for just such an application. There are also sheer make-up products, suitable for women who don't want much coverage.

5) Powder— a dusting of loose powder is essential if you have oily skin and you use make-up. Today's powder can absorb excess oil, help moisturize, and control oil on your skin.

Just Out: Vitamin E Oil
May Reduce Skin Cancer Risk Up To 50%

Recent research at the University of Arizona at Tucson has revealed that vitamin E oil may reduce skin-cancer risk by up to 50 percent. According to the study, vitamin E oil seems to counteract the dangerous immune system suppression caused by the sun. The study was conducted with the alphatocopherol form of vitamin E oil and other forms may not work as well. Also, some people are allergic to vitamin E oil.

Free Brochure
On Preventing & Detecting Skin Cancer

A new brochure which provides information on detection and prevention of skin cancer is available from the Skin Cancer Foundation in New York.

To get a free copy of the brochure titled, "Skin Cancer: If You Can Spot It, You Can Stop It", send a SASE (business-size envelope) to: the Skin Cancer Foundation, Dept. SE, Box 561, New York, NY 10156.

Secrets To Get Rid Of Dry Skin

Both sun and wind can drain your skin of its moisture. Air conditioning can also be a problem because when air is cooled and its humidity level sinks too low, moisture quickly evaporates from your skin. Here are some measures you can take to fight dryness and keep your skin both soft and supple:

1) Use a humidifier when your air conditioner is on in order to help boost the air's moisture level.

2) Don't take long, hot baths. Such baths will induce a great amount of water loss through sweating. Take quick showers and warm sponge baths instead.

3) Either cut down on soap when you bathe or switch to a moisturizing soap like Vitabar in the Vitabath Plus formula.

4) Use a rich lotion or cream on damp skin after showering, to seal in moisture.

5) Use an emollient-rich sunscreen. Two such sunscreens are Vaseline Intensive Care's Moisturizing Sunblock and Coppertone's Moisturizing Sunblock Lotion.

Tanning Pill Warning

If you plan to use tanning pills because you've heard they are a healthful alternative to sun exposure, you've been misled. Tanning pills are actually anything but healthy, and they're illegal. These pills can cause nausea, diarrhea, severe itching, skin eruptions, hepatitis and night blindness. And instead of creating a realistic tan, they leave the skin an unappealing shade of orange. Tanning pills were actually outlawed by The Food and Drug Administration back in 1981, but due to indifferent law enforcement, they are sometimes still sold by mail or in tanning salons.

Secret To Heal Skin Problems

Some skin conditions such as poison ivy or runny eczema can be successfully treated by a starchy bath created by soaking or boiling a potato in water. This bath in "potato water" can dry and smooth wet and blistery skin inflammations, but before using such a remedy, it's best to consult your doctor. Sometimes, a potato water bath can further irritate dry, itchy skin or fungal infections.

The Best Ways To Eliminate Acne

Acne tends to be more of a problem during warm-weather months because the sweat glands are more active. The more you sweat, the more the mixture of perspiration and oil spreads on the skin's surface and clogs pores.

You can fight acne by washing your face more often, especially after working out. If adequate facilities aren't always available, you can carry a sealed plastic bag, containing cotton balls soaked in astringent.

Another method of minimizing clogging is to use an oil-free sunscreen. Choose one that's labeled "non-comedogenic" and lists alcohol as one of its main ingredients. Also make sure it is water-resistant.

4 Blemish Fighters

Witch hazel— removes excess oil.

Sulfur— dries up oil.

Benzoyl peroxide— speeds up the healing process by acting as a peeling agent.

Salicylic acid— removes debris from the pores.

Best Way To Washing and Drying Your Hair

To remove the buildup of dirt and oil, regular washing with a mild shampoo is necessary. Dry hair should be washed every 4 to 6 days. Oily hair can be washed as often as necessary, sometimes every day. Rinse your hair thoroughly after every washing. A final rinse that contains the strained juice of a lemon is of special benefit to oily hair.

The outer surface of the hair can be made smooth by using a conditioner. The conditioner should be applied only to the ends if your hair is oily. If you have dry hair, leave the conditioner on a few minutes before rinsing. If you regularly use a hair dryer or a curling iron, you should use an extra amount of conditioner.

Since hair is at its weakest when it is wet, extra-hard rubbing can cause it to break and tangle. It is best to wrap your head in a towel and let it absorb the moisture before drying your hair. To finish drying your hair, comb it with a wide-toothed comb.

The Best And Worst Shampoos For Your Hair

Almost all hair problems are caused by harsh hair products, the chemicals used for permanents, and overheating caused by blow-drying, heated rollers, or exposure to the sun. You can cut down on the risk of damaging your hair if you choose the right shampoo. Here is what one experienced hair stylist recommends as the two best shampoos: 1. Faberage Organics and 2.Pantene.

You should take special care when buying shampoos. Some contain harsh ingredients that can damage your hair. The shampoos that contain more natural ingredients are the best.

Zinc Deficiency Linked To Hair Loss

Low levels of the mineral zinc have reportedly been associated with an unexplained loss of hair. If you've had such a hair loss, you may want to check for a zinc deficiency. To get more zinc in your diet you can eat more meat, particularly organ meats such as liver, or take a zinc supplement.

AMA Dietary Guidelines

Here are the American Heart Association's dietary recommendations, designed to reduce blood cholesterol and prevent or control high blood pressure. If the guidelines are carefully followed, and combined with regular exercise, the result is not only a healthful diet, but one that is also effective for weight control.

1) Your total fat intake should be less than 30 percent of your daily calories.

2) Saturated fat intake should be less than 10 percent of your daily calories.

3) Polyunsaturated fat should not exceed 10 percent of daily calories.

4) Cholesterol intake should not surpass 300 milligrams per day.

5) Carbohydrate intake should make up 50 percent or more of your daily calories. (mostly complex carbohydrates).

6) The rest of your daily calories should be provided by protein.

7) Sodium intake should not exceed 3 grams (3,000 milligrams a day).

8) Alcohol consumption should not exceed 1 to 2 ounces of ethanol a day. Two ounces of 100 proof whisky, 8 ounces of wine or 24 ounces of beer each contain 1 ounce of ethanol.

9) Your total caloric intake should be enough to maintain your recommended body weight.

10) You should consume a wide variety of foods in order to get a proper balance of nutrients.

To help you follow such a dietary plan, the AMA has published a pocket reference book, THE AMERICAN HEART ASSOCIATION FAT AND CHOLESTEROL COUNTER, which lists the amount of fat, saturated fat, calories, cholesterol and sodium contained in hundreds of foods. You can get this handy reference book at most bookstores and supermarkets. You can also get more information by calling your local American Heart Association or 1-800-AHA-USA1.

Alcohol And Weight Control

Limiting your consumption of alcohol is not only important to your general health and well being, it's also essential if you wish to maintain your desirable weight. Each gram of alcohol has 7 calories (there are about 200 calories in one ounce), compared to 4 calories in carbohydrates or protein. Even more significant is that calories from alcohol are considered "empty calories", because they don't add any nutritive value to the diet. If alcohol is served in a mixed drink, such as a whisky sour or a Manhattan, the amount of calories is even higher.

It is known that alcohol stimulates the appetite, and according to some recent tests, people on restricted-calorie diets may be more likely to eat more after consuming alcohol. That's why most experts advise dieters to limit their consumption of pre-meal alcoholic drinks.

Another recent study, conducted by Stanford University researchers, provides some rather interesting news. In the study, several middle-aged, overweight men were furnished food and an average of two alcoholic drinks per day. While the men consumed more calories due to the added alcohol, and ate slightly more food, compared with non-drinkers, their basal metabolism experienced a pronounced increase after one drink per day, thus burning off some of the excess calories. The faster metabolism rate also appeared to counteract some of the excess alcohol calories in men who had one to three drinks a day compared with light drinkers or non-drinkers. The results seem to indicate that alcohol calories may not turn into fat as readily as other calories. While the study is not conclusive, and while alcohol consumption may turn out to be somewhat less fattening than traditionally believed, moderation is still recommended.

6 Common Weight Loss Mistakes

Before beginning any weight-loss, diet or exercise program you should consider the following:

1) You should consult your doctor before you begin any weight-loss, diet or exercise program. This is especially true if you are overweight, or suffer from a medical problem such as diabetes or heart disease.

2) Avoid crash diets and other rapid-weight-loss programs that drastically cut the number of calories you consume.

3) Extremely low-calorie, liquid-formula diets should not be used without the recommendation of your doctor and then only under his or her supervision.

4) The only drugs you should use to lose weight should be prescription drugs, which are recommended by your doctor and used only for a short time.

5) Avoid diets that call for restricting fluid intake. This can lead to dehydration.

6) Using dieting aids that contain laxatives or diuretics will not lead to a significant weight loss, and may harm your body.

12 Weight Loss Ideas That Work

Here are several insider tips on how you can achieve and maintain a desired weight:

1) Make a long-term commitment. Too often, losing weight is a "spur-of-the- moment" reaction to a superficial set of circumstances (being able to get into a new outfit or looking thin to impress old friends at a class reunion are short-term, and essentially superficial reasons to

lose weight.) If you need to lose weight, make the commitment not only to lose the weight, but to keep it off.

2) Keep a food journal. By keeping a written record of when, where, and what you eat, you determine your major problem area. Your journal should be a precise record of where your calories and nutrition are coming from. With this type of information you will be better able to change your eating habits.

3) Be patient. Don't expect to lose ten to fifteen pounds of fat in one week. Also make sure your long-term goal is realistic. Ask your doctor for guidance on setting and achieving a desired weight. With your doctor's advice, you should choose a weight that is safe and healthy for your height, age and lifestyle.

4) Stay away from crash diets and other "quick-fix" schemes for losing weight. Most of these diets don't work and result mostly in water-weight-loss. Also, many people coming off a rapid-weight-loss diet cave in to the tempation to go on an eating binge, resulting in weight-gain. The best, safest and most effective way to lose weight is gradually. You should choose a diet that you can live with for the rest of your life.

5) Get regular exercise. A regular exercise program, combined with a sensible diet, will make it much easier for you to maintain a desired weight. The exercise(s) you choose should be something you enjoy and will continue to do. (see chapter 5).

6) Don't skip meals. If you skip a meal you will be more inclined to overeat at the next meal. Also, choose specific times to eat your meals and snacks, and don't eat at any other time.

7) Eat slowly. If you take your time eating, you will be better able to realize you're full before you overeat.

8) Avoid eating foods out of their original containers. While you may think you're only having a small amount, you'll probably end up eating more than if you had served the food in measured portions.

9) Don't be discouraged if you "backslide". An occasional "sweet attack", eating binge or lapse in exercising is only natural. The important thing is what you eat on a regular basis. One food indiscretion will not ruin your regular healthful diet.

10) Weigh yourself no more than once a week. Record your weight in your food journal. This will allow you to evaluate how well your weight control program is progressing.

11) Drink more water. Drinking six to eight glasses of water a day is not only good for you, it also curbs your appetite.

12) If you're not hungry, don't eat. Don't feel that you have to eat everything on your plate just because it's there.

Little-Known Weight Management Facts

You will gain one pound of body fat if you consume 3,500 calories more than you expend. You can lose a pound of body fat by walking five miles each day for a week, provided you don't increase your food consumption. It should be obvious from those two facts, that the key to weight control is not consuming more calories than you expend. Therefore, even if you follow a well-balanced diet and don't overeat, an inadequate amount of physical activity will still result in increased body fat.

If Your Weight-Loss Diets Never Work Or Last, Here's What They Are Probably Missing

The "Missing Ingredient" in most weight loss attempts is regular excercise. It has been proven conclusively that even moderate physical activity improves health, and reduces stress. Even doing things around the house can be helpful. Lawn-mowing, although not as regular an activity as cycling usually is, burns just as many calories, and routine gardening uses almost as many calories as moderate swimming. Regardless of what you do—ordinary physical labor or extensive aerobic workouts—performing some regular physical activity is important to your general health and well being.

Regular exercise benefits every part of your body, helping it to perform more efficiently. If you get regular exercise you are likely to have lower levels of cholesterol in your blood and you are less likely to develop hypertension or heart disease. But just as important, you need regular exercise to give you vitality and a sense of physical well-being, which leads to your being more relaxed and secure. Regular exercise will improve the quality of your sleep and your ability to deal with stress.

6 Incredible Effects Of Exercise, Walking And Running

Extensive studies over the last few years have increased our knowledge of the amazing benefits to be derived from exercise. While most people know that exercise is good for them, few can say exactly why. In general terms regular exercise not only improves the overall development and efficiency of our bodies, it also improves the quality of our lives. Still, many people find it hard to stay motivated and maintain a regular exercise program. If you are one of those people, here are several specific benefits derived from regular exercise that can also serve as motivation:

1) Weight-reduction— if you are overweight and you want to loss extra pounds, along with a balanced diet you must get regular exercise. Exercise increases your body's need for energy, and some of this requirement is provided by reserves of stored excess fat. The facts are simple, without regular exercise you will not be able to maintain a desirable weight.

2) Reduced risk of heart disease— even a moderate amount of exercise done on a regular basis can significantly reduce your chances of having a fatal heart attack. Apparently, exercise reduces the risk of coronary heart disease by helping to prevent obesity and high blood pressure. It also helps improve blood flow through the arteries. It can also help to reduce the level of low- density lipoproteins, which are responsible for depositing fat into the lining of the arteries, and increase the level of high-density lipoproteins which help prevent heart disease.

3) Relief From Stress And Depression— for most people, regular exercise serves to enhance their sense of well being and improves their self-images. It can also provide a natural "high" caused by the release of endorphins, which are morphinelike substances, inside your brain.

4) Relief Of Menstrual Problems— many women experience a reduction in the severity of premenstrual symptoms and an easing of menstrual pain, when exercising on a regular basis.

5) Better posture— the more you exercise, the more you increase the strength and the tone of your stomach muscles. You also start to lose fat. Stronger stomach muscles help give you better posture, which may help reduce back pain.

6) Cancer prevention— some studies suggest that regular exercise may protect against certain cancers. In one of those studies, the death rate from cancer was much lower in men and women who were physically fit. Other studies have confirmed a possible link between cancer rates and levels of physical fitness. That doesn't mean you won't get cancer if you exercise regularly. But it appears that the risk of getting cancer is significantly less for those people who do exercise.

Free Hotline For Questions On Heart Disease, Diet And Exercise

The Arizona Heart Institution and Foundation has established a nationwide toll-free information line called "Hartline". Trained nurses are available from 8 a.m. to 5 p.m. (MST) to answer callers' questions on all aspects of heart disease. In addition, Hartline can provide information on such topics as diet and exercise. The Hartline number is 1-800-345-4278.

Exercise And Diabetes

According to a recent study, middle-aged men who exercised regularly had a lower risk of developing adult diabetes, which is the most common form of the disease. The study showed that the men reduced their risk of developing adult diabetes by as much as 6 percent with every 500 calories they burned off each week by exercise. The findings also suggest that the positive effects of regular exercise seem to apply regardless of such health risk factors as obesity, high blood pressure, aging, and/or family history of the disease. And while the study used men as its subjects, it is believed that the findings could probably hold true for women as well.

Diabetes affects men and women in almost equal numbers. In all, over 12 million Americans suffer from the disease. And, according to the study, vigorous exercise such as jogging or playing tennis, provided more protection than did less vigorous activities such as golf. Also, of the men who participated in the study, those at the highest risk benefited most from exercise. In fact, men who participated in vigorous activity, burning about 3500 calories each week, cut their risk nearly in half when compared with men who were inactive.

If you have diabetes, you may need to drink a sweet liquid or eat a food containing sugar just before you begin exercise. It may also be wise for you to carry sugar or candy with you in case your blood sugar level drops as a result of vigorous physical activity. Consult your doctor for his or her recommendations before you begin any exercise program.

Build Strong Bones With Regular Exercise

Recent studies show that weight-bearing exercises, such as walking, retard bone loss and in some cases may even help bone growth. One study, at Washington University in St. Louis, found that women with osteoporosis—a progressive thinning of the bone caused by calcium depletion—who took an adequate amount of calcium and walked for one hour a day three days a week for 22 months actually increased, by six percent, their bone density at the spine.

Weight-bearing exercises strengthen the bones by increasing their mineral content, especially their calcium content, and can make a great difference in bone density. It is especially important for children and young adults to get adequate exercise and eat right to prevent bone loss in later life. The more dense your bones by age 35, the less your risk of developing osteoporosis. But, as the studies indicate, it's never too late to slow down bone loss and promote increased bone density. Exercise and an adequate amount of calcium in your diet can work wonders.

Exercise— A Natural Antidepressant

Recent studies conducted at California State University indicate a significant reduction in tension is possible with exercise. Both the California State study and a study conducted by the Florida Department of Health and Rehabilitative Services showed that walking greatly reduced tension and stress. In the Florida study, people in a two month walking program reduced the stress they felt at work by as much as 30 percent.

Most experts feel that walking helps relieve tension and depression because of the repetitiveness of the walker's footfall and the cadence of his or her breathing. Both of these factors help distract a person from his or her worries. Studies also suggest that people who suffer from depression feel better when they exercise regularly as well. Just a moderate increase in aerobic activity seems to have a powerful antidepressant effect.

Some experts speculate that the exercise-induced release of brain chemicals that seem to produce a feeling of well-being (endorphins) are responsible for the positive change in mood. Whatever the reason, most scientists agree that exercise can be a very effective antidepressant.

Exercise And Arthritis

There is strong evidence which indicates that swimming or aquatic exercise provides relief from arthritis pain. As many as 70 percent of the people who participated in a recent study appeared to get a good deal of relief from arthritis pain after they went into the water. The participants engaged in swimming and/or aquatics, which can include walking in a pool and other range- of-motion exercises.

Aquatic exercise, while not as familar as land exercise, is a good way to improve and maintain flexibility in the joints and increase muscle strength. Body weight is displaced by the water, resulting in much less stress on the joints. Also, exercising in water is less painful for people who suffer from arthritis, so they should find it more appealing than other forms of exercise.

You can get more information on aquatics by contacting your local Arthritis Foundation, YMCA or YWCA.

Exercise And Cholesterol

Exercise combined with other healthful lifestyle choices, such as weight control and being a non-smoker, can help raise high-density lipoproteins (HDLs)—also known as "good cholesterol"—and as a result reduce certain health risks, including heart attack.

Medical experts say that even though HDL levels are to some extent genetically determined, they can be raised several ways, without using medication. In studies at Stanford University and Medical College of Virginia, losing excess weight and kicking a smoking habit have both been shown to lead to an increase in HDL levels. Postmenopausal women receiving estrogen replacement therapy also tend to have higher HDL levels.

Regular exercise is another method of ensuring high HDL levels. Experts say that regular muscle contractions stimulate the production of HDL. And while vigorous exercise produces the greatest effect, studies indicate that even mild exercise is of some benefit in raising HDL levels.

Sex Is The Best Cure For A Cold

Sex is just what the doctor ordered to help you recover faster from a cold or flu. That's because getting turned on gives your immune system a boost so you heal more quickly and also releases hormones that make you feel better, according to Dr. Miriam Stoppard, author of "The Magic of Sex"

Electrocardiogram, Recommended For Some People Before Exercising

Experts recommend an electrocardiogram or heart stress test for men and women over 40 who are about to begin an exercise program and who have not been active. This also applies to those who have a history of medical problems, such as high blood pressure, diabetes or premature heart disease (before age 55) in parents or brothers and sisters. The test is also recommended if you are over 40 and have a history of cigarette/tobacco use.

Possible Health Hazards Of Exercise, Walking Or Running

Studies have shown that strenuous exercise causes physiological stress and strain on the body. And without adequate time for the body to rest, recover and rebuild, injury or illness can result. That's why experts agree that moderation is the key to safe and effective exercising.

According to the American College of Sports Medicine most healthy adults should workout 3 to 5 days a week, with no more than 2 days between workouts. Exercising an average of less than 2 days a week doesn't result in any significant improvement in your overall physical fitness. But, if you exercise more than five times a week, you increase the risk of injury. That's why 3 to 5 times a week is the recommended "course of action".

You should take care to monitor the intensity of your workouts. Work your heart rate at 60 percent to 90 percent of capacity and exercise nonstop for 20 to 60 minutes. You can calculate your ideal training zone by determining your maximum heart rate, using the following formula: Subtract your age from 220; then multiply that number by the percentage of how hard you plan to work out. For example, the maximum heart rate for a 40 year old is 180 (220 minus 40 equals 180); 60 percent of 180 is 108, and 90 percent is 162. Therefore, the ideal training zone is a pulse rate between 108 and 162.

For nonathletes, or people who haven't exercised in quite some time, the American Heart Association recommends working at a target heart rate of between 60 and 75 percent of the maximum rate. Older people or those in poor health should start out at the low end of the range, while better-conditioned people can start at the high end. And after 6 months or so, exercisers may want to increase up to 75 to 85 percent of maximum heart rate. Most people can stay fit working out at 75 percent of maximum heart rate.

Another key to safe and effective exercise is to "listen to your body". Many times we may experience pain, stress or exhaustion from the whole body or from particular joints and muscles. The concept of "working through the pain" is, at best, foolhardy. To avoid injury, you must acknowledge and respond to pain and/or discomfort swiftly and positively. This means changing your pace or switching to another activity that uses different muscle groups, or stopping the activity altogether.

Here are some signs of a high-stress workout. The symptoms may indicate that an individual is exercising too hard, too long or too often, and should take the necessary steps to modify his or her exercise routine:

1) Muscle aches and pains 2) Muscle cramps 3) Pain in the feet, knees or hips 4) Generalized fatigue 5) Chest pains 6) Light-headedness

or confusion 7) Loss of appetite 8) Sleeping difficulty 9) Nausea or vomiting 10) Pale or bluish skin tone 11) Shortness of breath (lasting for more
than ten minutes) 12) Palpitations

5 Ways To Prevent Injury While Exercising

1) Balance your body weight—your body should be aligned and
centered so that your weight is properly balanced. Properly balanced,
your body is stable, comfortable and ready for exercise.

2) Breathe steadily— try to exhale as you contract a muscle and
inhale as you release it. This will help prevent muscle fatigue.

3) Protect your spine— you can do this by contracting your stomach muscles during all exercises.

4) Take regular breaks to rest— you should pause for a brief
moment to replenish your energy levels after every series of 10 repetitions. A pause of no more than 5 to 10 seconds should be sufficient

5) Exercise slowly— a slow, steady effort creates strong, hard
muscles. You risk injury by speeding through a routine.

Exercising In Hot Weather

The main concern when exercising at high temperatures is heat
exhaustion or heatstroke. To avoid succumbing to either condition, you
should drink plenty of water before, during and after exercising. Don't rely
solely on thirst as a guideline for water requirements. Also, be sure to
wear lightweight, breathable clothing, and stop exercising if you notice
any signs of dizziness, nausea, or if you have difficulty breathing.

Synthetics, such as polyproplyene, are good as a first layer of
clothing because of their ability to draw perspiration away from the skin,
keeping it dry. Other synthetics, such as Gore-Tex and Thintech, are used
frequently for outer layers because they are both wind- and water-resistant.

5 Tips For Winter Exercising

The cold inclement weather of winter need not interfere with your exercise program. Here are several suggestions that will help you maintain your outdoor exercise routine, even in the coldest weather:

1) Dress with the weather in mind. In cold weather, layered clothing keeps your comfortable as your body heats up. Also wear a hat or hood to prevent loss of body heat through your head. Keep your hands and ears covered to avoid frostbite. You should also apply sunscreen on any exposed skin.

2) Warm up before you begin exercising. Take five to ten minutes to complete you stretching and warm-up routine before you go outdoors. The step becomes even more important the older you are, and the colder the weather.

3) Drink lots of water. If you exercise strenuously, try to drink water every 15 minutes. Even in cold weather, your body will become dehydrated during exercise.

4) Keep dry. You should always wear a water-repellent jacket when you are out in inclement weather. Wet clothing is not only heavy, it also robs the body of heat.

5) Move indoors on extremely cold days. Mall walking has become a very popular and inexpensive alternative to health clubs. You don't even have to shop, just walk.

Stretching: How To Do It Right

Regular stretching exercises should be performed before and after any form of vigorous physical activity to help you warm up and cool down. They are also necessary if you are performing regular muscle strengthening exercises. Knowing the proper stretching techniques is also essential. Statistics show that most common sports injuries—walking, running, and so on—are the result of improper warmups. Properly done, stretching will help you increase your flexibility, and could become a healthful daily routine as well as a warmup for sports or other exercise.

Here are six effective stretching exercises, designed for regular routines and/or pre-vigorous-exercise warmups: (To avoid injury during stretching you should use only slow, careful movements. Don't jerk or bounce while you are stretching because you could easily injure the joint ligaments of the discs in your spine. Be sure to get your doctor's approval before you begin any exercise routine.)

1) You can stretch the hamstrings by raising a leg onto a raised surface, such as a table, then bend down toward the outstretched leg. Repeat the stretch with the other leg. You should be careful not to jerk or bounce the movement. Also, don't be foolish and stretch to the point of pain. In fact, if it does hurt, you should stop immediately, because you are most likely doing something wrong. Remember, incorrect stretching can be dangerous. Also, use common sense and consider your age and degree of fitness before you begin doing this or any other exercise. If done properly, this is an effective stretch for the hamstrings at the back of the thigh.

2) You can stretch your shoulders by standing tall (no slouching) and stretching both your arms straight behind you. This will help improve the flexibility of your shoulders.

3) To stretch the inner parts of your thighs, stand with your legs apart and then move one leg away from you to the side. Lean the upper part of your body away from your outstretched leg. This stretch should help improve flexibility in your inner thigh muscles.

4) To stretch the quadriceps muscles at the front of your thigh, while standing, hold one leg behind you and pull on it gently. Be careful when doing this stretch because using an arm to help you stretch your leg can cause you to overstretch. You could also easily lose your balance.

5) To stretch the lumbar spine, lie on your back, with your knees up and your hands clasped behind your head. Try to bring your shoulders off the floor and down toward your pelvis.

6) To stretch your abdominal muscles, lie flat on your stomach, with your hands underneath your shoulders, palms on the floor and elbows bent. Slowly push your shoulders and chest up off the floor until you feel a pull across your stomach. Keep that position for several seconds, then lower yourself back to the floor.

16 Things You Sould Have
In Your Medicine Cabinet

1) A thermometer for taking temperature. If you have children younger than 5, a rectal or ear (tympanic) model is also good to have on hand.

2) Self adhesive bandages to treat minor wounds. Also a larger bandage to wrap pulled muscles or twisted ankles which do not require emergency attention.

3) An eye cup, used with water to float off foreign particles in the eye, is also useful, as are cotton swabs.

4) Acetaminophen tablets to reduce fever and pain. Keep acetaminophen syrup on hand for children. (Children younger than 15 should not take aspirin because of its link to Reye's syndrome.)

5) Oil of cloves for temporary relief of toothaches.

6) Liniment containing methyl salicylate for relief of muscle aches and pains.

7) An antiseptic liquid, such as hydrogen peroxide, for cleaning out cuts and scrapes.

8) An antibiotic ointment or cream for preventing infection in minor cuts and scrapes.

9) Calamine lotion for treating itchy skin conditions, including insect and plant stings.

10) Petroleum jelly to provide relief from some types of skin dryness.

11) Ipecac to induce vomiting of swallowed, non-corrosive, poisonous material in an emergency. Although you should have ipecac on hand, don't use it until you have been directed to do so by a local poison control center.

12) Antacid to relieve heartburn and indigestion.

13) Antidiarrhea medication, such as Pepto Bismol.

14) Antihistamine to reduce allergic reactions.

15) Throat lozenges for easing the pain of a sore throat.

16) Key medical phone numbers.

4 Ways To Be Prepared For Home Emergencies

1) Know where to call— this means locating and posting telephone numbers for your local emergency medical service, your local poison control center, your doctor, and the nearest hospital emergency department, next to your telephone. Many communities now have the 911 phone number for emergency response, but in some communities you must dial a seven-digit number to call for an ambulance.

When you call for an ambulance, give your name, address, and telephone number, and then clearly and calmly explain the situation and describe any obvious injuries. Stay calm and follow exactly all the instructions you are given.

2) Keep a well-stocked first-aid kit— your first-aid kit should contain several basic items usually required in emergencies. A good first-aid kit includes such items as a first-aid manual; disposable, instant cold packs; antiseptic wipes; antibiotic cream; aspirin and acetaminophen; gauze and adhesive tape; a triangular bandage (for making splints); a roll of cotton; an adhesive bandage; waterproof bandages; an elastic bandage; a thermometer; scissors, tweezers, safety pins; and syrup of ipecac. Such basic kits are available at most drug stores.

3) Know your medical history— this requires keeping a record of the medical history of each member of your family. The information you should have recorded includes all medications being taken (including dosages); any allergies, such as medications and/or insect bites; and when immunizations were given.

4) Get training in basic first-aid and CPR— such training will help ensure that your actions in an emergency situation will be both appropriate and effective. Groups such as the American Red Cross, the American

Heart Association and the National Safety Council offer first-aid and CPR courses and information. You can find your local ARC and AHA by looking in your telephone directory. To get information on first-aid programs offered by the National Safety Council, call 312-537-4800.

Ten Basic Emergency Procedures

1) Choking (obstruction to the airway)

If the victim cannot breathe and is unable to speak, there is most likely a complete blockage of the airway that must be removed quickly to prevent suffocation. You should have someone else (if you are not alone with the victim) call for an ambulance while you perform the Heimlich maneuver on the victim. The Heimlich maneuver produces an artificial cough to help an individual who is choking force the obstructing object out of the trachea. Here are the steps involved in the Heimlich maneuver:

Conscious choking victim

A) Stand behind the victim, putting your arms around his or her waist. Place your fist with the thumb side against the victim's stomach just above the navel and below the ribs and breastbone.

B) Hold your fist with your other hand and give several quick, forceful, upward and inward thrusts into the abdomen until the obstruction is expelled. Dn not squeeze the victim's ribs with your arms— be sure to use only your fist.

C) You may have to do six to ten thrusts before the victim coughs up the object or becomes unconscious.

D) If you are home alone and you are choking, give yourself abdominal thrusts by pressing your abdomen onto the back of a chair or some other solid object.

Unconscious choking victim

A) If the person who is choking is or becomes unconscious, you should place the heel of one hand on the victim's stomach, just above the navel and below the ribs. Place your free hand on top of your other hand.

Keeping your elbows straight, give several quick, forceful, downward and forward thrusts toward the head.

B) If the above maneuver fails, you should attempt to remove the obstruction with your index finger. Hold the victim's lower jaw and tongue between the thumb and fingers of one hand and lift up the jaw. Look for anything that may be obstructing the airway. With the victim's face up, insert your index finger down inside the cheek toward the base of the tongue. Using a "sweeping" motion, move your finger across the back of the victim's throat to dislodge any obstruction. Be careful you do not push the obstruction further down the victim's throat.

2) Breathing Emergencies

Such emergencies may be caused by a variety of things including airway obstruction, ingestion of poison, injury to chest or lungs, heart-attack, allergic reactions, and electrocution. If a person is not breathing, there will not be an up-an-down movement of the chest or abdomen, and you will not be able to hear or feel air being exhaled. Listen and feel at the nose or mouth for breathing. If the victim is not breathing, gently tilt his or her head back and lift the chin. This reopens the airway by moving the tongue away from the back of the throat.

Mouth-To-Mouth Resuscitation

The method of artificial ventilation used most often to restore breathing is mouth-to-mouth resuscitation. Here are the basic steps involved:

A) Place the palm of one hand on the victim's forehead and the fingers of your other hand under the bony part of his or her chin and tilt the head back.

B) Pinch the victim's nose shut. Open your mouth and take in a deep breath.

C) Seal your lips around the victim's mouth and give two full breaths of 1 to 1 1/2 seconds each. Remove your mouth after each exhalation and take a deep breath.

D) Turn your head toward the victim's chest, with your ear just above his or her mouth. Listen for air being exhaled and watch the victim's chest. Continue breathing into the victim's mouth at a rate of 12 breaths per minute for an adult, 15 per minute for a child.

If you are alone with the victim, call for an ambulance after one minute and then resume resuscitation efforts. Check for a pulse and breathing every minute.

3) Absence of a pulse

This can be caused by many things including cardiac arrest from a heart attack, suffocation, severe blood loss, or electrocution. It is vital to act quickly because permanent brain damage can occur in as little as 4 to 6 minutes. If you are home alone with the victim, do one minute of CPR, then call for an ambulance. Otherwise, have someone call for medical help while you begin CPR.

Place your hands in the center of the victim's chest—between the nipples— and compress the chest to a depth of 1 1/2 to 2 inches for an adult and 1 to 1 1/2 inches for children. Perform the compression 15 times and then give two breaths. Repeat this technique three more times, then recheck for a pulse. If there is still no pulse, continue CPR until medical help arrives.

While CPR is invaluable in such situations, it can also be harmful to the victim. Inexpert application of the technique may cause fractured ribs or even rupture of the heart. That's why it is important to be thoroughly trained in the proper CPR procedure.

4) Severe external bleeding

If you are not alone with the victim, have someone call for an ambulance while you apply pressure to the wound. Place a thick, clean compress, such as sterile gauze or a soft, clean cloth directly and firmly over the entire wound. Don't try to remove any objects that may be embedded in the wound, because that could worsen the bleeding.

Unless doing so causes the victim pain, you should elevate the wounded area. Cover the cloth or gauze with a bandage, tying or taping it in place. If blood soaks through the compress, do not remove it— instead, add another pad over the first compress, and continue to apply pressure.

5) Poisoning

Act quickly to find out what type of poison was taken. Look for objects such as empty medicine bottles or household cleaner containers. If you suspect an inhaled poison, get the victim outside into the fresh air and then call for an ambulance.

As long as the victim is conscious and you know that the poison taken was a corrosive or caustic substance such as ammonia, immediately give him or her a sip of water or milk to dilute the poisoning. Do not try to induce vomiting until you have received specific directions to do so from your local poison control center or other emergency personnel.

6) Serious burns

Severe burns may be caused by dry heat, such as fire; by moist heat, such as hot liquids and steam; or by electricity; corrosive chemicals; or friction. Burns that are critical and require prompt professional attention include third degree burns which leave a charred area after destroying skin and underlying structures; blistering burns on a child or on an elderly person; all burns to the head, face, neck, hands, feet, or genitals; inhalation burns; electrical burns; chemical burns; and burns covering large areas of the body.

The treatment of burns and scalds depends on the severity of the injury. In general, the first treatment involves reducing the temperature of the burned area. This will help prevent further injury to the skin and underlying tissues as well as to stop the burning and reduce pain. The initial cooling of the burned area can be done by immediately flushing the area with cold water. The injury should then be covered with a dry, clean cloth. Do not put any pressure on the burned surface.

Never apply ointments, sprays, antiseptics, or home remedies such as butter to a burn. And don't break blisters.

7) Fractures

A fracture can be a crack or a complete break in a bone. If the victim's head, neck or back is injured, if he or she cannot walk or has trouble breathing, or if you suspect multiple injuries, don't move the victim. You should call the Emergency Medical Service immediately.

If the injury does not involve the head, neck or back, help the victim rest in a comfortable position. Apply ice or a cold pack to the injury, and immobilize it with a splint or a sling. A splint can be made from objects such as boards, sticks or branches, or several rolled newspapers. To ensure that a broken bone is completely immobilized, the splint should extend beyond the joint above and the joint below the fracture. The victim should also be transported to a medical facility for X-rays.

8) Bites and stings

Many different insects, snakes, and other animals are capable of inflicting injury through biting or stinging. Each type of injury requires slightly different treatment.

A) Insect stings— the most common stinging insects are honeybees, hornets, wasps, and fire ants. If such an insect "nails" you or a member of your household, look for a stinger. If you find one, remove it by scraping the skin carefully with a clean knife, a plastic card or a fingernail. Wash the area with soap and water and apply a cold pack to reduce swelling. Applying calamine lotion or a water and baking soda paste may help relieve discomfort.

Once you have removed the stinger and have cleaned the sting area, watch for signs of an allergic reaction. If you are going to have a reaction, it should happen within 30 minutes or so. Symptoms include difficulty breathing, wheezing, tightness of the throat or chest, nausea and dizziness, severe itching, and swelling of the tongue or mouth. If any of these symptoms occur, call the EMS or take the victim to a hospital or some other medical facility.

B) Scorpion stings and spider bites— keep the area of the sting lower than the victim's heart. Wash the area of the sting or bite, cover it, and apply a cold pack. Also maintain an open airway and restore breathing and circulation if necessary.

Try to capture and/or identify the spider and call the poison control center or your doctor.

C) Ticks— using tweezers, remove the tick by grasping at its head and pulling steadily and slowly. Do not try to pull the tick out with your fingers. Clean the area with rubbing alcohol or an antiseptic and apply a cold pack to reduce swelling. If the tick head remains embedded in the skin, see your doctor immediately. Otherwise, watch for flu-like symptoms to develop. Such symptoms usually develop within two weeks. If the symptoms develop,see your doctor.

Ticks can spread bacterial infection, Lyme disease and certain types of viral encephalitis.

D) Snake bites— clean the bite area with soap and water and immobilize the part of the body that was bitten. Try to keep the wound lower than the victim's heart. Do not apply cold water or ice to the wound. In most cases, it is not recommended that you apply a tourniquet, or suck or cut the wound.

Try to identify the snake and its size. Call for an ambulance or take the victim to a medical facility immediately.

9) Animal bites

Bites by domestic pets and wild animals can become infected. They also carry the risk of tetanus and rabies.

Clean minor wounds with soap and water. Do not clean major wounds as they should be cleaned at a hospital or medical facility. Control any bleeding by applying direct pressure. If the bite is serious, or there is any possibility that the animal had rabies, call for an ambulance or transport the victim to the nearest medical facility.

Report the incident to your local health department or animal control service.

10) Other conditions requiring immediate emergency medical treatment

Many common medical symptoms can be treated safely at home for the first 24 to 48 hours, but there are some other conditions in which you should call for an ambulance without delay.

A) Severe central chest pain that is not relieved by rest. This symptom may signal a heart attack, especially if it is accompanied by weakness, moist, pale or bluish skin, breathing difficulty, sweating, changes in heart rate, and a pain in the arm.

B) Sudden, unexplained drowsiness or loss of consciousness. Possible causes for either condition may include an overdose of drugs, a biochemical disturbance such as uncontrolled diabetes, or a brain disorder such as meningitis.

C) Severe abdominal pain. If such pain is not relieved by vomiting, or if it is accompanied by sweating or faintness, or any abdominal pain which is centered on one side of the body and persists for 3 hours, it could signal a serious problem such as appendicitis. The symptoms require immediate medical attention.

How To Prevent Hot Water Burns When Showering

To prevent hot-water burns when you take a shower or bath, always turn on the cold water first and turn off the hot water first.

If your shower releases a sudden rush of hot water whenever a cold water tap is turned on or a toilet is flushed, you are at risk of a potentially dangerous scalding. Many times fluctuating water temperature is merely a nuisance, but there are times when the resulting thermal shock from a rush of scalding hot water or a burst of cold water can cause serious accidents and injuries.

According to the National SAFE KIDS Campaign, more than 5,000 children are scalded each year, with more than two-thirds of those victims under the age of five. Since their skin is so delicate, children who are exposed to 140 degree water for only 3 seconds, can receive third-degree burns. You can correct fluctuating water temperature and reduce the risk of thermal shock by installing a temperature-control or pressure-balanced mixing valve.

Pressure balance valves control water temperature and eliminate shocks by compensating for pressure variances in the water line. This type of valve works best if there are no fluctuations in the temperature of the water supply itself.

Thermostatic valves use a thermal element which adjusts water flow based on temperature fluctuations. A thermostatic valve will maintain water temperature regardless of whether a temperature change is due to pressure fluctuations or to a change in the temperature of the water supply. If there is a complete loss of either hot or cold water pressure, thermostatic valves will shut down.

Home Fire Prevention And Escape Tips

It doesn't take long for a fire to get out of control. Even a small flame can grow into a virtual inferno in under one minute. Most fatalities in home fires occur between 10 p.m. and 6 a.m., when most people are sleeping. Having smoke detectors on every level of your home, including the basement, will give you an "early warning system" so you and your family will be able to make a safe emergency exit.

Your first line of defense against small household fires is a fire extinguisher. You should keep a fire extinguisher on every level of your home, including your basement. Make sure you read all the instructions and know how to use the extinguisher, and check each extinguisher evey month to make sure they are ready to use in case of fire.

You and your family should have occasional fire drills in order to practice the safest and quickest way of escape. If fire strikes, try to remain calm and remember to follow these procedures:

1) Alert everybody in the house.

2) Don't try to extinguish the fire if you can not do it without endangering life.

3) If your clothes catch on fire, drop to the ground and roll over and over.

4) Crouch down below the smoke in a room and crawl to safety.

5) Test the warmth of all doors before you open them. If a door feels cool, open it a crack to check for smoke. If there is no smoke, keep going. Close the doors behind you as you go.

6) Go straight to a predetermined meeting place outside your home.

7) Always use a neighbor's phone to call the fire department.

The facts are clear, there are plenty of health hazards around the house. They can have a definite impact upon your overall health if you don't watch out. You should avoid unecessary exposure to chemicals. Some common houshold chemicals can be harmful to your health.

The important fact is that you should be well prepared for any emergency. This would include having an emergency first aid kit, a book that details first aid procedures, and being familiar with emergency phone numbers.

The Common Vitamins & How They Can Help

Vitamin A

This is a fat soluble vitamin, of which the most active form is retinol. Vitamin A is essential for normal growth and for the formation of strong bones and teeth in children. It also plays a major role in vision and cell structure, and it provides protection for the linings of the respiratory, digestive, and urinary tracts against infection. It is also essential for healthy skin.

A vitamin A deficiency occurs only in people who have an exceptionally poor diet. The effects of such a deficiency include poor night vision, dry, inflamed eyes, and dry, rough skin. In extreme cases, vitamin A deficiency can result in severe corneal damage that can lead to blindness if left untreated.

Vitamin A is available in many foods, including liver, oily fish, dairy products, egg yolk, margarine, and various fruits and vegetables, such as carrots, kale, broccoli, spinach, apricots, and peaches. The recommended daily allowance for adults is 0.8 to 1 mg.

B- Complex Vitamins

Vitamin B1 (Thiamine)

This is a water-soluble vitamin that is present in many animal and plant foods. It plays a vital role in the proper functioning of the nerves, muscles, and the heart.

While a balanced diet usually provides sufficient amounts of thiamine, those people most susceptible to deficiency include people with a poor diet, people with above average energy requirements, and people with severe alcohol dependency. Extreme thiamine deficiency may result in beriberi, abdominal pain, constipation, depression, and loss of short-term memory.

Especially good sources of thiamine include wheat germ, bran, whole-grain or enriched cereals and breads, brown rice, pasta, liver, pork, fish, eggs, beans, and nuts. The recommended daily allowance of thiamine is 1.1 to 1.5 mg.

Vitamin B2 (Riboflavin)

This vitamin is essential for various biochemical reactions involved in the breakdown and utilization of carbohydrates, fats, and proteins, and in the production of energy in the cells. It is also essential for the production of hormones by the adrenal glands.

A serious deficiency of riboflavin may cause chapped lips, soreness of the tongue and corners of the mouth, and certain eye disorders.

Riboflavin is present in a wide range of foods, including milk, cheese, eggs, green, leafy vegetables, whole-grains, enriched breads and cereals, and liver. The recommended daily allowance is 1.3 to 1.7 mg.

Vitamin B3 (Niacin)

Niacin is essential for the utilization of energy from food. It also plays a major role in the functioning of the nervous system, the manufacture of sex hormones, and the maintenance of healthy skin.

A niacin deficiency, while extremely rare, can, in severe cases, lead to diarrhea, soreness and cracking of the skin, and certain mental disturbances.

The primary dietary sources of niacin include lean meat, liver, fish, poultry, dried beans, nuts, and whole-grains. The recommended daily allowance of niacin is 15 to 19 mg.

Pantothenic Acid

As a member of the B-complex vitamin group, pantothenic acid is required for the release of energy from food, the manufacture of some hormones, and proper functioning of the nervous system.

Deficiency of pantothenic acid is rare, but can occur as a result of severe alcohol dependence, severe injury, or severe illness. The most extreme cases of deficiency may result in a peptic ulcer.

Pantothenic acid is present in almost all vegetables, cereals, and animal foods. While there is no recommended daily allowance, the suggested daily intake is 4 to 7 mg.

Vitamin B6 (Pyridoxine)

This is a water-soluble vitamin that has many essential roles, including regulating the synthesis of proteins from amino acids.

A deficiency of pyridoxine may cause weakness, irritability, depression, skin disorder, and anemia.

Good sources of pyridoxine include meats and poultry, fish, whole-grains, wheat germ, bananas, most fruits and vegetables, potatoes, and dried beans. The recommended daily allowance is 2 mg.

Biotin

Biotin serves to aid the action of enzymes involved in the synthesis of substances in the cells.

A deficiency of biotin may result in poor appetite, hair loss, depression, and eczema.

Biotin is present in many foods, including liver, peanuts, dried beans, egg yolk, mushrooms, bananas, grapefruit, and watermelon. The suggested daily intake of biotin is 30 to 100 mcg.

Folic Acid: The Little-Known Vitamin You Need For Anemia Problems

Sometimes called "vitamin M", this water-soluble vitamin is involved in growth and reproduction, the production of red blood cells, and in the healthy functioning of the nervous system.

Mild folic acid deficiency is relatively common, but it can usually be corrected by increasing the intake of food containing folic acid. The main effects of folic acid deficiency include fatigue and anemia.

The primary dietary sources of folic acid include green, leafy vegetables, broccoli, spinach, mushrooms, nuts, dried beans, peas, egg yolk, liver, and whole-wheat bread. The recommended daily allowance is 200 mcg.

Vitamin B12 (Cyanocobalmin)

This vitamin is water-soluble, and it contains the mineral cobalt. It is essential for forming blood and the fatty sheath which surrounds the nerves, and in the construction of genetic material.

Strict vegetarians may become deficient, since meat is the primary source of this vitamin. The effects of vitamin B12 deficiency may include anemia, depression and loss of memory.

Foods rich in vitamin B12 include liver, beef, pork, lamb, poultry, fish, dairy products, eggs, oysters, and yeast. The recommended daily allowance is 2 mcg.

Vitamin C (Ascorbic Acid)

This is a water-soluble vitamin that plays an important role in the growth and maintenance of healthy bones, teeth, gums, ligaments, and blood vessels. It may even strengthen the body's natural defenses against infection.

A mild deficiency of vitamin C may cause weakness, swollen gums, and nosebleeds. Severe deficiency leads to scurvy and anemia.

Recent research suggests that vitamin C—taken directly or through orange juice—may reduce the harmful effects of low-level radiation. The study— conducted on field mice—showed that vitamin C protected against the harmful effects of low-level X-rays, which are the type used in medical diagnosis. It is still unclear, however, if humans can also benefit from those protective qualities of vitamin C.

Other recent studies suggest that fruits and vegetables high in vitamin C and carotenoids—orange, yellow, and red pigments—may help prevent cataracts, as well as play a protective role against certain cancers. These studies, taking place at the USDA Human Nutrition Research Center on Aging at Tufts University in Boston, while neither definitive nor conclusive, should serve as positive reinforcement for a healthy addition of fruits and vegetables into the average daily diet.

Vitamin C can be found in fresh fruits and vegetables. Citrus fruits, tomatoes, green, leafy vegetables, broccoli, potatoes, sweet red peppers, strawberries, and cantaloupe are especially good sources. The recommended daily allowance is 60 mg.

Vitamin D

This is a fat-soluble vitamin which actually encompasses a group of related substances, including ergocalciferol (also known as vitamin D2) and cholecalciferol (vitamin D3) which play several important roles in the body. Vitamin D helps regulate the balance of calcium and phosphate, helps form bones and teeth, and aids the absorption of calcium from the intestine.

The body needs only small amounts of vitamin D, which can be provided by a balanced diet and normal exposure to sunlight. A deficiency of vitamin D may lead to low blood levels of calcium and phosphate, which results in a softening of the bones. In children this condition is known as rickets— in adults, it is called osteomalacia.

The best dietary source of vitamin D is fortified milk. Other good sources include butter, cheese, margarine, oily fish, liver, eggs, fortified cereals and breads, and cod liver oil. Normal exposure to sunlight is the non-dietary source. The recommended
dietary allowance of vitamin D is 5 to 10 mcg.

Vitamin E (Tocopherol)

Vitamin E is a fat-soluble vitamin which is essential for normal cell structure and the formation of red blood cells. It also protects the lungs and other tissues from damage by pollutants and helps prevent red blood cells from being damaged by poisons in the blood.

A deficiency of vitamin E may lead to the destruction of red blood cells, which ultimately results in anemia.

The primary dietary sources of vitamin E are vegetable oils, eggs, fish, green, leafy vegetables, cereals, wheat germ, meat, and dried beans. The recommended daily allowance is 8 to 10 mg.

Vitamin K

This is a fat-soluble vitamin which is essential for normal blood clotting.

A deficiency of vitamin K reduces the ability of the blood to clot. This condition may cause nosebleeds, bleeding from the gums, intestines, and urinary tract, and seeping of blood from wounds.

The main dietary sources of vitamin K include green, leafy vegetables, vegetable oils, pork, liver, egg yolk, cheese, potatoes, fruits, and grain products. Vitamin K is also manufactured by bacteria which normally live in the intestine. Newborn infants lack such intestinal bacteria and are therefore given vitamin K supplements to prevent deficiency. The recommended daily allowance for adults is 60 to 80 mcg.

Should You Take Vitamin Supplements?

Studies conducted by the Food and Drug Administration reveal that about 50 percent of Americans take vitamin and/or mineral supplements. The percentage seems high, especially considering the fact that if your diet is balanced, supplements are not required. Most of the vitamin deficiency disorders have been eliminated by today's varied and fresh food supply.

Eating a variety of foods should provide you with sufficient amounts of all vitamins. Excessive amounts of some vitamins, such as A and D, may actually be harmful. That's why supplements should be taken only on the advice of a physician. Some multivitamin supplements contain as much as five times the recommended daily allowance of certain vitamins.

In certain circumstance, a doctor may recommend vitamin supplements. Such circumstances might include a person who is taking certain drugs which reduce the intestinal absorption of vitamins, or for some women who are pregnant or who are breast-feeding. In any case, even though excessive amounts of most vitamins may not be harmful, you should consult your doctor before you use a vitamin supplement.

Potassium Power-Your Heart Needs It

The importance of potassium in the diet is underscored by the American Heart Association's acknowledgement that people who consume adequate amounts of the mineral are less likely to suffer from the major risk factors for stroke and heart attack. Eating raw fruits and vegetables that are high in potassium appears to help protect individuals against high blood pressure and blocked arteries.

Bananas are good sources of potassium as are beets, potatoes, yams, and other root vegetables are all excellent To get the full benefit of the potassium in these foods, they should be eaten raw as often as possible because cooking tends to remove the mineral.

Healing Tips For Gout

This is an arthritic-type condition developing from excess uric acid in the tissues. Most gout patients tend to both overproduce and under-excrete uric acid.

While gout can attack any joint or combination of joints, doctors say that in 9 out of 10 gout victims the big toe is affected. It usually causes inflammation, swelling, redness, and severe pain. Usually such an attack of gout will occur suddenly, progress rapidly, last several days and then disappear. It may recur at intervals of weeks, months or years.

If you are a middle-aged man who is somewhat overweight and have a family history of the affliction, you're a likely candidate for gout. However, in almost every case the disease can be treated and controlled. Here are some medical experts' suggestions for dealing with gout:

1) Rest and elevation— the intensity of the pain during an acute attack of gout can be excruciating. Doctors recommend that you elevate the throbbing joint and try to rest.

2) Use a painkiller— the excessive pain you feel during an attack of gout is caused by inflammation around the afflicted joint. A painkiller that can reduce inflammation, such as ibuprofen, can give you some relief. If you use such a pain killer make sure you follow bottle directions. Don't increase the directed dosage without first talking with your doctor.

Painkillers such as aspirin and acetaminophen should be avoided because aspirin will most likely make the condition worse by inhibiting the excretion of uric acid, and acetaminophen's ability to reduce inflammation isn't strong enough to have a significant effect on gout.

3) Make it cold— applying cold is a good idea only if the affected joint is not too tender to touch—which it often is. If you can stand to touch the joint, you can try applying a crushed-ice pack. Leave the pack on the affected joint for about ten minutes. You can cushion it with a towel or sponge. Repeat the treatment as often as needed, or as often as the tenderness will allow.

4) Avoid high-purine foods— increased levels of purine which is a product of DNA, can raise the level of uric acid in the blood. While a strict low-purine diet is not necessary, victims of gout should avoid foods that are high in purine, such as liver and other organ meats, poultry, and legumes.

5) Drink plenty of water— always a healthy idea, drinking lots of water can help people with gout by flushing excess uric acid from the system before it can be too harmful. Herb teas can also be helpful.

6) Avoid alcohol— if you are susceptible to gout, you shouldn't drink alcohol. For someone who is prone to gout, alcohol consumption can trigger an acute attack.

7) Slim down— if you are overweight and prone to gout, it is essential that you gradually lose your excess weight. People who are overweight tend to have higher uric acid levels. Don't try to lose a lot of weight in a short time. The weight loss should be gradual.

Hemorrhoids: 5 Keys
For Their Treatment And Prevention

Some people consider them an embarassment, but experts say that 70 to 80 percent of all adult Americans have hemorrhoids. Some people aren't even aware that they have them. They only notice them when they begin to itch, bleed, or protrude, and then it's time to fight back.

1) Watch your diet— the best way to deal with hemorrhoids is by eating lots of fiber and drinking plenty of fluids, ensuring soft and easy bowel movements. You should not have to strain to have a bowel movement. If you do, you're most likely producing hard stools and subsequently, hemorrhoids.

2) Apply a lubricating oil— an application of petroleum jelly to the area will protect it when hard stools pass. If you prefer, you can use one of the many over-the-counter hemorrhoid products.

3) Sit in a sitz bath— fill the bath tub to a level so that when you sit the water will come up to your navel. Once you're in the tub, carefully raise your feet above the water. You can rest them on the sides of the tub. Warm water will help ease the pain while increasing the flow of blood to the area. That can help shrink the swollen veins.

4) Don't do any heavy lifting— if you are prone to hemorrhoids, any type of heavy lifting or vigorous exercise could cause straining which might make the problem worse.

5) Cut down on your use of salt— too much salt in your diet tends to retain fluids in your circulatory system, which could lead to a worsening of your hemorrhoids.

7 "Hiccups" Cures

The hiccup sound we hear is caused by a sudden involuntary contraction of the diaphragm followed by rapid closure of the vocal chords. While no one knows for sure what causes the contractions, some doctors speculate that they occur when nerve centers which control the muscles of respiration become irritable. Most cases of hiccups last only a few minutes. If they last longer than a day or two, you should seek medical attention.

Whatever "cure" is tried, the general goal is to increase carbon dioxide levels in the blood or to disrupt the nerve impulses causing the hiccups. However it's done, hiccups cures sometimes work and sometimes they don't. But since there's really nothing to lose in trying, here are several home-tested ways you can "cure" hiccups:

1)Hold your breath— try holding your breath for at least 30 seconds— longer if you can.

2) Swallow some sugar— a teaspoon of sugar, swallowed dry, reportedly works for some people.

3) Bend over and drink— you may find this one hard to do but there are those who swear it works. Get a glass of water and instead of drinking the usual way, try bending forward and drinking the water from the opposite side of the glass.

4) Gargle with water.

5) Put a paper bag over your mouth and nose, then inhale and exhale into it repeatedly.

6) Pull your knees up to your chest.

7) Chew slowly, then swallow some dry bread.

How To Prevent And Get Over Flus

Fever, headache, muscle ache and weakness are commonly experienced symptoms of influenza or the "flu". This nasty viral infection comes in a variety pack of three main types: A, B and C.

Whichever letter of the alphabet you get can make you miserable. There are some precautions you can take to reduce your vulnerability to the flu, but once you get it there's nothing to do to get rid of it until it's ready to leave. Antibiotics don't work because it is a virus. There are, however, certain things you can do to make a bout with the flu a little less miserable. Here are a few suggestions:

1) Stay in bed— in all but the mildest of cases, a victim of the flu is usually better off in bed, resting in a well-ventilated room.

2) Get lots of liquids into your system— this is especially important when you have a fever because of the possibility of dehydration. Liquids can also provide essential nutrients when you feel too sick to eat solid food. Try thin soups and fruit and vegetable juices. Warm fluids can also soothe a sore throat.

3) Make use of a painkiller— an analgesic such as ibuprofen, aspirin or acetaminophen can help reduce the fever and the body aches and pains caused by the flu.

4) Get steamed— steam heat has a soothing effect on the lungs, helping to reduce the discomfort caused by a cough, sore throat, or dry nasal passages.

5) Soak your feet— if you have a headache or nasal congestion, soaking your feet in hot water may help.

6) Get vaccinated— protect yourself against the flu by getting a flu shot in the fall or very early winter. Because the vaccine takes about two weeks to get into action, you shouldn't wait until the flu is all around you before getting your shot.

7 Ways To End Motion Sickness

This includes everything from air sickness to car sickness to sea sickness. Regardless of whether it's land, sea, or air, this is unpleasant stuff. It causes sweating, pallor, and nausea, often progressing to vomiting. The sickness is triggered by the effect of any constant pronounced movement on the organ of balance in the inner ear, although psychological stress seems to play a role. To avoid motion sickness, or to reduce the effects of its symptoms, try some of these expert recommendations:

1) Avoid any strong odors and foods that unsettle your stomach.

2) Steer clear of smoke— either active or passive cigarette smoking can trigger impending motion sickness. Non smokers should be sure to sit in the non-smoking sections of trains, planes or buses.

3) Travel by night— you won't be able to see the motion as well in darkness as you do in daylight, so you may reduce your chance of getting sick if you travel by night.

4) Avoid alcohol— even if you are only a passenger, too much alcohol can help set off motion sickness symptoms. Consume enough alcohol and you won't even have to be in motion to experience symptoms similar to motion sickness.

5) Sit up front— when you're traveling in a car, be sure to sit up front and focus on something in the distance, such as the horizon.

6) Take a pill before you travel— the most popular antihistamine drugs for motion sickness are Dramamine, Benadryl, and Bonine. Taken a few hours in advance, any of these drugs can prevent motion sickness symptoms from occurring. However, these over-the-counter drugs can also cause drowsiness and might not be a wise choice if you plan to drive.

7) Try a natural remedy— in some studies, powdered ginger was found to be more effective than some over-the-counter medications. It is an old remedy for stomach disturbances and doesn't cause drowsiness.

How To Stop A Nosebleed

Most nosebleeds are more-messy-than serious conditions. Knowing what to do to stop the flow of blood doesn't take a degree in medicine. All it takes is some common sense and the ability to follow a few basic steps.

1) Sit upright and gently blow your nose to remove any clots.

2) Pinch your nostrils together and squeeze for 5 minutes or so, breathing through your mouth. Keep your head tilted down so the flow of blood won't go down your throat.

3) If that procedure doesn't work, insert into each nostril a small piece of sterile absorbant cotton or gauze made wet by nose drops, white vinegar, hydrogen peroxide, or water. Press the nostrils firmly together for another 5 to 7 minutes. The bleeding should stop by the time you slowly and gently remove the cotton or gauze.

4) If none of the above procedures work, consult your doctor.

5) It sometimes takes a week or longer for your nose to heal com-

pletely after a nosebleed. Be very gentle with your nose during the recovery period.

How To Get Rid Of Poison Ivy And Poison Oak

About half the population in America are susceptible to allergic reactions from poison ivy and poison oak. Those reactions are anything but pleasant— a nagging itch and red rash , caused by the toxin urshiol.

The best defense against poison ivy and poison oak is avoidance. The next best defense is to know how to treat the symptoms if avoidance fails. Here are some timely suggestions:

1) Recognize the plants— the only way to avoid poison ivy or poison oak is to know what they look like so you can keep your distance. Both plants have three leaflets and white berries. Some people remember this by reciting these two old rhymes: " Leaflets three, let it be", "Berries white, poisonous sight". If you recognize poison ivy or poison oak, you should avoid contact with any part of the plants.

2) Wash the area of contact immediately— you may be able to avoid becoming infected if within 1 to 3 minutes after exposure you can remove the irritating oil by washing the affected area with rubbing alcohol, or if none is available, lots of water.

3) Use a lotion— some over-the-counter lotions containing calamine or zinc oxide can help relieve itching. However, you should avoid lotions containing diphenhydramine hydrochloride, an antihistamine, and benzocaine, a topical anesthetic.

4) Don't scratch— although it's difficult to keep from doing it, you should not scratch the itchy area, and you should also avoid using hot water on affected areas.

5) Try a cool compress— take a piece of cotton cloth soaked in cool water and place it over the affected area. Let a fan blow over the area also.

6) Jewelweed to the rescue— some people report that an effective herbal treatment involves rubbing the crushed leaves and stems of the orange-or yellow-flowered jewelweed over the affected area.

7) Wash everything— if your clothing or equipment has touched poison ivy or poison oak, clean them as soon as possible.

Post Nasal Drip How To Dry It Up

This annoying condition arises from abnormal accumulations of secretions in the upper throat, behind the nose. When that happens, there is a watery or sticky discharge, which is affectionately called post nasal drip. Here are some expert suggestions on how to dry up the drip:

1) Blow your nose— while this may be an obvious thing to do under the circumstances, it is often overlooked. By blowing your nose regularly, you will get rid of some of the drainage from the front of your nose.

2) Use a saltwater gargle— add 1/2 teaspoon of salt (1/3 if you have high blood pressure) to 8 ounces of water, and gargle. This solution should help clear your throat.

3) Go easy on the spicy foods— some "hot" and "spicy" foods such as hot peppers and curry, can act as irritants and make the condition worse.

4) Drink lots of fluids, except milk— warm fluids such as tea or warm water with lemon can help keep the mucus lining moist and get rid of post nasal drip. Milk, however, may promote excess mucus production, making the condition worse.

5) If your post nasal drip is persistent, consult your doctor. You may have a genuine sinus infection. Your doctor may prescribe decongestants and suggest that you increase your household humidity.

Self Healing For Psoriasis

This is a mysterious, although common skin disease which is characterized by thickened patches of inflamed, red skin, sometimes covered by silvery scales. It tends to recur in attacks of varying severity. the exact cause of psoriasis is unknown, and treatment varies. While there is no cure, there are a number of things you can do for self-treatment.

1) Let there be light— mild cases of psoriasis may be helped by exposure to sunlight or an ultraviolet lamp. Consult your doctor before you try either treatment and get his or her recommendations.

Some studies suggest that over 90 percent of people who suffer from psoriasis report improvement with regular doses of intense sunlight. However, this type of exposure also increases your risk of sunburn and skin cancer. One way to reduce this risk is to use a potent sunscreen on areas where you don't have psoriasis and only expose the affected areas to the full intensity of the sun's ultraviolet waves.

2) Use an emollient— many dermatologists recommend emollients as an over- the-counter treatment for psoriasis because they help your skin retain water. Any non-irritating body oil or petroleum jelly can be effective. For best results, apply the emollient right after you bathe and before you dry off.

3) Coal tar may help— ointments containing coal tar are available over-the- counter and while they are less potent than prescription coal tar ointments, they can be effective in mild cases of psoriasis. If you try such an ointment and it causes burning or irritation, stop using it.

4) Maintain your ideal weight— medical experts say that people who shed excess weight seem to experience some improvement in their skin condition.

5) Relax— evidence indicates that psoriasis is another health problem in which stress can play a part. Find ways to relax and make your life less stressful.

6) Try cold water for itching— many people find relief from itching caused by psoriasis by soaking in a cold-water bath. You might also try applying it to affected areas of the skin.

Stop Drinking This If You Have Psoriasis Problems

According to a report in the British Medical Journal, excessive alcohol consumption worsens psoriasis. The researchers say that the amount of alcohol consumed and the frequency of intoxication contributed to a worsening of psoriasis among those people being studied. Based upon this research, people who suffer from psoriasis are encouraged to stop drinking alcohol.

5 Ways To Get Rid Of Sinusitis

This is a particularly unpleasant affliction, caused by infection spreading to the sinuses from the nose along the narrow passages that drain mucus from the sinuses into the nose. It usually creates a feeling of tension or fullness in the affected area, sometimes accompanied by a throbbing ache. There's also usually a nasty nasal discharge of yellow or green mucus. What can you do to relieve these symptoms? Here are 5 expert-recommended treatments for sinusitis:

1) Try steam— steam inhalations moisten the secretions and help to remove them. Allow your bathroom to get steamy, and then stand in a hot shower for several minutes, at least 2 times a day. You can also create a "steam tent" by placing a towel over your head and leaning over a pan full of steaming water.

2) Buy a room humidifier— this will help keep your nasal and sinus passages from drying out. Be sure to change the water daily and clean it once a week to prevent the growth of fungus.

3) Use decongestants— single-action tablets containing only decongestant are usually effective in drying up the sinuses. They work by constricting the blood vessels and by helping to alleviate pressure.

4) Drink plenty of fluids— whether the liquid is hot or cold it should help thin out mucus and keep it flowing. Hot herb teas may prove especially effective.

5) If your sinusitis persists even after 3 or 4 days of self-treatment, you should see your doctor. You may need to take antibiotics to get rid of the infection, or you may need to undergo surgical drainage of the affected sinuses.

Sunburn What You Should Know

Letting the sun burn our skin isn't the smartest thing we can do but we do it anyway— regularly. Even though we know that excessive tanning causes degeneration of the skin and is implicated in skin cancer, we often think only of the cosmetic benefits. Then, before we realize it, it's too late to think of anything but the pain. Next time, we'll take some precautions, but for now, what can we do for some relief? Here are some expert tips on easing the pain of sunburn and on avoiding it altogether:

1) If you must tan, do it slowly— this is the best way to tan without burning. About 30 minutes before you go into the sun, apply a potent sunscreen with a sun protection factor (SPF) of at least 15.

2) Avoid being in the sun during its most damaging hours— from about 10 a.m. to 2 p.m. (11 a.m. to 3 p.m. Daylight Savings Time) the sun's ultraviolet rays can be especially damaging.

3) Use painkillers if you burn— in many cases, aspirin can relieve the pain, itching and swelling of a mild to moderate sunburn.

4) Cool your skin— apply compresses of ice-cold water, skim-milk, witch hazel, or Burrow's solution for 10 minutes or so every few hours.

5) Get into yogurt— some people swear by plain yogurt. It is both cooling and soothing and should be applied to all sunburned areas. Rinse off in a cool shower, and pat your skin gently dry.

6) Drink lots of water— always good for you, drinking lots of water will help to reduce the drying effect of a burn.

7) Moisturize— after the sunburn pain is gone and dryness and itching develop, apply a moisturizing cream or lotion. You can also use an over-the- counter hydrocortisone cream after you bathe.

8) Give yourself time to heal— stay out of the sun until all signs of the sunburn, including any peeling and flaking, are gone. When you finally return to the sun, don't forget your sunscreen.

How To Get Rid Of Urinary Tract Infections

These infections are caused by one or more types of bacteria invading the bladder, urethra, or other parts of the urinary tract. Common UTI symptoms include a burning sensation on urinating and frequent urination. Backache and fever may also accompany the infection. Doctors say that at least 50 percent of all women will contract a bladder infection, sooner or later. Here are several expert recommendations for reducing the discomfort of UTI.

1) Drink a lot of water or juices— urologists say you should drink plenty of fluids— water and juices—to flush out the bacteria that are caus- ing the inflammation. While there's no conclusive evidence, some recent studies suggest that cranberry juice may indeed be an effective treatment for UTI.

2) Avoid coffee, tea and alcohol—these fluids may irritate the uri- nary tract.

3) Soaking in a hot bath— many women find this a good way to get relief from UTI.

4) Try an anti-inflammation drug— both aspirin and ibuprofen may help to reduce the inflammation in the bladder.

5) Get more vitamin C in your system— some doctors say that large doses of vitamin C can acidify the urine enough to disrupt the growth of bacteria. Before you begin taking vitamin C as a treatment for UTI, you should get your doctor's approval.

6) Urinate before intercourse— an empty bladder can reduce the likelihood of irritation in the pelvis by allowing more space. It also helps get rid of bacteria that may be present in the vagina.

Varicose Veins:
Get Rid Of Them Without Going To A Doctor

No doubt about it, most people can find nothing good to say about having twisted, distended, superficial veins just below the skin. Varicose veins are not at all popular. They affect 1 out of every 2 women over 40 and 1 out of every 4 men. If untreated they tend to grow worse. So how do you treat them?

1) Wear elastic support stockings— generally available in med- ical supply stores, elastic support stockings can help provide relief. You can consult your doctor about the weight and length of the stocking you need. While support stockings can relieve discomfort, they are not a cure.

2) Get your feet off the ground— whenever possible, elevate your legs above hip level. This should help relieve the discomfort whenever they are aching.

3) Avoid high-heels and cowboy boots— this type of footwear can only aggravate the condition.

4) Maintain a trim figure— excessive weight places more pressure on your legs. If you keep your weight down, you'll probably have fewer problems with varicose veins.

5) Walk, walk, walk— if you sit or stand for prolonged periods of time you wind up causing problems in your legs because the blood will most likely pool. Walking throughout the day is not only a way to prevent the blood from pooling, it's also great exercise.

7 COMMON CHILDHOOD ILLNESSES

1) Measles, German measles and mumps

Measles is one of the most serious and contagious of all childhood diseases. Medical experts say that about 1 out of every 6 cases of measles is followed by such complications as pneumonia, earaches, sinusitis, and encephalitis. In the first few days of a measles infection the symptoms will suggest that the child has a severe cold. They include a runny nose; red, watering eyes; a fever of 100 degrees or higher; and a dry, hacking cough.

Those symptoms are followed by a slight drop in temperature and the appearance of tiny white spots lining the mouth. Then the child's temperature rises again and an itchy, blotchy red rash appears first on the head and neck and then on the rest of the body.

The symptoms of German measles (rubella) are virtually the same as those described above but less severe. However, there is a more constant fever and swollen glands under the jaw.

When a child has mumps, the glands under his or her chin on one or both sides of the face become swollen. The child may also have difficulty eating, a general feeling of wooziness or nausea, as well as a fever of at least 100 degrees.

To treat all three of these infectious diseases (and chicken pox), you should keep the child at home until your doctor says the contagious stage is over. (Also try to keep the child away from any family members who have not been vaccinated). The essential treatments are bed rest and plenty of liquids. Measles or German measles may cause the child to be sensitive to light so keep the room darkened. The discomfort caused by the rash can be eased by applying cool water and calamine lotion.

Infants younger than a year old, children taking steroid drugs, and those with chronic diseases such as asthma or diabetes, are at high risk for complications from infectious diseases. If your child is in that group and has been exposed to measles, German measles or mumps, contact your doctor. Also remember that there are vaccinations that will give your children complete protection from those infectious diseases.

2) Croup

Croup is a viral respiratory infectious disease that causes swelling of the tissues of the larynx and of the air passages above and below. It is characterized by a barking cough or a crowing sound when inhaling. Croup occurs most commonly in children between the ages of 2 and 4, and in general is fairly common among children 3 months to 5 years old.

The best way to treat the symptoms of croup is to use steam to loosen the phlegm which has built up in bronchial passages. The croupy child should be kept near a vaporizer or a humidifier, or in a bathroom with a constant stream of hot water running into the tub. Sit in the steamy room with the child on your lap. The steam and the upright posture should help relieve the cough.

The child should be breathing more easily within 30 minutes or so after receiving the treatment. If he or she isn't, and has a fever higher than 100 degrees, call your doctor immediately.

3) Otitis Media

An inflammation of the middle ear, otitis media often follows a cold or the flu. Its symptoms are characterized by a sudden, severe earache, a fullness in the ear, slight hearing loss, ringing or buzzing in the ear, and a fever of 100 degrees or higher.

Acute cases of otitis media are treated with antibiotics and anal-
gesics. At the first sign of an ear infection, you should get in touch with
your doctor. Apply a heating pad to the ear to ease the pain and give the
child pediatric acetaminophen. If the earache persists, fluid in the
eardrum may have to be drained.

4) Lice

Lice are small, flat-bodied, wingless, bloodsucking insects that
cause itching on the head or body. They leave small red bite marks on the
neck and behind the ears. Both lice and their eggs (nits) are visible to the
human eye and are transmitted by human contact or shared clothing,bed-
ding, brushes, and combs.

Several over-the-counter shampoos, such as Nix, Endlice, Rid,
and A-200, will usually eradicate lice. There are also stronger prescription
products available. Machine wash on hot cycle or dry-clean all clothing,
bed linens, and towels which might have been infected. Articles that are
not easily washed or dry-cleaned, such as caps or leather clothing, can
be sealed tightly in a plastic bag in order to kill the lice.

5) Sore throat

Sore throat is a common symptom of many childhood illnesses
such as colds and the flu. However, if you see small white spots on your
child's tonsils or on the back of his or her throat and the swollen glands
under the jaw, it could signal strep throat or tonsillitis.

If there is a strep infection, your doctor will most likely prescribe
antibiotics. Otherwise you can give the child acetaminophen and ordinary
cough drops to ease the discomfort.

6) Colic

Colic is usually most severe in babies from 4 to 6 weeks old and
is characterized by the infant's being irritable, crying or screaming excessively, drawing the knees up to the abdomen, and sometimes, passing gas.

Treatment essentially involves waiting for the baby to grow out of
the condition, which usually happens by 3 to 4 months. There are no
cures for colic, but you can treat the symptoms in various ways, including:

A) Fennel tea— pharmacologists say that the oil in fennel seeds is a carminative— a substance that helps expel gas. To make fennel tea, boil fennel seeds in water, then strain and dilute the liquid.

B) Place the baby face-down on your knees while stroking his or her back.

C) Give the baby a pacifier.

D) Place a heating pad—set on a safe, comfortable setting—or a warmed wash cloth under the baby's stomach.

E) Take the baby for a ride in the car. Motion seems to be good for colic.

7) Rheumatic fever

This condition is not nearly as common as it was years ago before antibiotics, but recent evidence indicates it may be on the increase again in parts of the United States.

Rheumatic fever is an inflammatory condition that always follows a streptococcal throat. If allowed to become severe it can cause permanent damage to the heart. It may also affect a person's joints and nervous systom.

Children between the ages of 5 and 15, in a group setting, are most commonly infected. The symptoms of rheumatic fever include fever and pain, inflammation, and swelling of one or more of the larger joints. The symptoms may also include weakness or shortness of breath caused by inflammation of the heart.

As soon as the diagnosis of acute rheumatic fever is made, an antibiotic, such as penicillin, is used to eradicate the streptococci. Aspirin or corticosteroid drugs are used to control the joint pain and inflammation, and to try to minimize heart damage.

The best way to prevent rheumatic fever is to get prompt treatment if you have a streptococcal sore throat. A sore throat with fever, which lasts longer than 24 hours, should be cause for medical attention.

HERBS TO TRY FOR VARIOUS AILMENTS

Many people have reported excellent results from the following herbs - available in any good health food store. Try them - they could work wonders for you!

Aches

Catnip, peppermint, valerian, black haw

Anemia

Comfrey, dandelion, raspberry leaves

Bed-wetting

Plantain, hyssop, red sage, camomi

Boils

hops, comfrey, slippery elm, sorrel, wild cherry bark, burdock

Bronchitis

Coltsfoot, golden seal, mullen, white pine, red sage, chickweed,

Cuts

Comfrey, hyssop, goldseal

Constipation

ginger, blue flag, balmony, rhubard root, chickweed

Dandruff

nettle, sage, burdock

Diarrhea

birch, comfrey, peppermmint, red raspberry blackberry root, mullein

Eczema

Beech, bloodroot, strawberry, white poplar bark, nettle,golden seal

Gas

Anise, mint, dill, sassafras, yarrow, sage

Bad Breath

Golden seal, rosemary

Headache

Catnip, coltsfoot, peppermint, rosemary, camomile

Heartburn

Beech, poplar, majoram, resemary, wild cherry bark, golden seal

Hiccoughs

Dill, orange juice

Hoarseness

Golden seal, mullein, wild cherry

Insect Stings

Parsley, balm, borage, fennel, hyssop, penyroyal, black cohosh

Itching

Yellow dock, borage, marjoram, chickweed

Nerves

Camomile, dill, golden seal, red clover, rosemary, thyme, red sage, wild cherry, sage, peach leaves, Solomon's seal

Obesity

Chickweed, white ash, sassafras

Pimples

Gentian, plantain, valerian

Poison Ivy

Golden seal, myrrh, bloodroot, lobelia

Arthritis

Blue flag, elder, willow, wintergreen, lobelia, nettle, poplar, black cohosh, cayenne, wild yam, yellow dock

Ringworm

Golden seal,lobelia, blood root

Burns

Bitterseet, chickweed, elder

Sinus Problems

Plantain, golden seal

Sore throat

Ginger, hyssop, mullein, sage, sassafras, borage, golden seal, wild alum root

Swellings

Burdock, comfrey, white oak bark, yellow dock, camomile, mugwort

Toothache

Pennyroyal, plantain, cloves, savory, balm

Urinary Problems

Squaw vine, peach leaves, dandelion, comfrey, chicory, carrot, poplar bark, white ash, marjoram, yarrow, burddock

Vomiting

Spearmint, clover, peach leaves (small doses)

Warts

Mullein

Worms

Bitterroot, lobelia, red clover, red clover, coltsfoot

Improve Appetite

Red raspberry leaves, peppermint, clover, sweet basil

Improve Sleep

Hops, mullein, peppermint,

Stimulants

Cayenne, ginger, peppermint, nettle, rue, penneyroyal

4 Herbal Teas
That Can Improve Your Health & Heal Problems

1) Goldenseal

This herbal tea fights germs and infections. It also stimulates the immune system. Some recent studies indicate that goldenseal may also help to combat tumors. To make goldenseal herbal tea, use one-half to one full teaspoon of powdered goldenseal root in one cup of boiling water and allow the mixture to steep for ten minutes. For best results, you should drink about 2 cups a day. To improve the flavor, you can add lemon or honey to the tea.

2) Alfalfa

Studies suggest that alfalfa can help reduce cholesterol and reverse the accumulation of plaque depsits on artery walls. Alfalfa tea can be made by using one or two teaspoons of dried alfalfa leaves per cup of boiling water. Let this brew steep for ten to twenty minutes.

3) Celery seed

Often used as an aid to weight loss, controlling blood pressure, and by diabetics, celery seed tea contains one to two teaspoons of crushed celery seeds per cup of boiling water. Allow this tea to steep for ten to twenty minutes and drink at least two cups a day.

4) Black Haw

Studies show that the chemical salicin—an aspirin-like sub-stance—found in black haw helps ease the pain of arthritis, headaches, and may be effective in lowering fevers. You can make black haw tea by boiling two teaspoons of dried bark per cup of water. Allow the brew to boil for ten minutes. Add lemon or honey to improve the taste and drink two to three cups a day.

Insider's Health Insurance Buying Tips
- Save Up To 40%

Health Insurance Policies can vary widely. It pays to examine several kinds before making a selection. Here are a few things to look for:

(1) Use an independent insurance agent. They can get policies and ates from dozens of health insurers - instead of just one. You could save up to 40%.

(2) Is the policy renewable? You should only purchase insurance that is guaranteed to be renewable as long as you pay your premiums. You should reject any policy that can be canceled if your health fails or if it must be renewed each year.

(3) Check nursing home benefits. Some policies place restrictions on nursing home payments — such as requiring that they be "medically necessary". The best policies pay benefits if the doctor simply orders the patient to nursing- home care.

(4) Does the policy offer inflation protection? You should determine if the policy increases nursing-home benefits as inflation rises. What looks like good insurance now may not look so good in 10 to 15 years.

(5) Check out the insurance company. More insurance companies went bankrupt last year (22) than in the previous five years. So it is highly important to check the financial stability of the company before buying a policy.

There are several ways to check on the stability of an insurance company. Here are some tips:

Find out how long the company has been in business.

Look in the library for ratings agency directories.

Contact your state insurance department and ask about the company.

Read business publications to keep abreast of which companies are having financial problems.

(6) When do your benefits begin? Some insurance policies have waiting periods before they began to pay. Other policies place limits on the amount of money or length of time that they will pay. The best policies are those that begin coverage as soon as you start receiving medical treatment.

(7) What does the insurance cover? Most insurance salesmen will tell you all about the many things that the policy covers. However, many neglect to tell you what the policy doesn't cover. So you may need to read the fine print and ask some questions.

Here are some items to look for:

Many nursing home policies won't cover custodial care costs.

They also won't pay unless a doctor states that the stay is medically necessary.

Pre-existing medical problems are often not covered when you get a new policy. You should carefully study any coverage restrictions on medical problems that have occurred before you bought the policy. Some policies have a "waiting" period built in before they begin to cover pre-existing health problems.

Some policies also restrict coverage for certain types of illnesses or medical procedures. You'll want to determine what these restrictions cover.

(8) How large are the benefits? Some policies have very high deductibles before the policy begins to pay. Other policies have low total payments and then coverage stops. So you need to make sure the policy will not leave you financially liable in the event of major medical problems.

How To Get The Claim Paying Records
Of The Top 25 Health Insurance Companies

Here are the 25 largest Health Insurance Companies and the ratings agencies you can call to find out about the companies' financial health:

1) Prudential Insurance

2) MetropolitanLife

3) Aetna Life

4) Equitable Life Assurance

5) Teachers Insurance And Annuity

6) New York Life

7) Connecticut General Life

8) John Hancock Life

9) Travelers Insurance

10) Northwestern Mutual

11) Principal Mutual

12) Massachusetts Mutual Life

13) Lincoln National

14) Mutual Life Of New York

15) New England Mutual

16) IDS Life Insurance

17) Allstate Life

18) Mutual Benefit Life

19) Variable Annuity

20) Nationwide Life

21) State Farm Life

22) Hartford Life

23) Aetna Life and Annuity

24) Connecticut Mutual Life

25) Jackson National

You can contact the following ratings agencies to get the ratings of these companies:

A.M. Best — 908-439-2200

Duff & Phelps —312-263-2610

Weiss Research — 800-289-9222

Standard and Poor's — 212-208-8000

The Best Health Insurance
If You Are Self-Employed

If you are self-employed or contemplating going into business for yourself, health care costs can be a major headache. Health insurance costs can be astronomical if you don't make the right decisions about the type of coverage that's best for you. With that in mind, here are several insider tips on how to get the best health insurance coverage if you are self-employed:

1) Find out whether your spouse can get coverage through his or her job.

2) Contact other self-employed people, entrepreneurs and small-business developent centers at universities and get advice on acquiring insurance. You will find people who have shopped around for the best deal - saving you a lot of time.

3) Look for a group plan. You may find a good group plan available through a trade or professional group or your local chamber of commerce. Group plans are usually cheaper than individual plans.

4) Deductibles are another important consideration in how high or low your premium will be— the higher the deductible, the lower the premium.

5) If you are soon to quit your current job to become self-employed, consider the interim option of COBRA. This is a federal program that extends your current coverage, if you pay for it, for at least 18 months if you are currently employed by a firm with 20 or more employees.

How To Get Your Insurance Company To Pay Your Claim When They Don't Want To

Millions of Americans have learned the hard way that collecting on insurance claims can be a nightmare. The procedure features a myriad of confusing forms, numerous phone calls and letters, and an intimidating bureaucracy. What can you do when your insurance company doesn't seem willing to pay your claim? Insiders say that the key to getting your insurance claim(s) paid is in knowing how to cut through all the confusing red tape.

Here are several insider tips for getting your insurance claims settled to your satisfaction:

1) Try to stay one step ahead of the bureaucracy. One way to do this is to make sure that you fill in every blank properly when filing a claim. Some companies will reject your claim simply because you omitted your date of birth.

2) Do not take "no" for an answer. Insiders say that every medical procedure has a code and that claims are sometimes rejected because of a computer mistake, resulting in the wrong code. It is estimated that as many as 30 percent of insurance claims are rejected because such minor details are incorrect.

3) Know what your policy covers before you undergo any treatment. You need to know how much your insurer has agreed to pay.

4) If all else fails, turn your claim over to a firm that files claims for policy holders who haven't had any success in getting their claims paid. These firms can usually cut through the red tape and get the insurance company to pay the claim, or call your state's insurance department for free help or advice.

How To Choose The Best HMO

Here are some tips for choosing an HMO.

(1) Will you be penalized for going outside the network of approved doctors? If so — how much?

(2) How much does the plan pay? Does it pay a percentage of the actual medical charges or of the allowable charge? There could be a big difference between the two.

(3) Talk to a few members of the HMO. Find out if they are satisfied with the service, cost, and speed of payment?

(4) What happens when you see a specialist who is not part of your HMO? Must you be referred to a particular specialist by your doctor?

(5) What medical services are not covered by the HMO plan?

(6) Check out the doctors on the approved list. Are they reputable? Do they have plenty of experience? Are there a lot of complaints against them?

(7) How much notification must I give the plan before going to a hospital or when an emergency occurs? Many plans require approval before the medical service is performed.

(8) How good are the services provided by the doctors who belong to the HMO's. How fast can you get an appointment? Can they answer your questions quickly?

The best way to find out about a particular HMO is to talk to several of its members and doctors. You should also talk to the Better Business Bureau and find out if many complaints have been lodged.

A recent magazine survey rated 46 HMO plans. The top five plans were: (1) Heritage National Health Plan (2) Pilgrim Health Care, (3) Independent Health (4) Blue Choice (5) Preferred Care. Of course these plans may not be available in your area. Also the quality of service varies from one region to another. Therefore you must do a thorough study before committing yourself to any particular plan.

How to Avoid Bogus Health Insurance

There are a number of steps that you can take to check out the company behind the insurance policy. This can help protect you against poor coverage or companies that fail.

(1) Call your state insurance department. Find out if the company is licensed in your state and if it contributes to a state guarantee fund.

(2) If a small company states they are backed by a large insurance company find out if this is true. Call the large insurance company and find out what protection it has.

(3) Talk to your states insurance regulators about the company making the offer. Find out if they have had many complaints about the company.

(4) Find out how long the company has been in business. Small underfunded or under managed firms often fail in the first 15 to 20 months. Look for a plan that has been in business 3 or more years.

Secret To Save Big Money On Nursing Home Costs

The cost of supporting yourself, a spouse, or your parents in a nursing home can quickly wipe out your savings account. Often, medicaid will only pay for part of the cost. Therefore, it is smart to do some long term planning.

Medicaid planning involves changing a family's assets. One way this can work is by setting up a trust for older family members who may need nursing home care. This can allow the older family member to qualify for medicaid benefits while still preserving some assets in the trust.

An older family member (the donor), could set up an irrevocable Medicaid Trust. He donates part of his assets to this trust. A trustee (usually a child or spouse of the donor) manages this trust. There are many ways that these trusts can be set up. The overall objective is to prevent medical fees from taking all of the money out of an estate before the estate can be passed along to the heirs.

There are both pluses and minuses with this type of Medicaid Trust. Therefore, you should consult a lawyer who is familiar with your state's Medicaid law before setting up a Medicaid Trust.

When To Choose Outpatient Surgery And Save Hundreds Of Dollars A Day

A typical outpatient arrives at a "freestanding" ambulatory care center or a hospitals' outpatient facility at an appointed time, and the facility's medical staff attends to his or her needs— including same-day surgery. Following a brief recovery, the patient goes home the same day. Choosing to have treatment as an outpatient can easily help reduce a patient's medical bill by up to 50 percent. Some studies have revealed statistics which suggest that potential savings nationwide as a result of outpatient treatment is well over $1 billion dollars a year.

Here are some one-day surgeries which are now safely and effectively performed at outpatient facilities:

1) Tubal ligation

2) Breast biopsy

3) Tonsillectomy and Adenoidectomy

4) Hernia repair

5) Cataract extraction

6) Varicose vein removal

7) Dilation and curettage (D & C)

There are many other surgical (and nonsurgical) procedures which can be performed at oupatient facilities with relative safety and a great reduction in medical bills. Before you choose outpatient surgery, however, you should make sure your doctor and/or medical advisor agree that the surgery you need can be taken care of at such a facility. Here are several things you should consider before choosing to have outpatient surgery:

1) Is the outpatient facility a professional and accredited ambulatory health- care facility? You can get some idea of how the facility operates by paying a personal visit and making your own inspection. You should also find out how much the facility charges for the procedure you

need and what services are covered in the charge.

You can find out a facility's accreditation by contacting the Association for Ambulatory Healthcare, 9933 Lawler Avenue, Skokie, IL 600077-3702; Phone (312) 676-9610.

2) What happens if there are unexpected complications? Even if your outpatient surgery is relatively minor in nature, complications can occur. Make sure the outpatient facility is near a hospital emergency facility.

3) Does your health-insurance policy feature ambulatory-care coverage? Most health insurance policies recognize and approve outpatient surgery, but you should make sure before you choose such an option. Be certain your policy recognizes the surgery you plan to have as one that can be performed at an outpatient facility. You should also know whether or not your insurance company approves and deals with the outpatient facility you plan to use.

Monetary considerations aside, you should get competent medical advice before making the final decision to have outpatient surgery.

Don't Fall For These Unneeded Medical Tests. They May Be A Complete Waste Of Time And Money

While medical testing is a valuable tool in diagnosis and in monitoring health, test results can be misinterpreted or misused. In some cases, the tests may even be unnecessary, resulting in a waste of time and money. The more you know about testing programs, the better you will be able to make informed decisions about what tests to take and which ones to avoid.

You should check with your doctor to make sure a test or retest is necessary. Find out why the test needs to be done, and get a second opinion before you give the go-ahead. Here are some tests you probably should avoid:

1) If you need to be retested again and again, you might want to put a stop to the procedure. This is especially true if the testing involves

repeated exposure to radiation, or nuclear medicine. Before you allow the testing to continue, find out why it must be done over and over. Consult with your doctor and find out if such tests are still required. In some cases, repeated testing is the result of an incompetent or "overworked" technician.

2) The American College of Radiology (ACR) recommends that you should avoid chest X-rays as a routine part of hospital admissions, and as part of a pre- employment physical. According to the ACR, most such chest X-rays do not turn up anything of significance and are not really worth the expense or potential risk.

The ACR does recommend chest X-rays if a person's health or medical history warrant them, or if a person is exposed (on a regular basis) to chemicals or other health hazards which could affect the lungs.

3) In the hospital, don't undergo routine presurgical screening tests which have already been done within the previous year.

4) Tests that involve intrusion into your body are known as "invasive" tests. Such tests are complicated and are designed to obtain a sample of tissue or to get an image which cannot be obtained from outside the body. These tests are potentially painful and dangerous and are only justified if the required results cannot be obtained by a simpler, safer method. Before you agree to an invasive test, you should get a second medical opinion, and be certain that the potential benefit from the procedure is worth the money and the potential risk.

7 Ways Emergency Rooms
Can Be Dangerous To Your Health

When you need the services of a hospital emergency room, your need is almost always sudden and unexpected. Far less frequently, people use such facilities for primary health care rather than maintaining a continuing-care relationship with a family doctor. In effect, these people use emergency rooms as their "doctors".

While emergency rooms have their advantages, such as easy access and not requiring an appointment before being examined and treated, there are also some potential dangers involved. Here are some

of the most common problems associated with emergency room treatment:

1) If the emergency room is busy (and they usually are) a patient
may have to wait up to several hours before being able to consult a doctor. Call a head to see the wait - you may be able to see your regular doctor sooner.

2) There is the possibility that you won't even be treated by a doctor. In some cases, emergency room technicians recommend x-rays and
perform minor treatment, such as cleaning and bandaging wounds. This
can increase the risk of improper or inadequate treatment.

3) Most emergency room treatment does not involve any personal communication, such as a patient usually has with a family doctor or in
a hospital. There simply isn't time in an emergency room environment for
a doctor to discuss a medical problem with a patient and get his or her
medical history. As a result, the patient's own participation in his or her
medical care is very limited. In an emergency room situation, a patient
has almost no say as to what type of treatment he or she will receive.

4) Many emergency rooms, even those that are open 24 hours a
day, are often under-staffed. In some cases, new doctors, with little practical experience, moonlight in emergency rooms, meaning the patient
does not get the benefit of being treated by an experienced physician.

5) While some ER's are staffed by board certified emergency
physicians, with qualified surgeons, anesthesiologists, cardiologists, and
pediatricians on duty, others are not.

6) Because of the often "frantic pace" in emergency rooms, treatment is usually superficial and arranging for needed follow-up care is difficult. Such arrangements are usually left up to the patient.

7) Emergency rooms offer little if any privacy. Patients with all
sorts of ailments and injuries may be crowded together. There may be an
increased risk of coming into contact with "tainted" blood from open
wounds, cuts and/or abrasions.

Do You Know Your Medical Rights?

Patients have certain medical rights when they are dealing with doctors or hospitals. Most patients are unfamiliar with these rights and simply go along with whatever the medical provider says. But several studies have shown that you can get better care by being familiar with your rights. Here is an outline of your medical rights:

(1) If you are a competent adult you can refuse medical care that you don't want.

(2) As a patient you have a right to be told the true nature of your illness. the doctor cannot lie or withhold information from you.

(3) You can leave the hospital any time you wish. You don't need permission from the doctor.

(4) You are free to refuse to be examined by any doctor, intern, or medical student.

(5) Once you have been admitted to a hospital, you cannot be discharged simply because you can't pay.

(6) A doctor can treat a child without the parent's permission in emergency situations.

(7) Hospitals and doctors are required to provide parents with information about a child's condition.

How To Sue A Doctor
Or A Hospital If You've Been Wronged...And Win

If you sustain a severe injury as the result of clearly inadequate medical treatment by a doctor or a hospital, you do have the recourse of getting satisfaction in court. Suing a doctor or an institution for malpractice is a serious matter which, if to be successful, requires undeniable evidence of improper treatment, and a competent malpractice attorney. If you do choose to get legal satisfaction, take extreme care in selecting a qualified attorney who is right for your particular case, and one who will get paid only if you collect money from your case.

If your case is strong, backed up by solid evidence, there is a good chance your attorney can get an out-of-court settlement. You should know, however, that malpractice suits can take years to resolve, so be prepared for a long battle. Many malpractice suits are settled out-of-court in order to avoid a long, drawn-out affair.

Quite often the very threat of a malpractice suit, backed up by solid evidence, is enough to encourage doctors and hospitals to reach an out-of- court settlement. However, the doctor or hospital must be convinced that your case has merit before they will "give in". You and your attorney can meet with the doctor and hospital representatives and present your case. Be reasonable, but firm. Explain that you demand satisfaction and that you are ready, willing and able to take the matter to court if a settlement can not be reached. If you have a solid case, you'll most likely end up with a satisfactory settlement without ever having to go to court.

You can also refuse to pay your bill. When the doctor or hospital demands payment, have your attorney respond with a complete outline of your case and the wrongs you suffered, and the threat of a malpractice suit. Once again, if you have been clearly wronged and you can prove it, the threat of a malpractice suit is often enough to force the offending parties into settling your case to your satisfaction.

One other option for careful consideration is arbitration. In some states a patient can sign (but is not required to sign) an arbitration agreement before being treated. In this type of agreement, the patient agrees to forego his or her right to a jury trial should there be a later claim of malpractice and a subsequent lawsuit. Instead of going to court, the case is heard by a largely neutral panel made up of one arbitor of the patient's choosing, one arbitor chosen by the doctor, and one "disinterested" arbitor. The arbitors then decide if the case is warranted and, if so, determine an award. It isn't advisable to sign an arbitration agreement without first discussing the matter with qualified legal counsel.

Finally, it should be stated that suing or threatening to sue a doctor or hospital should never be used simply as a tactic to avoid paying justified bills, or getting undeserved compensation. The only time you should ever consider such action is if you have suffered a real injury or malpractice has clearly occurred. There are too many frivolous suits clogging up the court system as it is. There are also too many competent doctors and fine hospitals that can be unjustly damaged by unwarranted claims.

How To Cut Your Medical Bills By Up To 50% And Still Get VIP Treatment

There are a number of ways to cut the cost of your medical needs. These can result in significant yearly savings.

(1) Use generic drugs if possible rather than name brand. Generic drugs can cost significantly less.

(2) Many pharmacies offer discounts to people over 62 years old. So shop around for the best buy.

(3) Some drug companies offer guaranteed low prices for certain drugs. One such company is CIBA-GEIGY — call them at 1-800-955-9100 for more information.

(4) Some large pharmaceutical companies offer price reductions plans for low income people. Sometimes your doctor will need to fill out an application for you. Talk to your doctor or contact the pharmaceutical company for more information.

(5) Contact your insurance company prior to any major medical procedures to find out what is covered.

(6) Make certain that you are not undergoing any unnecessary tests.

(7) Talk to your doctor and get a detailed explanation of costs before you agree to any major treatments.

(8) Don't be afraid to challenge your insurance company for bills they say are not covered. Often you can get at least partial coverage if the treatment was truly needed.

How To Get Free Or Discount Medical Care

There are a number of private, state government, and federal government organizations that make cash grants to help cover medical expenses. These grants sometimes are restricted to people who have low income or other special circumstances. Some of these fund sources also have other restrictions such as, living area, type of medical problem, age, and so forth. Here are some tips that can help you locate these funding sources:

State Government Sources

Most states have an office called the Department of Health and Human Services. It is usually located in the state capitol. Often they have funding programs and can also point you to other money sources. Look in the telephone book for the phone number of these offices.

Federal Sources

Medicare — covers persons who are receiving social security, certain disabled people, and people with chronic renal disease. Contact your local social security office.

Migrant Workers Programs

This program is for migrant agricultural workers who suffer seasonal unemployment. Grants are supplied to institutions and individuals. Call (202) 535-0500 for more information.

Veterans Hospitalization and Home-Based Care

The Veteran's Administration provides a wide range of excellent medical services. These benefits can be obtained by veterans who have been honorably discharged, receive a VA pension, or have a service connected disability. In some cases a spouse or child could also qualify for benefits. Here are some phone numbers for VA benefits:

Hospitalization — (202) 535-7384

Home Care — (202) 535-7530

Nursing Home — (202) 535-7179

Outpatient Care —(202) 535-7384

Prescription — (202) 5335-3277

Corporate Funding

Many corporations provide some medical grants for individuals. Sometimes you have to be an employee to receive these grants. Here are a few foundations which give medical grants.

Child Health Foundation — Box 530964, Birmingham, AL 35253 (205) 251-9966 - - childrens diseases

FHP Foundation — 401 E. Ocean Blvd., Suite 206, Long Beach, CA 90802 (Covers S. California, Utah, New Mexico, and Arizona programs for the elderly.

Anschutz Foundation — 2400 Anaconda Tower, 555 17th St., Denver, CO. 80202 — for the elderly and poor.

Monsanto Fund — 800 n. Lindbergh Blvd., St. Louis, MO 63167 (for midwest states).

Keebler Company Foundation — One Hollow Tree Lane, Elmhurst, IL 60126.

Ryland Group — 10221 Wincopin Circle, Box 4000, Columbia, MD 21044

Donaldson Trust, Durfee Attlebroro Bank, Trust Dept., 10 N. Main St., Fall River, MA 02720 — cancer treatment.

There is also a book that lists additional funding sources, FREE MONEY FOR HEART DISEASE AND CANCER CARE by Laurie Blum published by Simon & Schuster.

10 Delicious, Healthy Vegetarian Recipes

These vegetarian recipes are well balanced meals that are low in calories and fat but high in nutrition.

1) Potato Casserole

4 large potatoes, 1 onion, 4 cups fresh green beans, 1-28oz. can of pureed tomatoes, 2 cloves of garlic, 2 tsp. italian herb seasoning. Cut

potatoes into large chunks, add onion and green beans into a large casserole dish, mix tomatoes with seasoning and pour over vegetables. Cover and bake at 380 degrees for 80 to 90 minutes.

2) Asparagus Soup

1/2- 1 onion, 1 tbs. olive oil, 1 potato (diced), 2 cups water, 2 ibs. fresh asparagus (sliced), 4 stalks of celery with leaves (chopped), salt and pepper to taste. Saute onions in the oil, add potato and water, simmer 15 to 20 minutes, add other ingredients, and cook until the vegetables are tender. Puree in a blender and milk to thin if desired.

3) Lentil Burgers

1 cup lentils, 3 cups water, 1 onion (chopped), 1 clove garlic, a stalk celery (chopped), 1 carrot (grated or finely chopped), 1/2 cup bulgur wheat, 1 tsp. each of mustard & chili powder. 2 Tbs. Tomato sauce. Bring lentils to a boil, add vegetables and simmer for 30 minutes, Add other ingredients and cook for 15 minutes. Cool shape into
patties and brown on a griddle.

4) Stuffed Bell Peppers

1 cup rice, uncooked, 1 small onion, 1 stalk celery, 4 green bell peppers, 4 ounce can tomato sauce, 1 tsp garlic powder, 1 tsp onion powder. 1/2 cup to 1 cup spaghetti sauce. Cook rice as recommended on box, saute onion and celery in 1 tbls. butter or margarine, par-boil green bell peppers for 5 or 10 minutes until fork tender but not mushy or fall apart stage. Mix rice, onion, celery, tomato sauce, garlic powder and onion powder. Drain bell peppers, and stuff with rice mixture. In a baking pan or glass baking pan pour spaghetti sauce to cover bottom of pan, add green peppers, sprinkle with shredded mozzarella cheese. Bake in 350 to 375 degree oven for 30 to 45 minutes.

5) Cheese Patties

1 - 8 oz. pkg. cream cheese, 6 eggs, sage to taste, 1 c cracker crumbs, 3 Tbls. chopped onion. Put cream cheese in a bowl & add sage & onions. Scramble eggs without any milk & add hot eggs. Mix well. Add 3/4 cup cracker crumbs, mixing well. Cool slightly & form into patties. Roll patties inn remaining crumbs. May be kept in refrigerator over night or

longer. When ready to use fry to golden brown. They may be fried immediately if you want to use them right away.

6) Mock Chicken Loaf

1 - 1# box cottage cheese, 1 cup cracker crumbs, 3 Tbls chopped
onion, 1 cup quick oats, 1 stick oleo, 2 envelopes Dark brown George
Washington seasoning (may be found in most large grocery stores), 2
cup water, 3 eggs. Boil water & add oats. Remove from heat to cool.
While oats cool put the cottage cheese, onion, seasoning & eggs in a
bowl. Melt oleo & stir in crumbs. When oats are cool, add oats & crumbs
& mix well. Bake at 350 degrees for 1 hour in a loaf pan.

7) Spinach cassarole

1/2 stick margarine, 4 Tbls flour, 2 cups milk, 1 pkg frozen
spinach (thawed), 1/2 pkg herb dressing. Cook margarine, flour, milk until
thick. Place thawed spinach in casserole dish. Pour thickener over
spinach. Put layer of 1/2 pkg. herb dressing over spinach. Mix 1/2 cup hot
water and 6 Tbls. of butter. Melt butter in water. Spoon over dressing.
Bake in 350 degree oven for 45 min.

8) Oatmeal Meatballs

1 cup ground walnuts, 2 eggs, tsp. poultry seasoning, 1 cup quick
oats raw, 4 Tbls. milk, 1 medium onion (grated). Mix all ingredients, Roll
into balls. Roll balls in bread crumbs and fry. Simmer in 2 Tbls. oil, 12 oz.
water, 2 pkg. Brown George Washington Broth. Simmer meatballs in
broth until most of liquid is absorbed. Cover with gravy or spaghetti
sauce. Bake at 350 degree for 1/2 hour.

9) Squash Casserole

4 yellow squash (sliced), 1/3 cup of chopped onion, 2 cooked
eggs (chopped),1/2 cup cheddar cheese, 1/3 cup melted margine, 1 cup
cracker crumbs.

Cook squash in boiling water — 10-15 minutes, saute onion in
margine, combine other ingredients, sprinklee crumbs on top, bake in
casserole dish 20-30 minutes at 350 degrees.

10) Parsnip Patties

1 large parsnip (shredded), 1/2 cup soaked garbanzos beans, 1/2 tsp. salt, 1 Tbl. oil, 1/4 cup water.

Blend garbanzos in water till fine, add other ingredients, Drop onto hot oiled skillet, cook 5 minutes til brown, cover and reduce heat for 10 -15 minutes. You may also make these into a regular patty.

Walking Lowers Your Risk Of Heart Disease

A recent study conducted by researchers at the Cooper Institute for Aerobics Research in Dallas suggests that regular walking may be one of the best exercises for overall fitness. The results from the study indicate that walking can help reduce the risk of serious illnesses such as heart disease, cut blood cholesterol levels, and help raise "good" choles-terol— HDL, the high- density lipoprotein that helps prevent heart attacks.

The research involved over 100 inactive women who were other-wise in good health. All of the women were between 20 and 40 years of age. None of them smoked. The women averaged fewer than three alco-holic drinks a day and did not exercise more than once a week. None of the women had high blood pressure or blood cholesterol levels.

The women were randomly placed in four separate groups— a control group which didn't exercise, and three groups that walked 3 miles a day, 5 times a week for a minimum of six months. One of the three groups walked at a 20-minute-a-mile pace. Another walked a more brisk 15 minute mile. A third group walked a fast 12 minute mile.

All of the "walking" groups showed significant improvement in risk factors associated with the development of heart disease. Apparently, even at low intensities, walking can provide a dramatic reduction in the risk of coronary disease. Plus, all three groups showed an increase of at least 6% in their blood HDL levels. Even a strolling pace, if it is done on a regular basis, appears to substantially increase high-density lipopro-teins or HDL.

Circulation Problems?
This Cure Is Free And Works Better Than Anything

A regular program of walking can help decrease levels of artery-clogging blood fats, and at the same time help increase the level of HDL, according to the findings from a recent study. It also appears that regular walking can help take the pressure off varicose veins in the legs and reduce the pain of clogged leg arteries by creating better circulation. All in all, studies show that better circulation, relief from varicose veins, weight-loss, reduced cholesterol levels, lower blood pressure, and relief from stress can all be accomplished, in part, with the help of a regular program of walking.

It should also be noted that anyone who has varicose veins and takes part in vigorous exercise is advised to wear elastic support hose to minimize the congestion of blood in veins and the subsequent accumulation in muscles.

3 Things To Do
For Better Health Benefits From Walking

One of the most common mistakes beginners make when starting a regular routine of walking is pushing themselves too hard. The key to building up your stamina and increasing your walking speed is to slow down. If you try to go too fast, or push yourself too far, you increase the risk of soreness and injury. You also increase the chances of getting discouraged because your "walk to fitness" is not having immediate results. The most important thing to remember when walking for fitness is to find and maintain a pace at which you are comfortable.

Gradually, as you build your stamina and become used to the new movements involved with brisk walking, you will begin to increase your speed. If you are in good health, you should, after a while, be able to walk a comfortable 12- minute mile. But don't press it. If you begin to feel physically or mentally stressed and/or strained you are trying to do too much, too fast.

Your posture is also important in effective fitness walking. For best results you should stand up straight— don't lean forward from the waist. Hold your head up high and let your shoulders relax. Many people look down when they walk and that puts an undue strain on the neck and the back. Walking "tall" with your head held high eliminates that pressure and automatically lifts your rib cage and frees your hips, allowing you to walk in a new, more comfortable and more effective way.

This new way of walking will help you to straighten your legs, land on your heels and roll forward to your toes, instead of lifting your leg and landing flat-footed as you may have been doing with incorrect posture. The better your technique, the less your risk of injury, and the more effective your routine of walking for fitness.

Still another important part of proper technique when walking for fitness is hip movement. The proper movement should be the same as the movement of your hips when you are shifting a medium-sized object you've been holding, from one hip to the other. One leg should straighten, while the other relaxes. When the knee bends, the hip should drop. You should maintain this hip movement—back and forth—every time you walk for fitness. Also, let your arms swing at your sides naturally. Once you've picked up a little speed, you may want to bend your arms at the elbow, but keep them swinging. The key is to let them swing naturally and don't pump them. Pumping your arms tends to make your shoulders tense up.

Each Mile You Walk Adds 21 Minutes To Your Life

According to a theoretical model developed by the Rand Corporation, you can add several years to your life by walking for fitness. Each additional mile walked by a sedentary person will add 21 minutes to his or her life, or an extra year of living for 25,028 miles, according to the Rand Corporation's theoretical model.

People who plan to take up jogging for fitness are advised to build up to it gradually. You can do that by walking until you can cover two miles with no discomfort. Then you can begin alternating between walking and jogging in 100 to 150-yard stretches. As you begin to build up your endurance, you should increase the distance you jog until you are running exclusively. Your goal shouldbe at least 3 or 4 twenty-minute runs a week.

Secrets To Buying The Best Exercise Shoes

Different exercises require different types of movement and therefore, different types of exercise shoes. Although there are a seemingly limitless number of different designs available, many athletic shoes are designed with fashion in mind, rather than as protection for your feet. In order to exercise safely and effectively you need to wear appropriate shoes. Here are four expert suggestions for choosing the right exercise shoes:

1) Walking shoes— these should have sturdy soles in order to absorb the wear and tear of walking on pavement and other rough surfaces. The soles should also provide good support for your arches.

2) Running shoes— the best shoes have rigid heel support and flexible fronts which will allow the feet to bend. Some styles provide elevated heels which absorb much of the impact of the feet when they hit the ground.

3) Aerobic shoes— these shoes must be designed for activities that require movement in different directions. They need to have a strong pad underneath the ball of the foot and material that will accommodate the heel so that it is not held rigid. Aerobic shoes should also be lightweight and have flexible soles.

4) Tennis shoes— since the foot moves in all directions during tennis, the best shoes are designed to provide maximum grip on the playing surface. The upper sole should also be cushioned for added protection.

A 20-Minute Home Aerobic Workout
That's Both Fun And Easy

A collaborative study by the University of North Carolina, Stanford University and the University of California at San Diego shows that any aerobic activity —even done on a moderate scale—can reduce the risk from coronary disease. Many people enjoy aerobic dance workouts as part of their exercise regimen. The following exercise, set to music, can be an effective part of any dance workout:

1) Stand with your feet wide apart and your toes turned slightly outward.

2) Bend your right knee, making sure you allow your hips to shift naturally left. Then, bend your arms at the elbow while at the same time moving your right forearm up and your left forearm down.

3) Reverse the movement, beginning with bending your left knee and shifting your hips to the right. Raise your left forearm as your right forearm falls.

4) Change positions—from the right side to the left side—about 30 times to the music.

You can combine the above exercise movement with other dance movements to create an excellent 20 minute aerobic workout. That's fun and easy - so you will stick to it even thought you are busy!

5 Easy Exercises That Help Prevent Back Pain

A strong back means fewer back problems. In order to strengthen your back, you have to exercise your back muscles, putting them through all their actions and movements. You also need to develop your abdominal muscles so that you will have proper posture, which relieves pressure on the spine.

Once the muscles of your back have been sufficiently strengthened, they will hold the vertebrae and discs in place, which will help prevent slipped discs and poor posture. Also, strong muscles will help you withstand sudden movements, such as twisting or turning, that can cause serious injury.

Before you begin any back strengthening exercises you should consult your doctor. Once you have your doctor's approval, you should begin your strength exercise routine with flexibility exercises. You should be warmed up and loose before you start doing the actual strength exercises, otherwise you increase the risk of injury. The strength exercises themselves must be done slowly without any fast or jerking actions. Stop exercising immediately if you feel any pain or discomfort, and visit your doctor.

Here are five exercises, designed to stretch and strengthen your back muscles:

1) To stretch your back muscles, get down on your hands and knees. From that position you should arch your back upward while bending your head down. Lift the knee of one leg up toward your forehead. Extend that leg straight out behind you and raise your head at the same time. Repeat this exercise with each leg.

2) You can strengthen your back muscles by lying on your stomach with your arms along your sides. Lift your head and shoulders off the floor and hold that position for several seconds before relaxing.

3) Repeat the steps in the above exercise but clasp your hands behind your head, extending your arms in front of you. Raise your head and shoulders, but no higher than is comfortable.

4) This muscle-strengthening exercise requires you to lie on your stomach with your arms in front of you and your elbows flexed. Lift each leg in turn, being careful to keep your knees straight. Then repeat the exercise, lifting both legs together.

5) Lie on your stomach, with your arms extended straight out in front of you. Lift your head and shoulders and at the same time raise both of your legs.

Insider Secrets To Having A Firm, Flat Stomach, Without Strenuous Exercise

Here's an insider method for achieving a flatter stomach in less than one month:

1) Maintain a low-fat diet. Consume little or no red meat and dairy products.

2) Drink lots of water. At least eight glasses of water a day are recommended.

3) Eliminate sodium from your diet. Sodium can cause bloating and puffiness.

4) Try to strengthen the abdominal muscle you use to pull in your stomach. You can find this muscle by placing your thumbs on your navel and interlocking your fingers, and then flattening your stomach with your palms. Once you've flattened your stomach, cough— the in and out movement you feel gives you the location of the abdominal muscle upon which you need to focus . You'll need to practice pulling in and tightening that muscle until it is trained to tighten automatically.

5) Do the following exercises:

Lie on the floor with your knees bent and your feet flat on the floor. Put your hands behind your head, cradling your head in your hands. Then, bring in your elbows toward the sides of your head. Contract your abdominal muscle, and then bring your shoulders up just a bit— two counts forward and two counts back in tiny lifts.

6) The next exercise begins in the same position as that already described, but with your knees drawn in closer and your ankles crossed. Keeping your abdominal muscle tight, gently lift your backside toward the ceiling— two counts up and two counts down.

In order to be effective, you should perform at least 50 repetitions of these two exercises every day. It's also a good idea to perform other exercises, such as walking or running in combination with the low-fat diet and the two exercises described above.

How To Get Rid Of Fat In Tough Spots

Flabby arms can be a thing of the past if you are willing to spend about 20 minutes a day to firm them up. This type of exercising will get rid of the layer of fat that sits on top of the muscle. You should start by working out two days a week, alternating days so as not to fatigue the muscles. Gradually work up to three to five times a week.

Once you've become accustomed to regular exercise, you can begin to exercise two primary muscles—biceps and triceps. Begin with basic exercises, such as bicep curls, using dumbbells or a straight bar. You can exercise the triceps (which are located on the back of the upper arm) by doing a tricep pushdown exercise on a cable machine. You should focus more on correct form rather than how much weight you are using.

You can lessen muscle fatigue by alternating workouts— do the chest and biceps one day, and the back and triceps the next day. An effective arm routine can be performed at home with a set of 5-pound dumbbells or a straight barbell. Twenty minutes should give your arms an effective workout. You can do curls at home, while you're watching TV.

Insider Secrets To "Spot-Reducing" Fat On Your Thighs And Buttocks

Here are some easy exercises that insiders recommend to help you reduce fat in problem areas on the thighs and buttocks:

1) To trim fat from your thighs, lie on your side with both knees bent, creating a 45-degree angle with your upper body. Slowly elevate and then lower your top leg without letting your hip roll back. Do two sets and then reverse the movement of the top leg, squeezing down, then raising up. Do two more sets and then repeat the routine on the other side. Try to do 8 sets of 8.

Another insider method of tightening up the thighs and buttocks is to stand with your feet just a little more than shoulder-width apart. Your toes and knees should be turned out. Keep your back straight and bend your knees over your toes, then lower your buttocks. Straighten your legs, tightening your inner thighs and contracting your buttocks. Try to repeat this exercise 15 times.

2) To reduce fat and tone up your buttocks, lie on your back with your knees bent, and your feet and lower back pressed firmly against the floor. Squeeze your buttocks tightly together and up, with your hip bones rising toward the ceiling. Hold this position for two seconds and then release and lower your buttocks slowly to the floor. For best results, do 2 sets of 25.

Getting The Right Home-Fitness Equipment For Your Needs

Many people are opting for a home gym over health clubs as a method of staying in shape. Having your own home-fitness equipment is both convenient and private, making it much more attractive than waiting in line to use equipment and then being on "display" at most health clubs. However, before you make an investment in home-fitness equipment there are several things you should consider.

1) What kind of exercise will be best for you? You should know what type of exercise you will enjoy doing and will continue doing on a long-term basis. If you are easily bored, it's probably a good idea to stay away from such equipment as stationary bicycles. If your time for exercising is limited, you may be better off choosing equipment such as ski machines, rowers, or stairclimbers. A treadmill would be a good choice for anyone who enjoys walking or running.

2) How many pieces of equipment should you have? Obviously the more pieces of equipment you have in your home gym, the more varied and comprehensive your exercise program will be. Alternating between different equipment provides a variety of benefits as well as helping to prevent boredom.

3) Is the equipment both comfortable and enjoyable? The best way to determine the appropriate equipment for your needs is to make a personal test at the store. Wear your sweats when you go to look at the exercise equipment and try a 5 to 10 minute workout on several different models. If a particular store won't let you test the equipment, take your business somewhere else.

Don't Buy The Heavily Advertised Exercise Units. You Can Do Much Better And Save As Much AS $240.00

Here are some of the most popular exercise machines which are available for home gyms:

Rowers— these machines are relatively inexpensive— a good model will cost around $700. A rower also takes up very little room, so storage space won't be a problem. Rowers are good because they require more muscle involvement and greater technique than some other home-fitness machines.

Treadmills— you can get a good, low-priced treadmill for around $400. Of course, better machines will cost more. The lowest priced treadmills are best for walking because they are usually not built to withstand the steady pounding of running.

Treadmills may be self-powered or motorized, and by changing the incline or the speed, you can "power-walk" or run or hike uphill. Some people who have switched from jogging to treadmills have found they are less likely to be bothered with sore knees and back problems.

Stationary Bikes— the most basic stationary bikes provide effective exercise, but very few "extras". A basic bike with adjustable resistance, durable pedals and a seat that is high enough to support your body size will cost from $250 to $900. Of course, some bikes are priced well below $200, but they are not likely to be very durable, especially for every-day use. A general rule for stationary bikes and other home exercise machines is, the heavier and more expensive it is, the better the machine.

Stationary Bikes which feature more electronics than the basic models , as well as more comfortable seats, are usually priced from $500 to $1000. The best bikes are also the most elaborate— electronically and otherwise. For the best stationary bike to add to your home gym, you can expect to pay $1,200 to $3,500.

Stair-climbers— One of the best and most popular of all the exercise machines, stair-climbers provide excellent exercise for the hips and thighs. The most basic stair-climbing machines are made with shock-absorbers and are priced below $500. These basic machines provide a stair-climbing motion with some electronics. They also provide a relatively good workout.

Stair-climbing units that are motorized are good because they can be adjusted to different intensities. These units are priced anywhere from $2,000 to $3,400. Other stair-climbers use hydraulic systems which provide a smooth, quiet and effective workout. Expect to pay about $2,200 for this type of unit.

Ski Machines— these machines provide great exercise for the arms and legs. They're excellent if you want to burn off excess body fat with only a minor degree of discomfort. NordicTrack provides the best ski machines, which are priced from $299 to $1,299. The machines work all of the body's major muscle groups, burning calories and providing an excellent cardiovascular workout.

You can get more information about ski machines from NordicTrack, including a free video and brochure, by calling 1-800-328-5888 (ext 301J2), or you can write to NordicTrack, Dept. #301J2, 141 Jonathan Blvd. N. Chaska, Minnesota 55318.

Here are the addresses of some other manufacturers of the most popular home- exercise equipment:

Proform, Inc., 875 S. Main St., Logan, Utah 84321

Concept II, Inc., Box 1100, Morrisville, Vermont 05661

Schwinn Fitness, 217 N. Jefferson St., Chicago 60606

StairMaster Sports/Medical Products, 259 Rt. 17K, Newburgh, New York 12550

Stairobic, 670 N. Commercial St., Manchester, New Hampshire 03101

There are many other manufacturers who make good home-exercise equipment. And there are machines priced lower than the ones listed above. To make the best choice for your home gym, it might be wise to talk with a fitness expert at your local gym or health club. You can also find more makes and models of exercise equipment by browsing through fitness magazines and department store catalogs. Editor's choice: Buy a ski machine that works both your lower and upper body at the same time - and save money!

How To Save 50% Or More
On A Health Club Membership

While many people go to health clubs or gyms to perform various types of exercises, more and more people are joining health clubs specifically to exercise with weight-lifting equipment. The machines are designed to strengthen specific groups of muscles and are usually safer than free weights. A good health club will feature a selection of sophisticated equipment that will enable you to get a complete workout.

When you join a health club or work out at a gym you will most likely be able to exercise on a series of different weight machines, often called "stations", as well as perform aerobic activity such as cycling or running in place, between stations. Some health clubs feature "multistation" machines which enable you to perform various exercises. You can also use single-station equipment individually or in sequential order to work on specific parts of your body.

The best health clubs will have a staff trainer to supervise your first few sessions, enabling you to learn a sequence of exercises that works each muscle group of your body. The supervisor should also give you instructons on the proper execution of each exercise to ensure that you know how to use the equipment safely.

Prices for health club membership vary from one club to the next. Many clubs charge a one time initiation fee plus regular monthly "dues". Depending on where you live and the club you join, you can expect to pay from $100 to $1,500 per year.

The best way to save money on a health club membership is to determine how often you will use a club's services. If you know you will make it to the club only once a week or less, look for a club with low monthly rates. Also do some figuring— how much do you wish to pay for each visit? Generally, the best way to, save 50% or more is to simply say that is all you can pay for a membership they will usually accept your offer if you are persistent!

New Treatment Relieves Chronic Dizziness

A new computerized scanning machine developed by researchers at the University of Southern California is offering hope to the millions of people who suffer from chronic dizziness. The new computerized machine measures the response of the eyes to head movements, helping doctors pinpoint the precise cause of dizziness or balance disorders.

Once doctors have discovered what part of the brain or inner ear is affected they can design an exercise program that teaches a patient to regain his or her balance. With the help of the new computerized scanner, a significant number of people have found dramatic relief from their chronic dizziness. In fact, many hospitals with physical therapy facilities are now offering the treatment.

The new physical therapy treatment is good news for those people who can't be helped by surgery, change in diet or through the use of prescribed drugs.

5 Keys To Building Big Muscles, Fast

The human body contains hundreds of different muscles, and with a little dedication and desire, you can exercise to strengthen and build up each group. All muscles increase in size if exercised regularly, and some exercises have a "faster" and more pronounced effect than others. That means to establish a successful strength and muscle building program, you should get guidance from a professional strength trainer. Many strength training experts recommend that you round out a regular exercise program with at least two strength-training workouts a week. Those guidelines are also recommended by the American College of Sports Medicine.

Here are five keys for setting up a successful strength- and muscle-building program:

1) Initially, your muscles will need an excessive amount of stimulus in order to become strong. Once you've gotten used to the program, you should adjust the amount of stimulus (with the guidance of a strength-training expert) to continue improving.

For best results, your body will require variety. In order for your neuromuscular system to advance you'll need to vary the weight you lift, or the number of lifts.

2) Increase the amount of weight you lift at regular intervals, and get enough rest to avoid overtraining.

3) For optimal success, your muscle-building program should include regular repetition of similar exercises, and easy, recovery workouts as a way to follow-up more strenuous workouts.

4) Experts recommend that you plan your most strenuous or demanding workouts after a few days rest. About two days later your next workout should be a recovery-type session involving lighter weights and fewer repititions. Following another day of rest, you can workout at an

intensity that falls somewhere between your first and second session.

5) When building muscles by lifting weights, it's important that you learn to pace yourself. Strength-training experts say that the weights you use should be small enough for you to complete 8 or more repititions. Before you add more weight, you should increase the number of repititions. The suggested goal is 12 repititions per minute. The general rule is: if you can perform three sets of 15 repititions on one muscle group without any problems, you are ready to add more weight.

One of the best ways to build up your muscles is to go to a health club and take advantage of the various weight-lifting machines. These machines, if used properly, can strengthen specific groups of muscles and are safer than free weights. Good health clubs also provide a staff trainer to supervise your muscle-building program.

Exercise, Caffeine And High Blood Pressure Alert

People who are prone to high blood pressure may want to avoid caffeine before a workout. A recent study suggests that a cup of coffee just prior to exercising is likely to intensify the normally slight increase in blood pressure brought on by physical activity.

The study involved 34 men ages 21 to 35 who took either an amount of caffeine equal to that contained in 2 to 3 cups of brewed coffee or a placebo before exercising.

According to the researchers, the results showed that 44 percent of the subjects tested experienced a temporary increase in blood pressure. The number was more than twice that of those who experienced a short-term rise in blood pressure due to exercise alone. The study also suggests that caffeine may cause blood pressure to continue to rise throughout moderate to intense exercise.

While the study was conducted on men with normal blood pressures, experts say it is likely the results also hold true for people with high blood pressure. For that reason, the researchers recommend that people with hypertension avoid or at least limit their caffeine intake on those days they plan to exercise.

Amazing New, Easy Way
To Lower Your Blood Pressure

Researchers at Miami University in Ohio report that exercising with a handgrip for only a few minutes a week may be one of the simplest ways to lower borderline high blood pressure. According to the the Miami University study, people who did four brief handgrip contractions per day, three days a week, lowered their average systolic pressure from 134 to 121. The subjects also lowered their distolic pressure from 86.5 to 71.6. The research was conducted over a period of two months.

Reduce Your Heart Disease Risk Up To 30%

It isn't just running, rowing, stair-climbing, cycling and so on that keeps you in shape. Any regular activity—walking, bowling, gardening, and so on— can help protect you from heart disease and other health disorders. A 20-year follow-up study, involving about 3,000 railroad workers, found that those who avoided physical activity run almost a 30 percent higher risk of heart disease than the workers who do light activity. The message is clear, a little bit of exercise is better than none at all. While regular exercise is recommended for optimum health, whatever physical activities you can do will be good for you.

5 Important Health Tests Every Women Needs

Current guidelines for regular doctor visits by women place an emphasis on regular Pap tests to screen for cervical cancer, regular visits to discuss general health and lifestyle issues, and yearly mammograms beginning at age 50 to screen for breast cancer. Many medical experts recommend that the following health concerns should be included in every woman's regular checkup:

1) Pap smear— this is the standard screening tool to detect abnormal cells in the cervical lining which could develop into cancer. A woman's first Pap smear is recommended at age 18 or when she becomes sexually active, whichever comes first. After 2 or 3 annual negative evaluations, the test should then be repeated at least once every 3 years.

Annual Pap smears are recommended for women who have multiple sexual partners, smoke or began sexual activity at an early age (before 18). Doctors also recommend a yearly physical examination of the ovaries (pelvic exam) at least every 3 years between the ages of 20 and 40 and annually after age 40.

Many experts suggest that for the best results, women should schedule Pap smears midway between menstrual periods; avoid tampons, douching, contraceptive products, and sexual intercourse for 72 hours prior to the test. You should also postpone the test if you have an active vaginal infection. These recommendations are designed to help women get the most accurate test possible.

2) Breast examination— a self-examination to feel for lumps or nodules should be performed each month— preferably after the menstrual period or on the same day each month for postmenopausal women. A clinical breast exam should be done every 3 years between the ages of 20 and 39 and every year beginning at age 40.

A baseline X-ray or mammogram should be taken between the ages of 35 and 40 or earlier if there is a family history of breast cancer or breast disease among mother or sisters and every one to two years between the ages of 40 and 50. Annual mammograms are recommended beginning at age 50.

3) Blood pressure— monitoring should be every two years, beginning at age 20 in otherwise healthy adults. If the diastolic pressure is between 80 and 90 or if the woman has a history of high blood pressure, heart disease, obesity, or diabetes, monitoring should be more frequent.

4) Blood cholesterol test — used to detect people at high risk of coronary heart disease, this test should be performed every 5 years in otherwise healthy adults beginning at age 20. If you smoke, are taking medicines that affect fat levels in the blood, or if your parents or siblings have high blood cholesterol, high blood pressure or premature heart disease, your doctor will likely recommend more frequent tests.

5) Immunizations— these include a tetanus-diphtheria booster every 10 years beginning at age 25; a flu (influenza) shot yearly, beginning at age 65; and pneumococcal vaccine—for protection against pneumonia—at age 65 only.

6) Counseling and discussion— this is recommended as a major part of a regular doctor visit every two years. Your doctor is likely to ask about your job, family life, marriage, stress factors, exercise, eating habits, sexual issues, and mental health.

Little-Known Way
To Prevent Pregnancy Complications

Current studies suggest that women who get enough calcium may be able to avoid high blood pressure which is one of the most common complications of pregnancy. When hypertension develops during pregnancy it presents a serious risk of still-birth, but calcium can lower blood pressure in some pregnant women.

The Recommended Dietary Allowance of calcium for pregnant women is 1,200 milligrams, but according to the studies, most pregnant women get only about 75 percent of that recommendation. The studies also suggest that those who have high blood pressure may need twice that amount.

The research indicates that pregnant women should probably consume more calcium-rich foods, such as leafy green vegetables, low-fat milk and low-fat yogurt. However, you should consult with your doctor before taking a calcium supplement or before consuming large amounts of any nutritional supplement.

Hepatitis B Testing For Pregnant Women

The Centers for Disease Control in Atlanta recently approved funding to cover hepatitis B testing for pregnant women who receive care at public clinics, as well as vaccinations for their babies. The goal of the new testing program is to reduce the number of dangerous liver infections by vaccinating babies soon after they are born.

The latest estimates indicate that as many as 18,000 of the approximately 3.8 million women who give birth each year in the United States may carry the potentially fatal hepatitis B virus. The virus can lead to liver cancer and cirrhosis. And since babies of infected women have more than a 70 percent chance of becoming infected, the Centers for Disease Control recommends hepatitis B testing for all pregnant women.

7 Keys To Getting Through Morning Sickness

Women who experience it might not think so, but morning sickness may be a sign that the pregnancy is going well. In fact, some studies have shown that women who vomit during pregnancy are less likely to miscarry or deliver prematurely than women who do not. However, doctors caution that while typical morning sickness—usually limited to the first two or three months of pregnancy—is reasonably beneficial, women who have an excessive amount of morning sickness may be at high risk for small babies. If your morning sickness goes on and on after the first two or three months, make sure you tell your doctor.

Even though typical morning sickness is a good sign, it is still something most expectant mothers would rather do without. While that may be out of the question, there are some simple tricks you can employ to make morning sickness less discomforting.

1) Eat several small meals throughout the day instead of two or three large meals. Eat your largest meal of the day at noon rather than in the evening.

2) Don't eat fried, fatty foods. It takes the body a long time to digest fried foods, meaning that they sit in the stomach longer.

3) Drink plenty of fluids.

4) Eat a dry saltine cracker in bed before you get up in the morning. You should try to keep a carbohydrate in your stomach at all times.

5) Eating a snack at bedtime may also help alleviate early morning sickness.

6) Consult your doctor about taking large doses of vitamin B6. A recent study at the University of Iowa indicates that women with severe morning sickness experience much less nausea and vomiting when taking up to 76 mg of vitamin B6 every day.

Researchers say that even though B6 is found in many foods, getting 75 mg a day would almost certainly mean taking supplements. Medical experts caution pregnant women not to exceed the RDA for vitamin B6 (2.6 mg a day) without first consulting their doctors.

7) Ask your doctor if you can quit taking iron tablets. The tablets can cause nausea.

The Easiest Way To Lose Weight "After" Pregnancy

Being pregnant does not give you an excuse to avoid regular exercise. Several studies have confirmed that women who exercise during pregnancy experience fewer aches and pains, improved sleeping patterns, and less weight gain than those pregnant women who don't exercise. The women who exercise during pregnancy also tend to regain their pre-pregnancy figures more quickly than those women who become couch potatoes during pregnancy.

Walking and swimming are two safe and effective exercises for pregnant women. There are also exercise classes specifically designed for pregnant women. According to studies conducted by the Melpomene Institute in Minnesota, special exercise classes can provide both physical and social benefits to pregnant women. You can get more information and advice on classes by sending $1 and a self-addressed, stamped envelope to: Selecting a Prenatal Exercise Program, c/o The Melpomene Institute, 1010 University Avenue, Saint Paul, MN 55104.

Hot Tubs And Saunas
Increase Risk To Pregnant Women

In a study of almost 23,000 pregnant women, researchers at the Boston University School of Medicine have discovered that those who used a hot tub while in the first two months of pregnancy were almost three times as likely as others to have a baby with a neural-tube defect, such as spina bifida. Those women who used a sauna during the same stage of pregnancy faced almost 2 1/2 times the normal risk.

The new evidence suggests that women in the first few months of pregnancy who are exposed to heat from a sauna or hot tub may face a much higher risk of having a baby with a birth defect affecting the brain and spinal cord, leading to the recommendation that women in the first three months of pregnancy should avoid using either one.

Alarming Dangers Of Group B Strep And Childbirth

Every year, 12,000 babies suffer brain damage or die after being infected with the common bacteria known as Group B Strep (GBS) during delivery. Until now, most obstetricians did not regularly test women for GBS, but new guidelines from the American College of Obstetricians and Gynecologists (ACOG) may change that. The new guidelines encourage screening for GBS between weeks 28 and 30 of pregnancy. If a woman tests positive, ACOG recommends that she be given intravenous antibiotics during labor to protect the baby, but only in the event of another risk factor, such as premature labor or premature rupture of membranes, present during labor.

Since as many as 40 percent of all pregnant women carry GBS, and less than one percent of their babies get sick, not all mothers who test positive are treated. According to medical experts, giving antibiotics to all mothers carrying GBS would increase the danger that the bacteria would eventually become immune to the drugs, making it even more dangerous.

New Treatment May Mean Easier Childbirth

A new vaginal insert presently being studied may shorten induced labor and reduce the need for caesarean sections in women who have had a previous vaginal delivery.

Medical research statistics show that every year thousands of pregnant women need to undergo induced labor for a number of reasons. Some women are confronted with potentially dangerous complications such as diabetes, sickle- cell anemia or ruptured membranes— others have not delivered well past their due dates. For those women, the only labor-inducing drug option has been oxytocin, a strong medication that can cause uterine contractions so strong they can present a very real danger to the fetus.

Scientists have developed a new treatment which offers pregnant women some important advantages, including a vaginal insert containing prostaglandin E2 (PGE2)— a chemical which can shorten induced labor significantly by softening and relaxing the cervix, leading to a more rapid dilation. PGE2 is administered by doctors who, 12 hours before inducing labor, insert a medicated disk near the cervix of the mother-to-be.

The new treatment was tested in a recent study of 81 women at Johns Hopkins Medical Institution in Baltimore. In that study, researchers discovered that prostaglandin could reduce the needed dose of oxytocin by up to 50 percent for many women, and eliminate the need altogether in others. The chemical also reduced, by over 65 percent, the rate of caesarean sections in women who had had a previous vaginal delivery.

The new treatment is still awaiting governmental approval, but many experts expect it to be on the market in the near future. These experts say that once governmental approval is obtained, they expect PGE2 to become a regular treatment for women who need to undergo induced labor.

Advantages Of Breastfeeding:
What Your Doctor May Not Have Told You

One of the most important decisions a mother makes in the months preceding her baby's birth is how she will feed her baby. According to medical childcare experts, more and more mothers these days are choosing to breast feed. The decision seems to be a wise one because the American Academy of Pediatrics has labeled breastmilk as the "perfect" food for a baby during the first year of life. Moreover, breast milk is easy for the baby to digest, and it provides antibodies until the baby's body can make them on its own. Breastfeeding also provides a special closeness for mother and baby, and it helps restore the uterus to pre-pregnancy size.

Here are several things a mother can do to ensure successful breastfeeding:

1) Go to breastfeeding classes before the baby is born.

2) Try to nurse the baby as soon as possible in the delivery room. Research shows that babies who begin nursing almost immediately after delivery are more successful at breastfeeding.

3) Nurse your baby as often as 8 to 12 times a day for the first few weeks, and let the baby nurse as long as he or she wants. The more a baby nurses, the more milk a mother will provide.

4) Allow the baby to nurse from both breasts during each feeding. Nurse on one side until it appears the baby is losing interest, then offer your baby the other breast.

The next time you feed your baby, begin with the side you ended with the time before.

5) Don't give your baby supplemental bottles or a pacifier until you have been nursing successfully for more than three weeks and the baby is gaining weight.

6) The key to success for any breastfeeding mother is to pay attention to her baby, and having the support of those around her in her decision to breastfeed. Some experts even recommend joining breast-feeding support groups.

Any prospective mother considering breastfeeding her baby should consult a pediatrician who is supportive of breastfeeding and can help with any questions or problems that might arise.

New Study Supports BreastFeeding
- But Not After Exercising

Several Scottish scientists say they have discovered biochemical differences in the brains of breast-fed and bottle-fed babies. Even though the differences in the brain did not necessarily affect brain functions, the new information lends support to mounting evidence that mother's milk is better for baby than cow's milk.

The Scottish scientists studied the brains of 22 babies who had died within 43 weeks of birth. Five of the babies who had been breast-fed had a higher level of docosahexaenoic acid (DHA), which is a polyunsaturated fatty acid, in their brains, compared to five babies of the same age who were on formula.

Even though no one is sure of the exact role of DHA in the brain, scientists believe it may be a substance for nerve cell conduction and cell membrane fluidity. None of this means that higher levels of DHA yield smarter children, but researchers say the results of the study should encourage more women to breastfeed their babies.

New research suggests that mothers should nurse or collect milk before doing exercises, rather than after. That's because babies don't seem to care very much for breast milk produced after the mother exercises.

In a study at Indiana University in Bloomington, researchers discovered that working out increases a mother's level of sour-tasting lactic acid. Babies in the study reacted negatively or refused altogether to nurse when their mothers fed them post-exercise milk.

Lactic acid remains at an elevated level in breast milk for about 90 minutes or longer after vigorous physical activity. That's why mothers are advised to nurse their babies before working out.

How Mothers Can Improve
Their Babys Immune Systems

New research indicates that something in mother's milk may help to speed up the development of a baby's own immune system, giving the infant a better chance to fight off sickness. By examining white blood cells found in breast milk, researchers at the University of Texas Medical Branch at Galveston discovered that some immune cells appeared to be more developed, more mature and to move faster than those in the blood.

Researchers speculate that the heightened activity is due to a protein in the milk which stimulates the baby's immune system. The protein, called tumor necrosis factor-alpha, appears to have far-reaching beneficial effects on the baby's immune system.

Studies Show That Bran
Reduces The Risk Of Women's Breast Cancer

Scientists have announced some encouraging news of a possible link between bran and a reduction in the risk of women's breast cancer. New studies investigating which factors, including diet, might have an effect on estrogen levels in the blood, suggest that fat and fiber may be two useful dietary "tools" in helping to reduce the risk of breast cancer. Previous studies have indicated that a woman's exposure to estrogen might increase her risk of breast cancer.

The new research includes one study in which 62 premenopausal women were placed on diets containing 15 to 39 grams of fiber in the form of wheat, oat and corn. Their intake of fat was kept constant, and their serum hormone levels were measured before, during and after the diet phase of the study. The measurements revealed that after eight weeks on the wheat-fiber diet, there was a significant reduction in serum estrone, a type of estrogen which has been inconclusively associated with increasing some cancer risk. At the same time, oat and corn fiber appeared to have little effect on the estrogen levels.

In another study, at Tufts University, 44 healthy premenopausal women were placed on diets in which both dietary fiber and fat were modulated to study the effect on estrogen levels. And, unlike the previous study, specific sources of fiber were not separated out. The study's results revealed that even when the women were placed on diets which were high in fat content, the high-fiber component had a lowering effect on estrogen levels.

Researchers report that while the combination high-fat and high-fiber diet resulted in a "positive" lowering of estrogen levels—due to the high-fiber component—the low-fat and high-fiber combination produced the most favorable benefits. There was a 45 percent reduction in estrone sulfate with the high- fiber, low-fat diet. The fiber component of the diet was also responsible for a 14 percent decrease in estradiol.

The studies suggest that fiber helps to lower estrogen levels independent of fat intake. According to some scientists, that may explain why in many foreign countries where fat intakes are similar to those in the U.S., cancer rates are actually much lower. It could be due to their high intake of fiber.

While no one is certain why fiber—especially wheat fiber—may have such a beneficial effect, some researchers speculate that it may be because the fiber helps to lessen the absorption of estrogens from the intestine, leading to their increased activity in the blood. Whatever the reason, the evidence indicates that bran, as fiber, may provide protection against breast cancer in women.

How To Do An Easy
5-Point Self-Breast Examination

Statistics reveal that monthly breast self-examinations save thousands of lives each year. That's why doctors recommend that every woman over age 20 should perform such a monthly examination.

The best time to perform a self-examination is two or three days after your period ends, when your breasts are usually not tender or swollen. If you no longer menstruate, you can examine your breasts at any time of the month, just so you do it at the same time each month. Familiarity with your breasts will better enable you to notice any changes. You should report any unusual changes to your doctor immediately. Here are the main things you should look for during each self-examination:

1) A change in the contour of your breast(s), such as a lump or swelling.

2) An increase in the size of a breast.

3) A change in either the appearance or direction of a nipple.

4) Discharge or bleeding from a nipple.

5) Puckering or bleeding from a nipple.

6) Unusually pronounced veins.

7) A change in the appearance of the breast skin.

8) Any unusual rash.

Here are the basic steps involved in breast self-examination:

1) Stand in front of a large mirror, with your arms at your sides. Observe both breasts for anything unusual, including any change in size or contour.

2) Clasp your hands behind your head and press them forward. Sometimes lumps that are difficult to feel are easy to see. Study both breasts again, looking for any changes— a swelling, dimpling of skin, changes in the nipple, or scaling of skin.

3) Next, press your hands firmly on your hips and bow slightly toward your mirror as you pull your shoulders and elbows forward. Look at your breasts again. Do you notice any significant differences between them?

4) Raise your left arm. Use three or four fingers of your right hand to feel your left breast carefully and thoroughly. Beginning at the outer edge, make small circular motions with the flattened fingers of your right hand, moving the circles slowly around the breast. Gradually work toward the nipple. Be sure to cover the entire breast, and spend at least two minutes on each breast. Pay special attention to the area between the breast and the armpit, including the armpit itself. You should feel for any unusual lump or mass under the skin. Repeat the procedure, using your left hand on your right breast.

5) Look down at your breasts and gently squeeze each nipple between your thumb and index finger. A minimal whitish discharge is fairly common for some women, but you should report any unusual or bloody discharge to your doctor immediately.

You may also do steps 4 and 5 while lying down. To do so, place a folded towel under your left shoulder (or under the shoulder on the side you plan to examine first) and your left hand behind your head. This position flattens the breast and may make it easier to examine. Using the circular motion described in step 4, examine both breasts thoroughly.

What To Do Right Now
If You've Had Silicone Gel Breast Implants

With the current controversy about the use of silicone breast implants, many women are scared of undergoing reconstructive surgery at this time. This can cause further distress for women who face mastectomies, without the silicone breast implants as possible cosmetic compensation. Much of the news about implants has been confusing and misleading. The best way to get professional up-to-date information on implant safety and support groups is to ask your doctor to share materials he or she may have available on implants.

Specialists recommend that women who have had silicone gel implants consult a qualified surgeon before deciding to have their implants removed. The current recommendation is not to have implants removed, but if you are concerned, you should get as much iformation on the issue as you can before you make a decision. You should also tell your mammogram technician there is an implant because evidence indicates that implants can interfere with mammography.

Besides your doctor, Information is also available by contacting any of the following:

1) The Food and Drug Administration—prefers to have inquiries sent on a post card to: Breast Implants, FDA, HFE-80, Rockville, MD 20857.

2) American Society of Plastic and Reconstructive Surgeons, Inc., 444 E. Algonquin Road, Arlington Heights, IL 60005. Call, 800-635-0635.

3) Maryland Department of Health and Mental Hygiene, 201 W. Preston, Baltimore, MD 21201.

4) Public Citizens Health Research Group, 7000 P Street NW, Suite 700, Washington, D.C. 20036.

5) Command Trust Network (a consumer-information group for past and potential implant patients), P.O. Box 17082, Covington, KY 41017.

6) Y-Me National Organization for Breast Cancer Information and Support, 182220 Harwood Ave., Homewood, IL 60430. Call, 800-221-2141.

7) The National Coalition for Cancer Survivorship, 1010 Wayne Ave., Suite 300, Silver Springs, MD 20910.

Toll-Free Information Sources

Toll Free Phone Numbers

These toll free numbers usually operate during regular business hours. They can provide you with additional information and sources for their specific topic.

AGING

800-782-7777 Agency on Aging

800-634-7654 Elder Support Network

AIDS

800-822-7422 Project Inform

800-234-TEEN Teen AIDS information.

800-342-AIDS U.S. Public Health Service

ALCOHOL

800-NCA-CALL National Council on Alcoholism

800-854-0318 Careunit

800-457-6237 Dial a Sober Thoought

800-257-7800 Hazelden Foundation

800-344-2666 Al-Anon Family Group Headquarters

800-477-3447 Alcoholism and Drug Addiction Treatment Center

ALLERGY

800-842-7777 American College of Allergy & imunology

800-822-2762 American academy of allergy and Immunology

ALZHEIMER'S DISEASE

800-621-0379 Alzheimer's Disease and Related Disorders Association

AMYOTROPHIC LATERAL SCLEROSIS

800-782-4747 amyotrophic Lateral Sclerosis association

ANOREXIA/BULIMIA

800-BASH-STL Bulimia Anorexia Self-help

ARTHRITIS

800-283-7800 Arthritis Foundation

BIRTH DEFECTS

800-221-6827 National Easter Seal Society

BLIND/VISION IMPARIED

800-424-8666 American Council of the Blind

800-424-8567 Library of Congress services

800-AF-BLIND American Founddatioiion for the Blind

800-221-4792 (cassette tapes) Recording for the Blind Inc.

800-562-6265 NNational Association of Parents of Visually Impaired

800-451-1339 American Society of Cataract and Refractive Surgery

800-548-4337 Guide Dog Foundation for the Blind

CANCER

800-4-CANCER National Cancer Institute

800-525-3777 American Medical Center, Cancer Research

800-221-2141 Y-Me Breast Cancer Support Program

800-843-8114 American Institute for Cancer Research

800-227-8713 National Foundation for Cancer Research

CEREBRAL PALSY

800-USA-1-UCP United Cerebral Palsy

CHILDREN

800-433-9016 American Academy of Pediatrics

800-422-4453 Child Help USA

800-USA-KIDS Missing Children Help Center

800-843-5678 National Center for Missing and Exploited Children

800-422-4453 National Child Abuse Hotline

CLEFT PALATE

800—24-CLEFT National Cleft Palate Association

COCAINE

800-262-2463 800 Cocaine Information 800-992-9239 Cocaine Abuse 24 hour Hotline & Treatment Program

COLITIS/ILEITIS

800-343-3637 National Foundation for Illeitis and Colitis, Inc.

CRISIS LINE

800-866-9600 Crisis Line

CYSTIC FIBROSIS

800-3444823 Cystic Fibrosis Foundation

DIABETES

800-444-6443 National Head Injury Foundation

800-962-9629 National Spinal Coord Injury Association

800-526-7234 job accomodation

800-248-ABLE community projects & networking, National Organization on Disability

800-34-NARIC National Rehabilitation Information Center

800-452-19448 Advocates for the Developmentally Disabled

DOWN SYNDROME

800-221-4602 National Down Syndrome Society

800-232-NDSC National Down Syndrome Congress

DRUG ABUSE

800-662-HELP National Institute on Drug Abuse 800-554-KIDS National Federation of Parents for Drug Free Youth

800-241-7946 National Parents Resource Institute for Drug Education, Inc.

800-638-2045 National Institute on Drug Abuse Prevention

800-258-2766 Just Say No Clubs

DYSLEXIA

800-ABCD-123 Orton Dyslexia Society

ENDOMETRIOSIS

800-992-ENDO Endometriosis Association

EPILEPSY

800-332-1000 Epilepsy Foundation of America

HEAD INJURY

800-444-6443 National Head Injury Foundation

HEADACHE

800-843-2256 National Headache Foundation

HEALTH

800-336-4797 National Health Information Clearinghouse

800-821-6671 Consumer Health Information Resource Institute

HEARING/COMMUNICATION HANDICAPS

800-424-8576 Better Hearing Institute

800-638-8255 National Association for Hearing and Speech

800-237-6213 (captioned film loans) U.S. Department of Education

800-446-9876 National Crisis Center for the Deaf

800-535-3323 Deafness Research Foundation

800-424-8576 Hearing Helpline

800-521-5247 Hearing Aid Helpline

HEART

800-241-6993 Heart Life

HERPES

800-227-8922 Herpes Resource Center

HUNTINGTON'S DISEASE

800-345-4372 Huntington's Disease Society

IMPOTENCE

800-622-4372 Center to End Impotence

INCONTINENCE

800-23-SIMON Simon Foundation

KIDNEY

800-638-8299 American Kidney Fund

LUNGS

800-222-5864 National Jewish Center's "Lung Line"

LUPUS

800-558-0121 Lupus Foundation

MEDICAL SPECIALITIES

800-776-2378 American Board of Medical Specialities

MENTAL HEALTH

800-969-6642 National Mental Health Association

MULTIPLE SCLEROSIS

800-624-8236 National Multiple Sclerosis Society

MYASTHENIA GRAVIS FOUNDATION

800-541-5454 Myasthenia Gravis Foundation

PARALYSIS

800-225-0292 American Paralysis Association

PARKINSON'S DISEASE

800-344-7872 Parkinson's Educational Program

800-233-APDA American Parkinson Disease Association

800-327-4545 National Parkinson Foundation

RARE ILLNESS

800-447-6673 National Organization for Rare Disorders

RESPIRATORY

800-222-LUNG National Asthma Center

RETINITIS PIGMENTOSA

800-638-2300 Natioonal Retinitis Pigmentosa Foundation

REYES SYNDROME

800-233-7393 National Reyes Syndrome Foundation

SCHIZOPHRENIA

800-783-3801 American Schizophrenia Association

SCLERODERMA

800-722-HOPE United Scleroderma

SICKLE CELL

800-421-8453 National Association for Sickle Cell Anemia

SPINA BIFIDA

800-621-3141 Spina Bifida Association

STROKE

800-553-6321 Courage Stroke Network

SUDDEN INFANT DEATH SYNDROME

800-221-SIDS National SIDS Foundation

800-638-7437 National Center for the Prevention of SIDS

800-232-7437 American SIDS Institute

SURGERY

800-638-6833 second opinion referrals, U.S. Department of Health & Human Services

TOURETTE SYNDROME

800-237-0717 Tourette Syndrome

TRANSPLANTATION

800-ACT-GIVE American Council on Transplantation

VENERAL DISEASE

800-227-8922 American Social Health Association

800-227-8922 National Sexually Transmitted Disease Hotline

The Best Home Pregnancy Test & Those To Avoid

Our Research Staff talked with Gynecologists, Pharmacists and mothers to determine the best home pregnancy tests. The best one is E*P*T because it is extremely accurate, easy to use and easy to read the results.

You should avoid off-brand home pregnancy tests as many are made cheaply and can give you incorrect results. In this case, you get what you pay for.

Secrets To Overcoming Fear Of Needles Or Blood

There are two effective methods you can use to overcome your fear of needles or blood. The first is called "Visualization Therapy". You simply close your eyes, relax and picture a pleasant experience of a shot or blood. Do this over and over again until your fear subsides.

The second method is equally as simple. You take a shot, pin or ketchup and place it in front of you, concentrate on a peaceful feeling from the object, then relate them to a needle or blood.

Many people have written us that these mind-control techniques work - and they are no longer afraid.

The Best And Worst Sun - Blocking Lotions

After talking to Dermatologists and skin care experts, we have concluded that the best sunblocking lotions (i.e., sunscreen) contain the following ingredients: An SPF factor of 15, Aloe Vera, and Vitamin E.

You should make sure these ingredients are in any sunscreen you buy. Additional tip: If two or more brands have these ingredients, buy the cheapest one. All sunscreens are the same, except for ingredients, so save the money.

Mouthwash Warning: Some Can Increase You Risk Of Mouth And Throat Cancer

Mouthwashes that contain alcohol increase your risk of mouth and throat cancer, some experts believe. The acidic substances in mouthwash mixed with alcohol are a bad combination.

To avoid this problem, look for ingredients in a mouthwash before buying it - and avoid any that contain alcohol.

9 Little-Known Things That Are Dangerous To Your Health - Some In Medical Community Hide These

The following things that many people do could be dangerous to your health. Unfortuneately, some people in the medical community hide or deny these things for their own benefit.

1) DIETS UNDER 1,200 CALORIES A DAY. You need a minimum number of calories each day for your body to function properly.

2) TAKING TOO MANY PRESCRIPITION MEDICINES. People think they need a "pill" to solve every problem. What they don't realize is that too many medications can deplete the body of energy, and of it's nat-

ural disease-fighting functions.

3) THINKING THAT DISEASE AND ILLNESS ARE ALL NATUR-AL. Many people believe that illness and disease is natural, and they can't do anything about it, so they feel helpless and hopeless. You can use the tips in this book to prevent disease and illness - even help reverse it. Don't let anyone tell you "older people always have health problems" or "there is nothing you can do about it."

4) NOT USING NATURAL HEALING AND PREVENTION METHODS. Many doctors are famous for prescribing medicine or surgery, and overlooking natural health aids. This is due in large part to their training which is in medicine only. Many natural methods (foods, vit-amins, herbs, excercises, thinking) can work better than traditional medi-cine or surgery - for a fraction of the cost and risk.

5) NOT USING YOUR ATTITUDE AND MIND POWERS TO HEAL. The power of thoughts, health self-imaging and visualization and positive thinking can work wonders for your health - although most doc-tors overlook this.

6) THINKING THAT DOCTORS "KNOW IT ALL". Your health is too important to trust 100% to anyone. You should buy books and mag-azines on health, always keep a healthy mistrust of anyone, and thor-oughly question and sugget things to your doctor.

7) NOT USING VITAMINS AND MINERALS. Although many doctors scoff at vitamins and minerals, millions of people think or know they help. Use the vitamin and mineral tips in this book. Their power can be awesome.

8) LETTING NEGATIVE, SICK PEOPLE MAKE YOU SICK. The more you listen to negative people about their health problems, the more you can subconciously make yourself sick. Many people have found this to be true. Don't let negative people "bring you down."

In each case, the real problem was mental. One man had prob-lems with a co-worker. This caused him stress and anxiety, which led to feeling bad. Once he dealt with the co-worker problem, he regained good health. In another case, a woman went to a psychologist and uncovered that problems from her childhood -- still unresolved -- were tha cause of her health problems. After counseling, she feels like a new woman today.

If doctors can't figure out what's wrong with you, it would be wise to analyze your past and present life to see if the problem is mental, and then deal with it.

Exciting New Data
On Thinking Your Way To Better Health

We've said it for years, and now new studies prove it is true: You can think your way to better health!

You should maintain a positive mental attitude, tell yourself often to "be happe", not over-blow problems and vesualize yourself free from health problems - and feeling terrific

These simple mind-control tips could work wonders to improve your health - as they have for many other people. Please don't discount them before you try them!

Best Way To Get The Real Story
On Any Medical Condition Or Problem

It always amazes us that some people with serious medical conditions or problems dont't know all the facts about it. If you don't know the facts, how can you expect to gain relief?

The best way we have found to get the real story on any medical problem is to regulary buy health books, magasines and to use the health referance books in your local library - a store house of very, very helpful information you can read, or copy and take home and study.

How To Protect Yourself Around A Smoker

It is now common knowledge of the damage that second-hand smoke does to non-smokers. You can protect yourself around smokers with these tips:

1) Politely ask them not to smoke. Many people will oblige and not puff away.

2) Keep windows or doors open if possible.

3) Go outside often and breathe fresh air.

4) Take extra Vitamin C, which can negate some effects of inhaling tobacco smoke.

WARNING:
DON'T USE GENERICS FOR THESE PRESCRIPTIONS

Although we normally advise the use of generic drugs as being as good as their expensive counterparts, we suggest you avoid using generics on any drugs that have just come onto the market.

The reasons: Newer drug generics may not yet be perfected in their manufacturing process, and the Federal Health Administration, being understaffed, may not yet have watched their manufacturing and delivery processes carefully.

Sleep In This Position For Better Rest

As incredible as it sounds, many of our readers claim that your sleeping position has a great effect on the quality of your sleep.

The position for better sleep: On your stomach, head tilted to side that is most comfortable, legs curled up a little towards body, pillow under head in vertical (up and down) position.

6 Tips To Look Younger Than Your Actual Age

We all want to look younger, and here are six tips from experts to help you:

1) SLIM DOWN. The trimmer you look, the younger you look.

2) WEAR BRIGHT COLORED CLOTHES. Like a bright room, bright colored clothes tend to make you look younger.

3) SMILE. One famous plastic surgeon claims the best way to look younger is to smile often.

4) GET A YOUNGER LOOKING HAIRSTYLE. Your hairstyle can add or subtract many years from your looks.

5) EXERCISE FOR A YOUTHFUL GLOW. The more energy and "glow" you get from exercise, the younger you will look.

6) WEAR MODERN, IN-STYLE CLOTHES. If you dress like younger people do, you will look younger yourself.

People Over 90 And Healthy Reveal Their Secrets

Believe it or not, their "secrets" are really quite simple, yet many people don't practice them. Here is what people over 90 and healthy say are the keys to a long and healthy life: A positive mental attitude, staying active and interested in things you like, having good close friendships, learning new things and sexual enjoyment.

NOTES

NOTES